embodied posture

Your Unique Body and Yoga
A Guide for Student and Teacher

STACY DOCKINS

yp Publishing

All rights reserved. Copyright © 2018 by Stacy Dockins. No part of this book may be reproduced in any form or by any means, electronic or mechanical, including photocopying, recording, photographing, scanning, or by any information storage and retrieval system, without written permission of the copyright owner, Stacy Dockins, except in the case of brief quotations in articles and reviews.

www.stacydockins.com

For more information, contact YP Publishing: info@yogaproject.com

Book design by Julie Hatlem
Photography by Jake Dockins
Illustrations by Emily Evans
Book editing by Marie González

YP Publishing, Yoga Project, LLC
First edition published in 2018
Printed in China

ISBN 978-0-578-41137-8

> Disclaimer:
> This book is not intended to be a substitute for the medical advice of a licensed physician. The reader should consult with a doctor before starting new physical exercise. This book is written, published, and sold with the understanding that the author and publisher are not engaged in rendering legal, medical, or other professional services by reason of their authorship or publishing. Before beginning any new exercise program, it is always recommended that you seek medical advice from your personal physician.

I dedicate this book to Jake, Kera, and Luke.

May you always follow your hearts—even when it's scary, looks different, and others don't understand. I love you more than you will ever comprehend.

~Mom

Table of Contents

Foreword viii

With Gratitude ix

Introduction x

PART ONE: Embodiment

Chapter 1 – A Return to Embodiment 2

Chapter 2 – Yoga and the Posture 4

Chapter 3 – Road Map to Embodied Posture Methodology 10

PART TWO: The Body

Chapter 4 – The Body in Posture 17

Chapter 5 – The Spine 20

Chapter 6 – The Shoulder 40

Chapter 7 – The Hip 56

Chapter 8 – The Knee 72

Chapter 9 – The Ankle 80

Chapter 10 – The Elbow 86

Chapter 11 – The Wrist 94

PART THREE: The Postures

Chapter 12 – Navigating the Posture 101

Chapter 13 — Foundation Postures ... 113

Foundation Postures Overview ... 113

Child's Pose ... 114

Tabletop ... 118

Downward-Facing Dog ... 122

Mountain ... 128

Halfway Lift ... 132

Plank ... 136

Low Plank ... 140

Chair ... 146

Easy Pose ... 150

Final Rest ... 154

Chapter 14 — Standing Postures ... 156

Standing Postures Overview ... 156

High Lunge ... 158

Warrior I ... 164

Pyramid ... 168

Warrior II ... 172

Side Angle ... 176

Reverse Warrior ... 180

Triangle ... 184

Chapter 15 — Twists ... 188

The Anatomy of Twists ... 188

Chair Twist ... 190

Crescent Twist ... 194

Revolved Half Moon ... 198

Revolved Supported Leg Raise ... 202

Table of Contents

    Revolved Triangle 206

    Seated Twist 210

    Supine Twists 214

Chapter 16 — Standing Balance Postures 217

    Standing Balance Posture Overview 217

    Eagle 218

    Warrior III 222

    Supported Front Leg Raise 226

    Supported Side Leg Raise 228

    Tree 232

    Half Moon 236

Chapter 17 — Forward Folds 240

    The Anatomy of Forward Folding 240

    Standing Forward Fold 242

    Standing Wide-Leg Forward Fold 246

    Boat 250

    Seated Forward Fold 254

Chapter 18 — Backward Bends 259

    The Anatomy of Backbending 259

    Sphinx 266

    Cobra 270

    Locust 274

    Upward-Facing Dog 278

    Bridge 282

    Camel 286

    Floor Bow 290

    Wheel 294

    Dancer 298

Airplane 302

Chapter 19 — Hip Openers 306
   The Anatomy of Hip Opening 306
   Half Pigeon 310
   Full Pigeon 314
   Low Lunge 318
   Happy Baby 322
   Yogi Squat 324
   Frog 326

Chapter 20 — Arm Balances and Inversions 328
   An Approach to Arm Balances and Inversions 328
   Waterfall 330
   Crow 332
   Side Plank 336
   Headstand 340
   Handstand 346
   Forearm Stand 350
   Side Crow 354
   Running Man 358

PART FOUR: The Gifts

Chapter 21 — Teaching Embodiment and Portable Gifts 364
   Glossary 374
   Endnotes and Additional Resources 378
   Index of Postures 382
   Index of Anatomical Actions 383
   Index of the Body 385
   Index of Other Content 387

Foreword

"If your lifestyle involves moving and/or breathing, you should be doing yoga." For years I've told anyone who would listen about this powerful, effective practice. Now I add, "And if you are going to do yoga, you need this book."

On my first visit to Yoga Project, I decided to do yoga teacher training with Stacy and Dave. But just a few days into the 200-hour training, my mind was filled with questions we wouldn't have time to answer. One morning after practice, I told Stacy she should write a book. Tilting her head, she smiled and said, "You know, I've always wanted to write a book." "Well then do it!" I replied. "The difference between writers and wannabe writers is that writers write." My motives were selfish. Stacy's abundant knowledge would benefit my personal practice and my teaching.

Always keeping her students and teachers in mind, Stacy set out to create the clearest, most comprehensive yoga anatomy reference available. This invaluable tool is her gift to us. I've taken other yoga anatomy trainings and studied other yoga anatomy books, but memorizing muscles, bones, anatomical directions and terms overwhelmed me. What was presented was not what I needed. This book and this approach are different. In *Embodied Posture*, Stacy has connected the dots between what is happening in the body scientifically and what is happening in your body uniquely on the mat.

Stacy firmly believes that yoga is good for everybody and every body. As I use Embodied Posture Methodology in my classes, I see students falling in love with the practice. "I can't do this pose" quickly becomes "I can do this pose this way." We are not only growing together in functional musculoskeletal wellness, but we are also unwrapping the wonderful portable gifts that yoga offers.

So, if you want to practice yoga, you need this book. If you want to teach yoga, you need this book. And if you want to further your adventures by becoming a teacher, consider training with Stacy and Dave. For information on their trainings in Fort Worth, Thailand, Bali, and Costa Rica, or for information on their studios in Texas, visit www.yogaproject.com or www.stacydockins.com. You can also follow them on Instagram @txyogastacy and @txyogadave for daily inspiration and good vibes.

Marie González
Flowing Grace Yoga

With Gratitude

If I had known the immensity of this project prior to beginning, I might not have begun. But, I charged forth with the enthusiastic bliss of a beginner's mind, not knowing what this journey would entail. As I met the many obstacles along my path, I had the strength and love of an amazing team supporting me every step of the way.

My husband Dave has been an integral part of this book, as he is with everything that I take on. I could never express how grateful I am for his selfless love and support in my life. My kids, Jake, Kera, and Luke, have been my biggest fans from day one. Their unconditional love, attitudes, and belief in me have been fuel for my soul when I met doubts and insecurities. I will always be thankful for the example passed on to me from my mom and dad, Grace and Salvador. Their dedication to speaking their truths has impacted my life in inexpressible ways.

My editor Marie is the angel who showed up in my life at just the right moment. I could not thank her enough for her hard work, dedication, and passion for the book's content. All of the photography in the book is the work of my incredibly talented son, Jake Dockins. I am so grateful that he was willing to be a part of this project. My dear friend Susie supported us on set with styling, makeup, and emotional support. She also showed up at just the right moment! I was incredibly blessed to find our amazing anatomical illustrator Emily; she was a dream to work with. My graphic designer Julie did a phenomenal job of making the book look fantastic. With all of my heart, I thank these individuals for their time and for believing in me and *Embodied Posture*.

I honor and acknowledge all of the great teachers who have paved the way, courageously sharing their own experiences and opinions in ways that expanded my own. Lastly, I'd like to acknowledge the willingness and trust of my many students from over the years. You have been my biggest teachers along this journey called yoga.

Introduction

I've often said, "You may think Stacy is a wonderful, skillful, and knowledgeable yoga instructor, but I assure you, she's a much better student. Her learning never stops!" When I say "better student," I don't mean "perfect yoga student" on the mat who can do exactly what the instructor says. Rather, Stacy is a student who studies intently to learn and to master. This book is the result of twenty-five years of her relentless questioning, studying, and desiring to be more helpful. I've had the joy of witnessing her growth through this entire yoga journey as a practitioner and teacher.

We met when we were only sixteen years old, so we've practically grown up together; we have been blessed to be partners on this journey of life. In the early years, yoga was the farthest thing from our minds as we were in the throes of raising three kids and surviving newly entered adulthood. Back then there was no way to predict we would be teaching or even practicing yoga. Stacy's interest in finding ways to feel better physically and mentally led us into this journey; I curiously went along, initially intrigued by the physicality of the practice. I can honestly say that my own personal growth along the way was and still is fueled by Stacy's constant desire to learn more.

Practicing and teaching yoga over the years, we eventually realized that we, as humans, are designed to feel. As newborn babies, we purely rely on feelings. These physical sensations are our God-given road map to direct us through everything from "I'm hungry" to "Something doesn't feel quite right." We are designed to feel, to gather information, and then to respond. As we get older, our brains develop, and we begin to use thought along with these automatic reactions. We gain the ability to reason, evaluate, and pause before responding. Every person feels and responds all day, every day. We may not be aware of this, but that's what's happening. If left unexamined, our feelings can be an impetus toward fear and closing, rather than toward patiently responding. Together, Stacy and I noticed how different things were when we took the time to tune back in to the feeling-pausing-responding gift that we have been given. This has been a big discovery for us. Now, as a result, we always aim to tune in to this gift to guide the moments of our lives.

This is the origin of *Embodied Posture*. Stacy embraced her own yoga practice and teaching as a way to tap back in to the wisdom that resides within, a way to strengthen the neural pathways of feeling, pausing, responding. This changed everything for me. This approach to the practice revealed my natural limitations and weaknesses, as well as my strengths, in a way that enabled me to accept and allow them all. What I was feeling in a posture became a whole new source of information I could use to help guide my actions. I went from trying to make yoga postures look a certain way to feeling and learning what was happening in my body while on my mat.

Through the years, I've watched students come to Stacy with difficulties in postures. Time after time, I've seen her help them break down exactly what is going on, so they can better understand their own bodies in the poses. Most of the time students need a little guidance to feel more clearly within to make minor adjustments. Stacy doesn't just tell them what they need to do; she empowers them to awaken to their own answers. Being around this as a yoga practitioner and instructor, I found this contagious. I began to feel the postures differently and see them in my students differently. I became more aware of the uniqueness in practitioners' bodies, so I became a much more helpful teacher. *Embodied Posture* methodology has taken my understanding of the practice to a new level.

This book is a way of approaching yourself, from the inside out. As a yoga student, you will increase your ability to tune in and pay attention. As a yoga teacher, being more curious on your own mat will greatly enhance what you are already teaching. Whether you're new to yoga, a longtime practitioner, or a yoga instructor, *Embodied Posture* will guide you to become the best student of you that you can be. Enjoy the journey!

Dave Dockins
Yoga Project

At the center of your being

you have the answer;

you know who you are

and you know what you want.

—Lao Tzu

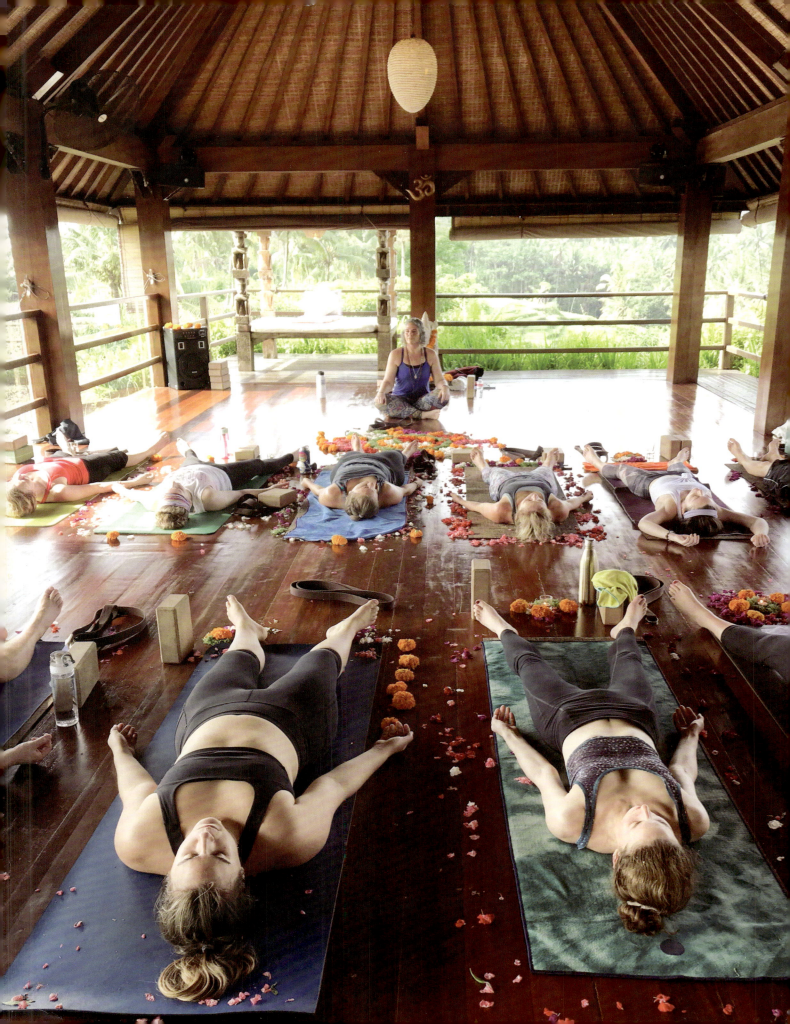

PART ONE
Embodiment

PART ONE | EMBODIED POSTURE

Chapter 1
A Return to Embodiment

Although this book is about your body, yoga, and anatomy, its true message is one of returning home. I want to encourage you to use the practice of yoga to return home within yourself. Since we continually live in our bodies while we are here on Earth, this may seem like an odd concept. But, in fact, we often abandon our connectivity to ourselves. In any given moment, we can choose to dwell on often-inaccurate thoughts of our pasts and futures, or we can be alive to what is true and happening now. Embodiment, or noticing what is felt within the body, is our most accessible doorway to the present. Through learning to feel again, we return home as the wholehearted human beings we were always meant to be.

Our miraculously designed bodies are constantly communicating with us. It's no accident that heart tugs and gut feelings are at the core of our strongest human experiences. If we are willing to be still and to feel, our bodies have much to tell us. We are created with an intelligent sensory capacity that invites us to interact with ourselves and the world around us. Within the quiet whispers of our bodies, there is constant communication beyond the level of words. Answers exist within; we must be willing to listen.

For many reasons, life conditions us to shut off this inner sense of knowing. We become numb to the sensory experience constantly alive within us. Instead of honoring our feelings as guidance, we develop subconscious patterns of avoidance and distraction, filling our hectic day-to-day schedules with doing, but not pausing. We forget to give ourselves the time and space needed to be with what arises. Strong feelings become triggers either to check out or to get busy. We tend to disconnect from the messages our bodies send us; therefore, we remain in a state of confusion. This confusion can lead us to seek refuge in all the wrong places—overeating, overdrinking, overworking, overtraining—partially due to our inability and unwillingness to accept all the facets of humanness. We have a hard time acknowledging that we are meant to feel discomfort, pain, sadness, anger, shame, and the entire array of emotions that make us completely human. It is not only acceptable to have these feelings, but they are absolutely necessary for experiencing a full life. In *Embodied Posture*, I ask you to use your yoga practice as a vehicle for returning home to sensory experience within your body. Embodiment becomes the first step toward embracing our wholeness.

Contrasting opinions on yoga alignment are plentiful. Even in one studio, an **asana** may be taught differently by various teachers. I think contrasting opinions are healthy, a sign that we are thinking outside the box and moving forward in our exploration of this ancient practice. Today hundreds of thousands of bodies are doing yoga, and each body's anatomy and experience is unique. Consequently, we should have different opinions and ideas about posture alignment. I also don't believe that any movement is inherently bad. However, we now have abundant information on biomechanics and anatomy which was unavailable in the past. The why behind our movement is key. With a tuned-in awareness and better understanding of how our anatomy moves through posture, we can make more intuitive choices about how we move our own unique bodies.

A RETURN TO EMBODIMENT | CHAPTER 1

My opinions on yoga and alignment have shifted tremendously over the many years I have been practicing and teaching. The more I understand, the grayer the lines become between right and wrong yoga alignment. As a matter of fact, the moment I feel adamantly right about something, I realize I need to question and explore it further. From my perspective, yoga cues aren't necessarily right or wrong; instead, sometimes they are relevant, sometimes not. Each practitioner will have their individual perspective. I didn't write this book to tell you how to do it "right." I'm simply sharing my ideas and understanding, hoping to shed some light on your own experience of embodying your posture.

For years, as I practiced yoga I tried to get my body to fit the pose. I was driven by how poses were "supposed" to look. Of course, this makes sense because yoga begins as a learned skill, and many of us are predominantly visual learners. But knowing what a pose looks like when someone else models it is only the beginning; finding our true and best alignment requires more than attempted imitation.

Somewhere along the way in my yoga journey, I discovered that instead of making myself fit a pose, I could adapt the pose to work for me. I discovered the tool of embodiment: feeling from my heart, my skin, my muscles, and my bones. I ultimately discovered that I was created with an inner guidance system helping me find my own alignment—not only in a pose, but also in my life. I learned that I can honor and embrace what I have learned from other teachers, books, and schools while ultimately allowing my personal experience to guide me. This book is designed with your uniqueness in mind. Please use *Embodied Posture* as a tool for getting to know yourself and your body better, and for powerfully adapting your practice to best serve you.

Yoga poses shouldn't hurt, and they should never degrade your body's structure. Embodied practice respects, honors, and fosters wellness on all levels. Your most effective alignment will arise from feeling within. If you've been practicing or teaching yoga for some time, take what you know, and investigate how it is currently working in your own body. Then go deeper. Discover when, how, and why the alignment cues you are using are relevant and when they aren't. As we cultivate the awareness needed to align yoga poses from inner experience, we gain awareness in the rest of our lives. And as we repetitively practice feeling from within on the mat, we have more and more access to this skill in our daily lives. Embodiment helps us be engaged, honest, and present in all the moments of our lives.

As I grow and learn, I may change my mind about some of the ideas included here, even before you read them. This is totally fine because I want this book to help you become a critical thinker, someone who isn't afraid of ebbing, flowing, and evolving. I hope that as yoga teachers and practitioners, we can move forward with greater understanding of how to honor each other's differences while embracing our sameness. It is through investigating our own internal experiences and openly listening to others that we grow together. This information can help bring more self-compassion and self-acceptance into your yoga and into your life, enabling you to have the same attuned, compassionate awareness of others. Together we can use this practice to promote wellness in all aspects of our lives.

PART ONE | **EMBODIED POSTURE**

Chapter 2

Yoga and the Posture

Yoga

Yoga has been practiced for millennia. Over time, yoga has changed, and views of it have changed. As individuals or groups have brought their unique experiences and perspectives to the practice, new ideas and meanings have developed. These viewpoints are invaluable. Our opinions don't exist in isolation; they only exist as threads woven into the entire fabric of humanity. Our journey here is truly one of togetherness, so the experiences of others can't be separate from our own. In *Embodied Posture*, I share my experience with you, not to invalidate other ideas, or to claim that I am "right," but rather to supplement the collective understanding of yoga and yoga posture.

What is yoga? My answer to this question is just my perspective, from my vantage point, at this moment in time. You may define yoga differently, and I respect and value that. Differing ideas, thoughts, experiences, and perspectives fuel our continual evolution as we approach this ancient practice.

Yoga has roots in ancient India. The word *yoga* translates, "to yoke or unite." Some might say that it is a yoking to authentic self, to true nature, to spirit, or to God. Others explain that it is a yoking between mind, body, and spirit. It has also been defined as yoking the differentiated parts of the body toward wholeness. For me personally, all of this is true. Furthermore, I believe that embodiment, feeling from within, is vital to yoga. I also believe that no matter what religious, spiritual, or life path you follow, yoga can enhance it. I have found that it doesn't serve my practice to cling too tightly to definitions of yoga.

The truth is, my understanding and experience of this practice change from day to day, depending on how I am seeing, who I am being, and my current life circumstances. Yoga gives me the opportunity to notice my body's physical sensations with clarity and compassion. It invites me to breathe with purpose. And it encourages me to pay attention to what is happening now. This seemingly simplistic practice is often the very thing that brings me back to the fullness of being alive. I practice and teach yoga as an embodied form of mindful awareness, a combined system of moving, breathing, and mental focus which cultivates this ability to be aware or to pay attention without judgement.

The Posture

Yoga posture is the vehicle through which we practice mindful awareness. It is also a tool for increasing musculoskeletal wellness. Both mindful awareness and musculoskeletal wellness play a role in balancing the **autonomic nervous system**, which plays a key role in our overall physiological well-being.

Mindful Awareness

Jon Kabat Zinn defines mindfulness as "paying attention in a particular way: on purpose, in the present moment and non-judgmentally."[1] Yoga poses provide an avenue for embodied mindfulness. In other words, yoga poses give us the chance to pay attention to the sensations within our own bodies. Yoga is a physical, moving practice which can be very different from practicing mindfulness in seated meditation. Noticing what we feel physically helps us relate to what's happening within ourselves as well as in our surroundings. Cultivating our ability to clearly observe what we feel can be a profound tool for self-discovery and for living a more whole life.

While moving through yoga postures, we have the opportunity for **interoceptive awareness**, or noticing what is happening inside our bodies. This might include body sensations arising from muscles strengthening or stretching, joints articulating together, breath coming and going, or our hearts beating.

Proprioceptive awareness is also cultivated in many yoga postures. This is an awareness of your body in space, such as sensing where your back arm is in Warrior II when attempting to get it parallel to the floor without looking. In Half Moon, moving to make more space between your lifted leg and the ground involves the sense of proprioception. Fine-tuning the skills of stacking your hips above your shoulders in Handstand is another example of using proprioceptive awareness.

At times our practice might require us to be more aware of what is nearby. This is **exteroceptive awareness.** If we wanted to synchronize our movement with other practitioners, we would need to increase our exteroception by listening to their breath and by noticing their movement pace. Additionally, we might practice listening closely to surrounding sounds or sensing the four walls around us. This is also exteroceptive awareness.

As we increase our interoception, proprioception, and exteroception on the mat, we increase our ability to be mindful in all aspects of life. Mindfulness, this purposeful awareness of ourselves and our surroundings, invites us to experience the full richness of the moments of our lives, increasing our ability to pay attention to all that's happening in the present. I often say that I practice yoga so that I don't miss out on life.

Many years ago, as a mother of three small children, I had a cathartic moment. Like many young mothers, I was in day-to-day survival mode. With a constant to-do list in my mind, all too often I allowed myself to stay in the grip of anxiousness and fear. Frequently I was a million miles away, caught in the trap of the virtual reality of my mind. I was stressed, tired, and unhappy. I vividly remember pulling into my garage in my minivan one evening, parking, and then pausing while I sighed heavily. In the rearview mirror, I caught a glimpse of my three beautiful children, two of them asleep. They looked like little angels. I stared at them for a

PART ONE | EMBODIED POSTURE

while, almost as if I didn't fully recognize them. I noticed a big freckle on my son's face that I hadn't seen before. They were growing and changing so quickly; it felt like it had been a long time since I had taken the time to stop and truly see them.

Life was rushing by me. In that moment, more than anything I desired not to miss out on the beautiful moments of my life. Eighteen years later, my children are all grown, and my youngest recently moved out to attend college. I'd like to say that I was mindfully aware of every single minute with my children from then on, but I am human. I can say that I am incredibly grateful for the gifts of yoga and mindful awareness, along with that awakening in my garage. Because of these things, my life tremendously shifted direction. Of course, I still have times of anxiousness and mental distraction, but now I have amazing tools that help me fully land in the present. I am learning every single day to recognize and move beyond the gripping anxieties and fears that arise. The tools of breath and self-observation I have gained on my mat have been paramount for me.

Musculoskeletal Wellness

Everyone wants to feel good physically. Not only do we want to be free of unnecessary pain, but it's also nice to have functional strength to get up from the floor easily, to carry a baby carrier or groceries without throwing out our backs, or to move rocks in the backyard. Physically, yoga promotes achieving and maintaining musculoskeletal balance. An effective yoga practice will help you find functional mobility with a balance of flexibility and strength.

Any joint's mobility depends on skeletal/joint structure, and soft tissue flexibility and strength. Many yoga practitioners don't realize that their skeletal structures can limit their ranges of motion in actions. When a specific movement or shape is hard to attain, most people think that they are too weak or too tight. This isn't always the case. The shape of our bones may be stopping us.[2] As a student of Paul and Suzee Grilley, I applied this understanding to my own practice and to teaching. Paul and Suzee are experts on this topic, and their teachings were instrumental in shaping me as a teacher.

We are all born with unique skeletal ranges of motion because our bones are shaped differently. It's even likely that your left humerus (upper-arm bone) has a slightly different shape than your right. Having differently shaped bones does not necessarily indicate that anything is wrong. This is the nature of organic life. When bone shapes limit range of motion, **skeletal compression** results. Basically, two bones are bumping, sometimes with corresponding soft tissues impinged between them.

You will never change skeletal range of motion with yoga postures. However, interoception can make you more aware of your limitations. Then, when you understand and experience your body more completely, you can feel when your bones are limiting an action instead of tight soft tissues. Plus, this awareness can positively influence your overall view of and approach to your practice. Chapter 12, "Navigating the Posture," goes deeper into distinguishing between skeletal and soft tissue limitations.

Although you will never change your skeletal structure, you can work toward balancing soft tissues which have been shortened or weakened due to life circumstances. Tight or lax soft tissues can create imbalance in overall structure, leading to pain and loss of functionality. To some degree, daily habits shape our soft tissue structures—fascia, muscles, tendons, and ligaments. If you spend lots of time at your computer or on your smartphone, the soft tissues of your upper back are probably overstretched while those of your front shoulders and chests are bunched and tightened. If you are seated most of the day, your hip fronts will tend to close while your back side becomes soft and weak.

We also develop set points in our ranges of motion. As a child, you could probably easily squat down and reach far under the couch to retrieve a dropped toy. However, our bodies work on a use-it-or-lose-it plan. As you age, if you rarely use these ranges of motion, you eventually lose them. If we spend our lives doing the same things with the same limited movements day after day, our physiology will adapt to accommodate only these movements. Remember, this applies even if you are physically active. If you run every single day without ever moving your body in different ways, you will lose certain ranges of motion. The same thing will happen if you only practice the same yoga postures day after day. But a well-rounded practice can help you regain healthy mobility where you may have lost it.

Contrary to popular belief, yoga is not about gaining excessive flexibility; rather, yoga encourages us to utilize all our natural, full ranges of motion. The stretching, reaching, twisting, folding, and extending are not for achieving pretzel status, but for helping us regain optimally functioning, mobile, sound structures. Stretching is beneficial if it's not taken too far and if it's always balanced with strengthening. Can you imagine how a joint would function if we only emphasized stretching to increase flexibility while ignoring strengthening? This would create instability and the perfect setup for injury. Unfortunately, this sometimes happens in yoga when a student strives to achieve an aesthetic ideal of a pose, focusing completely on the appearance of the pose and disregarding how it feels.

In yoga we want to improve *balanced functional strength*, strength that supports being resilient and capable in everyday life. Building functional strength necessitates movements requiring whole-body integration rather than concentrating on isolated parts. The use of Cylindrical Core (fig. 13.17) is an example of purposefully engaging different parts of the body collectively to support the spine. In contrast, if we focus solely on doing exercises like crunches or leg lifts for core strengthening (isolating and shortening the front body muscles), we could eventually create an imbalance in our structure, quite possibly making us more vulnerable to injury. The full-body actions of reaching, leaning, and getting up and down from the floor are wonderful movements incorporated into yoga that contribute to overall functional strength and healthy mobility.

Sitting on the floor and getting up and down are things we can take for granted, but we must have specific ranges of motion and strength to maintain these abilities. In our studio classes, we include playful movements of jumping, bounding, and balancing weight in the hands. As adults, we tend to stop playing. I personally believe that our bodies, minds, and spirits thrive on playfulness. And who doesn't want to keep up with their grandkids in the backyard? Some might try to convince you that yoga is a serious practice, but I think it's truly all experiential play. Learn to enjoy the experience of being in your body, feeling your heart pounding, your breath moving, and sweat droplets rolling. This is the true experience of aliveness.

Maintaining an overall balance of strength is also important. For example, in a vinyasa yoga practice, the pushing muscles of the front body are repetitively strengthened in poses like

PART ONE | EMBODIED POSTURE

Plank and Low Push-Up. This should be balanced with strengthening the pulling muscles of the back side. We can achieve this by incorporating more poses like Locust (fig. 18.10) while emphasizing back body engagement. Once again, varying movement is vital for balanced functional strength, no matter what physical regimes we follow. Yoga offers many ways to strengthen and release the body. As practitioners and teachers, we must intentionally take responsibility for not becoming too repetitive in our actions.

It is always good to change up poses by doing them differently. Simply mixing up your transitions between poses can create huge biomechanical shifts demanding different strengths and mobilities. This keeps your practice interesting and fun. I am also a big fan of cross-training. As much as I love the comfort of my yoga mat, I continually challenge myself to get off the mat and into other physical activities. Walking, jumping, running, cycling, lifting, and climbing all compliment yoga well, so combine yoga with the other physical activities you love.

Mindfulness and musculoskeletal wellness go hand in hand. Mindful awareness is required for understanding and experiencing our strength, lack of strength, and range of motion. We must pay attention to what we are feeling to grasp how far is far enough and to find the courage to challenge ourselves to grow. A dialed-in awareness is also essential for recognizing how and when to back off. Furthermore, this awareness is one of our primary tools for moving toward **autonomic balance**, a state of equanimity between our sympathetic and parasympathetic nervous systems.

Autonomic Balance

The autonomic nervous system controls our unconscious body functions. Some say that imbalance in this system is the leading cause of many chronic illnesses.[3] Part of the peripheral nervous system, the autonomic nervous system consists of the **sympathetic** and **parasympathetic** branches. Optimally, these systems work together in a balanced way since we need them both to survive and to be well. The sympathetic branch is invoked any time the body needs to deal with a physical or mental stressor. The parasympathetic branch basically acts as the brakes to any process triggered by the sympathetic. Working to balance stress-related responses, the parasympathetic nervous system is activated by slower, deeper breaths and mindful states.[4]

Sympathetic nervous system: fight or flight	Parasympathetic nervous system: rest and digest
Increased heart rate	Decreased heart rate
Increased blood pressure	Decreased blood pressure
Increased ventilation (breath rate)	Decreased ventilation (breath rate)
Slowed digestion	Return to normal digestive function
Increased use of available energy (blood sugar dysregulation)	Blood sugar regulation
Increased blood flow to core body muscles	Regulation of blood flow

YOGA AND THE POSTURE | CHAPTER 2

Whether we are aware of it or not, our hectic lifestyles put many of us in chronic stress. This stress creates over-toned sympathetic and under-toned parasympathetic systems. This imbalance can lead to dysregulated blood sugar, high blood pressure, endocrine imbalances, sleep disorders, digestive issues, anxiety, and depression.[5]

As we learn to notice what we feel inside, paying attention to our internal sensations, we can better discern what we need for the balancing act of wellness. Training our brains to be more mindfully aware reduces mental stress as we gain increased capacity to discern, re-evaluate, and self-regulate.[6] I believe that the combined effects of balanced musculoskeletal wellness, increased mindful awareness, and longer, slower breathing are some of the best medicine available on the planet.

Consider...

A student struggling with stress recently approached me after class. She wanted some suggestions of yoga postures she could do while at work when she noticed her stress level increasing. "The first thing I would do is focus solely on breath," I said. I told her to inhale for a count of four and exhale for a count of eight, continuing this pattern for at least a minute. While yoga postures are great, we can't usually pause a meeting to drop into Downward-Facing Dog. Scientific research strongly correlates longer, slower exhalation with increased parasympathetic response,[4] showing that the breath is a wonderful tool all by itself. I also recommended combining this breathing pattern with some simple movements like Cat/Cow and an easy inverted posture like Waterfall when she wanted to include postures and could. How amazing that some of our most powerful tools for physiological regulation are readily available at any moment in time!

PART ONE | EMBODIED POSTURE

Chapter 3

Road Map to Embodied Posture Methodology

Think of any given yoga pose as a collection of anatomical actions. Ask yourself what individual movements must occur to achieve the overall posture shape? This is the first vital step in tuning in to the pose's intricacies happening within your body.

Embodied Posture is designed as a reference book. As such, it contains many helpful features. Before you dive in, review these features.

"The Body," part 2, describes the major joints and their corresponding anatomical actions. Please don't be intimidated by the science here. While it may seem a bit deep at first glance, my goal has been to provide accessible information you can immediately apply on your mat. For every major anatomical action, I have answered these questions: What moves? What works? What stretches, opposes, or relaxes? Chapters on the spine, shoulder, hip, knee, ankle, elbow, and wrist provide clear and easy reference. You don't need to memorize bones or muscles and their actions, but when you are investigating postures, this detailed information will help you understand what you are feeling.

Part 3, "The Posture," covers individual poses. Each is presented as a collection of anatomical actions clearly labeled in a pose figure. I discuss possible limiting factors, modifications, and variations, along with cues and questions for investigation. All pose information is linked back through cross-references to the drawings and details in "The Body" chapters. You won't need all of this on every pose, so don't get bogged down with it. Use the "What am I feeling?" charts as needed. These charts require an overall understanding of **Embodied Posture Methodology**, or **EPM**, which may take some time to develop. So, be patient with yourself. I hope the information instills a deeper sense of inner experience, rather than an intellectual overload of technical data. Can you allow your learning to be in the form of feeling within?

All figures have two numbers, a chapter number followed by the figure's placement within the chapter. For example, figure 14.1 is a picture of High Lunge, the first image in chapter 14. In addition, you will see that some terms are in **bold type**. While these terms are defined within the text, you can also find them in the Glossary at the end of the book. I've included additional resources in the Endnotes if you would like to research further, as well as an Index.

EPM encourages aligning your yoga postures from within. This practice combines awareness, information, and exploration.

Awareness

The part I love most about EPM is that it doesn't work unless we tune in. We must shift from depending on external sources to trusting what we feel within our bodies. While we still gather knowledge from the outside, for example from teachers, books, videos, etc., heightened awareness of what we are feeling inside is key to using EPM.

Information

Knowledge is power. The better we understand our bodies, the more empowered we are to trust what we feel. Awareness and curiosity in your postures will lead you to want more. The information here will increase your knowledge and your ability to tune in. Our minds absorb information best when we are hungry to learn. Therefore, I suggest you focus on what you need as you need it; you will be more likely to retain what you learn when you are ready to apply it.

Exploration

Use the information you gather from this book along with your heightened awareness to explore the nuances of your own posture and movement. Play with varying approaches to the posture; notice how they feel. Try the modifications and variations I offer, and then consider even more ways to modify and vary the pose. Notice how the pose feels in the moment as well as how your body feels later.

Remember, your goal is not to find the ultimate alignment and then to continue practicing the pose in the same way forever. Our bodies and minds thrive on varied movement. Allow your idea of "correct" alignment to ebb, flow, and transform as your practice changes from day to day. Embrace an open and malleable perspective.

Ten Steps to Approaching Your Practice Using EPM

1. If you are new to yoga, begin with the pose images in this book or the cues your teachers give you; this is the only way to start. Be curious and open.

2. Tune in to sensory experience. Get used to feeling. Feel muscles working, muscles stretching, and bones stacking. Feel your breath and heartbeat.

3. Notice what you feel within your joints. Start with your spine, shoulders, and hips, and then consider your other joints.

4. Aim for a strong, stable posture in which you can maintain your **victorious breath**, (p. 111).

5. Notice anything that limits your strong, stable posture, such as inability to achieve part of the pose, tightness, "stuckness," weakness, fatigue, pain, or restricted range of motion. If nothing is in the way of your posture, remain open to expanding the experience of what you feel inside. Proceed to step 6 if you have questions about what you are feeling.

PART ONE | EMBODIED POSTURE

6. Focus on the location of sensation. Can you feel where the limitation is? Be patient if this is challenging; it will take practice.

7. Refer to the "What am I feeling?" chart for the pose. Here you will find quick answers to these questions: What is strengthening? Where could I notice tightness? Is compression possible? Here is a sample chart for High Lunge (fig. 14.1).

High Lunge. What am I feeling?

HOW DO I GET THERE?	WHAT IS STRENGTHENING?	WHERE COULD I NOTICE TIGHTNESS?	IS COMPRESSION POSSIBLE?
Axial extension	Axial extensors, fig. 5.10	Entire trunk	
Shoulder flexion	**Shoulder flexors, fig. 6.4**	Shoulder extensors, fig. 6.5	✓ Fig. 6.3
Scapular elevation and upward rotation	Elevators and upward rotators of the scapulae, p. 54 *Natural placement with arm positioning*	Depressors and downward rotators of the scapulae, p. 54	
Elbow extension	Elbow extensors, fig. 10.2	Elbow flexors, fig. 10.3	
Back-leg knee extension	**Back-leg knee extensors, fig. 8.2**	Knee flexors, fig. 8.3	
Back-leg hip extension	Back-leg hip extensors, fig. 7.6	**Back-leg hip flexors, fig. 7.5**	
Front-leg knee flexion	**Knee extensors, fig. 8.2** *Even though the knee is bent, extensors stabilize eccentrically and/or isometrically to oppose gravity.*		
Front-leg hip flexion	**Front-leg hip flexors, fig. 7.6** *While lowering into the lunge, hip extensors work eccentrically to oppose gravity. While holding, they work isometrically.*		
Back-leg ankle dorsiflexion	**Back-leg ankle dorsiflexors, fig. 9.3**	**Back-leg ankle plantar flexors, fig. 9.4**	✓ Fig. 9.2

My discoveries:

ROAD MAP TO EMBODIED POSTURE METHODOLOGY | CHAPTER 3

8. If you still don't have your answer, refer to the chapter about the joint you are investigating in part 2, "The Body." For each anatomical action, you will find a "Quick summary" providing the most helpful, minimal, relevant information needed to think critically about your body in posture. Use the three parts of the "Quick summary" as you investigate the following types of questions:

Quick summary — Questions you might investigate with this information

What moves? (skeletal reference)	??
These are the bones which might be moving toward each other, including any possible compression. Remember, skeletal compression is when two bones meet.	Does skeletal compression limit me in this pose? Am I aligning my pose in a way that fits my own joints? Am I feeling compression? If so, how can I change the angles of the pose to reduce this compression?
What works?	??
These are the primary movers, or **agonist** muscles, at the joint origin. Many other muscles work with the main movers, including those moving other joints.	What is strengthening in this pose? If this pose is challenging for me, what muscles or groups of muscles might be weak or limited? If this movement is painful, which muscles might be compromised? If I have a muscle/tendon injury, might that injury affect this movement? (For instance, if an injured hamstring has been diagnosed, which movements require the hamstring to work?)
What stretches, opposes, or relaxes?	??
These are the primary **antagonists**, or those muscles being stretched most directly at the joint origin. Muscles do not move and stretch separately from the other soft tissues connected to them. Everything is connected fascially. This is also known as **myofascial connectivity**, or connected muscle and fascia.	Which soft tissues are being stretched in this pose? Are soft tissues limiting me in this pose? If I experience pain with the stretch of a particular movement, which muscles might be compromised? If I have an identified muscle/tendon injury, might it affect this movement?

9. Refer to chapter 12, "Navigating the Posture," so you can better understand what you are feeling.

10. Using all of this, begin investigating modifications and variations from this book and from other sources. Be patient with yourself while you explore your most embodied posture alignment.

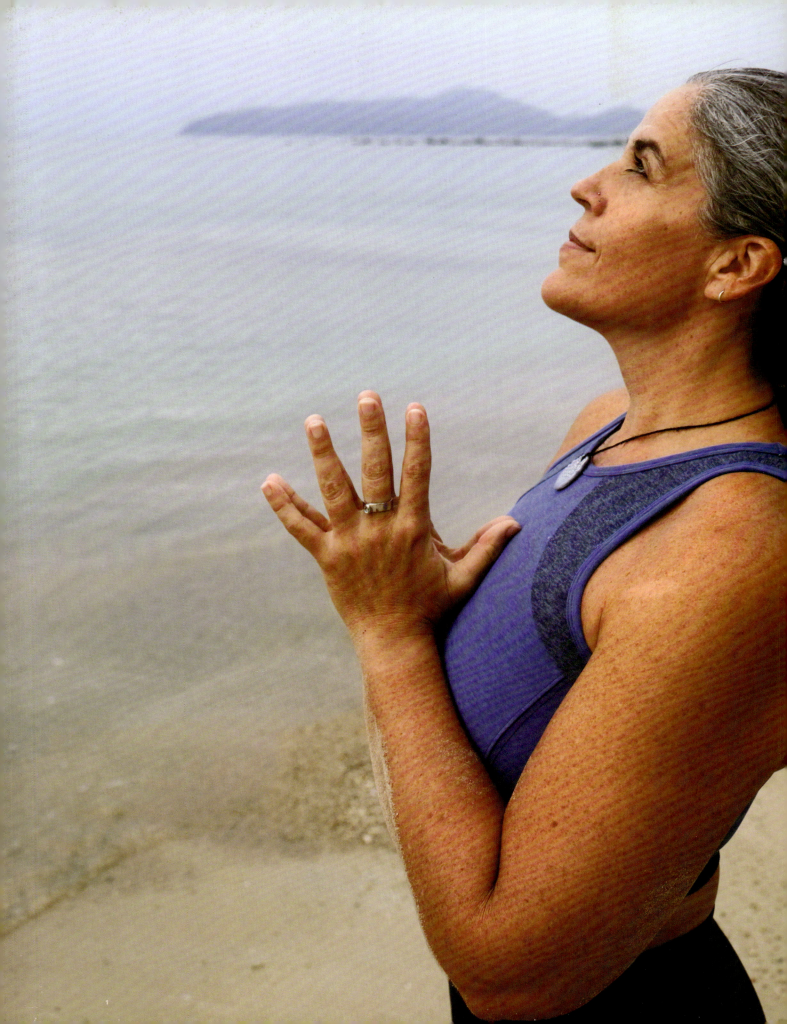

PART TWO
The Body

PART TWO | **THE BODY**

There is something wonderfully bold and liberating about saying yes to our entire imperfect and messy life.

—Tara Brach

Chapter 4
The Body in Posture

Although reducing the body into separate components makes it easier for us to study, this is not how the body works. The body functions as one continuous, complex, integrated network, not as individual parts and pieces. This is partially due to **myofascial connectivity**, or the interconnection between fascia and muscle.[7] For instance, if we feel tightness in Forward Fold, we can't be certain that tightness is only in the hamstrings because the hamstrings are fascially connected to the entire back side of the body. Noticing the hamstrings is a good starting point, but we should always zoom out and consider more. We also can't understand how the body is working by focusing on one isolated joint. All contributing actions must be considered.

Nonetheless, understanding the individual joints and how their corresponding muscle units work to move our bodies is extremely valuable. We can only grasp the body's holistic integration if we also understand the intricacies of the differentiated parts. Once we better understand how the body moves locally (at a specific joint) and regionally (through broader myofascial connectivity), we can begin seeing yoga postures as collections of movements. Examining these movements helps us understand how a particular collection of anatomical actions work together within a pose.

In referencing the body and anatomical actions, I occasionally use the following directional terms:

Lateral	The side of the body or of the body part
Anterior	The front of the body or of the body part
Posterior	The back of the body or of the body part
Superior	Toward the head
Inferior	Away from the head
Midline	Invisible line drawn down the body's center
Superficial	Toward the skin
Deep	Away from the skin, deeper into the body

PART TWO | THE BODY

As we study the body's major joints and how they move, I will refer to the following anatomical directions of motion:

Flexion	Decreasing the angle between two corresponding bones in a joint, closing the joint
Extension	Increasing the angle between two corresponding bones in a joint, opening the joint
Abduction	Moving an arm or leg away from the body's midline.
Adduction	Moving an arm or leg toward the body's midline.
Internal (medial) rotation	Rotating a body part toward the body's midline.
External (lateral) rotation	Rotating a body part away from the body's midline
Forearm supination	Turning the palm up or forward as in **anatomical position**
Forearm pronation	Turning the palm face down or backwards from anatomical position
Plantar flexion	Pointing the foot
Dorsiflexion	Flexing the foot
Scapular protraction	Sliding the scapula laterally on the ribs
Scapular retraction	Sliding the scapula medially on the ribs
Scapular depression	Moving the scapula down, away from the ear
Scapular elevation	Lifting the scapula up, toward the ear
Scapular upward rotation	The outward, upward rotation of the scapula that happens when the arm abducts or lifts
Scapular downward rotation	The downward rotation of the scapula that happens when the arm lowers down from a lifted or abducted position

THE BODY IN POSTURE | CHAPTER 4

It is important to note that I have referred to individual muscles only within their corresponding joint actions. If you are investigating a specific muscle, look up the muscle in the Index to find the anatomical actions associated with it. Then trace those actions through the Index back into the postures in part 3 of this book. The terms defined here and those in bold throughout the book are also included in the Glossary.

For each anatomical action, as **agonist** (working) and **antagonist** (opposing/stretching) muscles are mentioned, remember that only the primary muscles are included. Additional muscles are involved in these actions. I have focused on the information that will help you most as you tune in to your unique body in posture.

Additionally, I have included information on common injuries for each body part discussed. *This information should not be used for diagnosing or treating.* Instead, use it to further expand your insight into the body. I hope this helps you gain a basic, overall understanding of how the body moves most effectively and safely, as well as what the results of imbalanced movement can be. Once you grasp the nature of injury at one joint, you will see common themes in injury and degradation at all joints. These themes recur over and over with body mechanics and injury.

As you dive in to the details of how your body moves, use your mat as your personal laboratory. Tune in to the sensations of what moves, what works, and what stretches with particular actions. Be curious about what it takes to dial up or to dial down certain sensations. Learn to zoom in to micro actions. You will discover that the most interesting aspects of posture are revealed by these tiny incremental shifts.

PART TWO | THE BODY

Chapter 5
The Spine

The spine, the central framework for our bodies, consists of thirty-three bones integrated with a complex network of muscles, tendons, ligaments, and fascia. It surrounds and protects the spinal cord, the electrical highway linking our brains to our bodies, and in turn, connecting us to the environment. Thus, the spine's health is vital to our overall physical, mental, and relational well-being.

Seven cervical, twelve thoracic, and five (sometimes six) lumbar vertebrae, along with the five fused vertebrae of the sacrum and the four fused vertebrae of the coccyx, compose the spine. These vertebral bodies are separated by twenty-three intervertebral discs made of fibrocartilaginous material providing cushion and shock absorption for movement. The spine has **primary (kyphotic)** curves and **secondary (lordotic)** curves that are also essential for shock absorption as well as for weight bearing. Without these curves, we could not run, jump, stand on our hands, or land back on our feet without breaking.

> ### Consider...
> Learning fuels curiosity. In other words, the best way to become more curious about something is to begin learning more about it. Curiosity is vital in the practice of embodiment. The more we learn about something, the more aware of it we can be. Being aware of what is happening within our own bodies allows us to tune in and to feel. This incredibly beneficial shift helps us step out of the "virtual reality" we can sometimes get caught up in within our own minds, getting off the roller coaster of thoughts and emotions that may or may not be reality based. This is a key component of Embodied Posture Methodology.
>
> As a student on the mat, curiosity will be one of your most potent tools for awareness. If you are a teacher, the more you know about anatomy, the more you can articulate the intricacies of the body. Your capacity to clearly and confidently share your understanding of the body will help increase your students' abilities to be mindfully aware of what they are feeling. For both teachers and students, understanding the body is imperative for shaping relevant physical practices that support long-term musculoskeletal wellness.

THE SPINE | CHAPTER 4

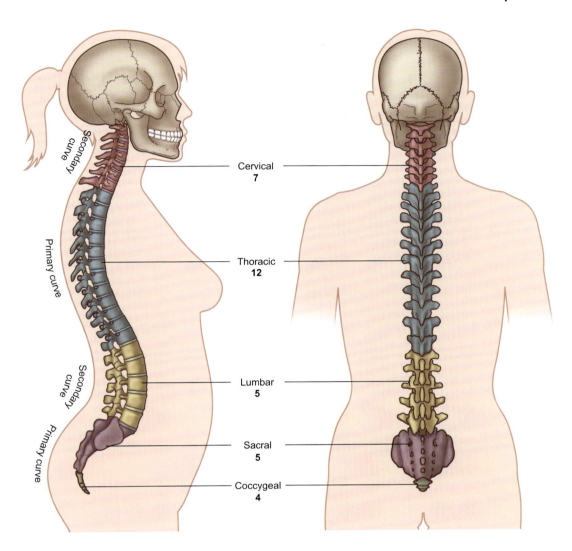

Figure 5.1. Overview of the spine.

Designed for five different movements, the spine can extend, flex, laterally flex, rotate, and extend axially. Regularly moving through each of these natural motions is crucial to sustaining long-term musculoskeletal health. Yoga is the only physical practice I know of that intentionally takes the spine through all its ranges of motion in one session.

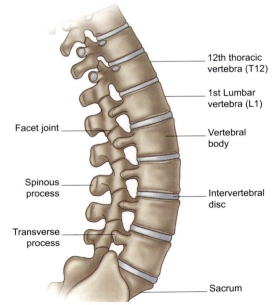

Figure 5.1b. Lateral view of the spine.

21

PART TWO | THE BODY

Spinal Extension

Spinal extension, or backward bending, offers a much-needed counter stretch to our predominant lifestyle actions and postures (fig. 5.2). Most of our repetitive daily activities (including sitting at a desk, working at a computer, driving, texting, etc.) happen in a forward-reaching plane. This can lead to forward rounding along the length of the spine. Repetitive or sustained forward rounding causes overstretched, weak back-body musculature and shortened, tight front-body musculature, creating imbalance. We need backward bending to maintain body balance. (See "The Anatomy of Backbending," chapter 18.)

An example of spinal extension in yoga posture is Upward-Facing Dog (fig. 5.3). *As we look at individual poses depicting certain anatomical motions, remember that no pose is just one action. Each pose is a collection of many joint actions. I am simply choosing to highlight a predominant action here.* For example, Upward-Facing Dog includes spinal extension, hip extension, knee extension, wrist extension, forearm pronation, ankle plantar flexion, and shoulder extension. We will eventually look at each of these anatomical actions.

As the spine moves into extension, the spinous processes move toward each other. This is the opposite of spinal flexion. A backbend reaches its maximum when the spinous processes meet. How and when they meet will vary, depending on one's spinal skeletal constitution. Remember, our bones are all shaped a little differently. Having more or less space between your spinous processes is a result of your unique body design. If someone has more space between their spinous processes, they will have more range to extend. Later I will discuss compression and navigating sensation, as well as how to determine whether your bones or your soft tissues are limiting your spinal extension. (See "Navigating the Posture," chapter 12.)

Compression and limitation are more likely with certain joint actions, depending on bone size, shape, and orientation. In figure 5.2, you can see that someone with less spaciousness between spinous processes will reach compression in backbend sooner than someone with more space, resulting in less spinal extension and a backbend that isn't as pronounced. *Skeletal compression causing limitation doesn't necessarily indicate an inherent problem. It simply reminds us that our bodies are each unique, and poses will feel and look different from person to person.* We will explore deciphering and navigating limitations in chapter 12, "Navigating the Posture."

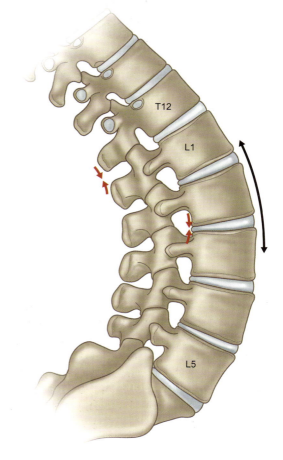

Figure 5.2. Lateral view of the lumbar spine in extension showing spinous processes moving closer together.

THE SPINE | CHAPTER 4

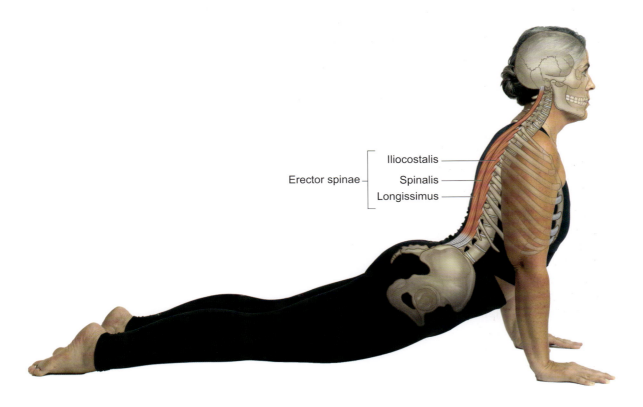

Figure 5.3. Primary spinal extensors in Upward-Facing Dog.

Spinal extension quick summary

What moves?	The spinous processes move toward each other as the vertebrae angle into extension.
What works?	**Spinal extensors** (fig. 5.3) erector spinae (iliocostalis, longissimus, spinalis)
What stretches, opposes, or relaxes?	**Spinal flexors** (fig. 5.5) rectus abdominis, internal and external obliques Or considering myofascial connectivity, the entire front of the body

PART TWO | THE BODY

Spinal Flexion

Spinal flexion is forward rounding of the spine. Although we want to be cautious not to habitually flex the spine forward like we do in a "slouched" posture, occasional, focused forward rounding can offer healthy back-body awareness and release. *Remember, a healthy spine is one that regularly moves through all its natural ranges of motion.*

As the spine moves into flexion, the anterior (front) edges of the vertebral bodies move closer together while the posterior (back) edges and spinous processes move farther away from each other. This is the opposite of extension.

While the spine flexors (agonists) are working, the nervous system is signaling the spine extensors (antagonists) to release, and they are being stretched. In Cat pose the spine is in flexion (fig. 5.5).

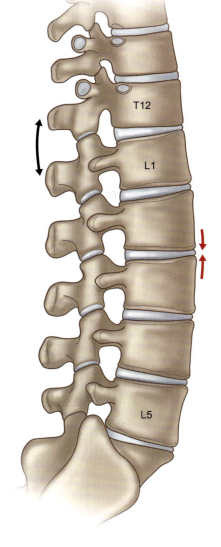

Figure 5.4. Lateral view of lumbar spine in flexion showing spinous processes moving farther apart.

Spinal flexion quick summary

What moves?	The fronts of the vertebral bodies move closer together while the backs of the vertebral bodies and the spinous processes move farther apart.
What works?	**Spinal flexors** (fig. 5.5) rectus abdominis, internal and external obliques
What stretches, opposes, or relaxes?	**Spinal extensors** (fig. 5.3) erector spinae (iliocostalis, longissimus, spinalis) Or considering myofascial connectivity, the entire back of the body

THE SPINE | CHAPTER 4

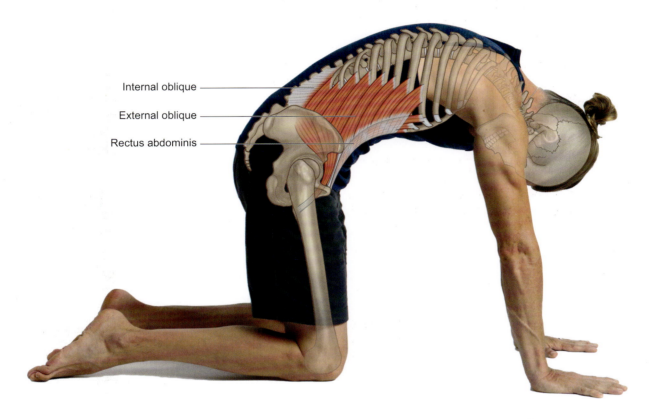

Figure 5.5. Primary spinal flexors in Cat pose.

Lateral Spinal Flexion

Because we primarily move in a forward-backward plane throughout our daily activities, including our structured fitness formats, we should purposefully maintain the spine's lateral movements. Lateral spinal flexion is bending the spine to the side (see fig. 5.6). As the spine moves into lateral flexion, the lateral surfaces of the vertebral bodies move closer together on one side and farther apart on the other side.

While the lateral flexors are working on the bending side, the lateral flexors on the opposite side are being stretched.

PART TWO | THE BODY

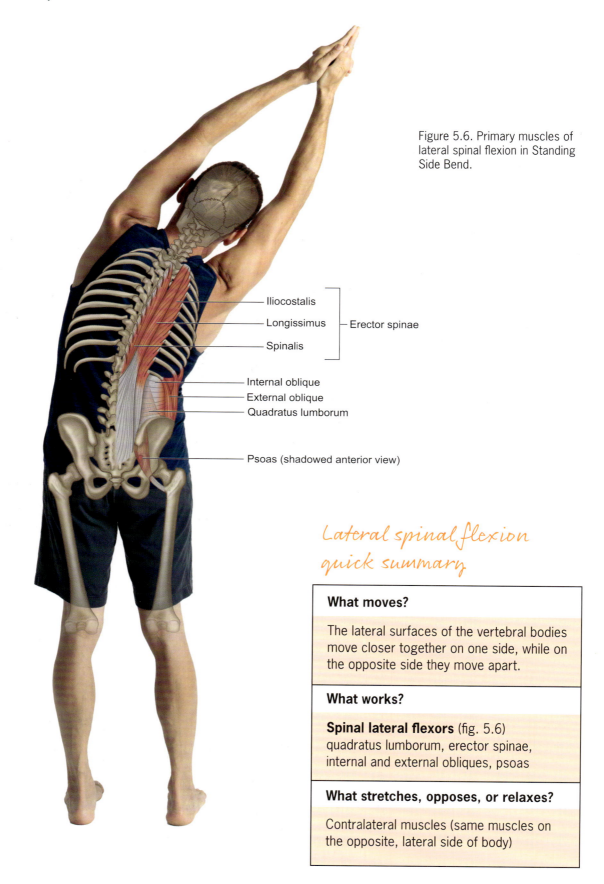

Figure 5.6. Primary muscles of lateral spinal flexion in Standing Side Bend.

Lateral spinal flexion quick summary

What moves?
The lateral surfaces of the vertebral bodies move closer together on one side, while on the opposite side they move apart.
What works?
Spinal lateral flexors (fig. 5.6) quadratus lumborum, erector spinae, internal and external obliques, psoas
What stretches, opposes, or relaxes?
Contralateral muscles (same muscles on the opposite, lateral side of body)

THE SPINE | CHAPTER 4

> *Consider...*
>
> Joints are where two or more bones articulate, or move, in relation to each other. The pulling action of muscles moves the bones. Muscles that move joints attach to one of the bones at the **origin,** and they attach to the corresponding joint bone at the **insertion.** When the muscles engage, activate, shorten, or pull, the bones move closer together.
>
> For every anatomical action (joint motion) there are primary **agonists**, the muscles working to move the bones. On the opposite side of the joint, the muscles relaxing and stretching are the **antagonists**. All muscles that move joints work in agonist-antagonist pairs. We will refer to them as the muscles that are working and the muscles that are stretching, opposing, or relaxing.
>
> Whenever a joint angle is getting smaller or closing in, the muscles on that side of the body are working. In contrast, whenever a joint angle is getting bigger or opening, the soft tissues on that side of the body are opposing the movement, stretching, and/or relaxing. So, in a backward bend, as the spinous process joints on the back of the spine move closer together, the muscles on the back side of the body are working, and the soft tissues on the front side of the body are opposing, stretching, and/or relaxing. As a protective mechanism, our spinal cord reflex demands that the antagonists let go when the agonists are firing. This is called **reciprocal inhibition.**
>
> Gaining an intimate understanding of your body and applying this knowledge in your practice can help you increase what you are feeling within poses. For example, working with reciprocal inhibition can be very useful when trying to encourage a particular part of your body to release.[8] In Seated Forward Fold, for instance, you can activate your quadriceps (knee extensors) to get your hamstrings and calf muscles (knee flexors) to relax. And in a backward bend, engaging the back-side muscles will encourage the front-side muscles to relax.
>
> Since muscle groups work in pairs, it helps to think of opposing pairs, so you can quickly and easily remember which muscles are working or stretching. The following are opposing muscle pairs:
>
> - extensors vs. flexors
> - medial rotators vs. lateral rotators
> - abductors vs. adductors
> - dorsiflexors vs. plantar flexors
> - supinators vs. pronators

Spinal Rotation

All twisting yoga poses entail spinal rotation. Maintaining the ability to rotate the spine is vital for a lifetime of sound, functional movement. Spinal rotation is facilitated by the articulation of the facet joints on the sides of the vertebrae. Thoracic facet joints (fig. 5.7) can glide

PART TWO | THE BODY

over each other enabling twists; these are planar joints. Lumbar facet joints (fig. 5.8) are reinforced planar joints; they are unable to glide over each other for twists. In fact, they block twisting action in the lumbar spine. Crescent Twist provides an example of spinal rotation (fig. 5.9).

The oblique muscles are the main agonists, as well as the main antagonists, in spinal rotation.

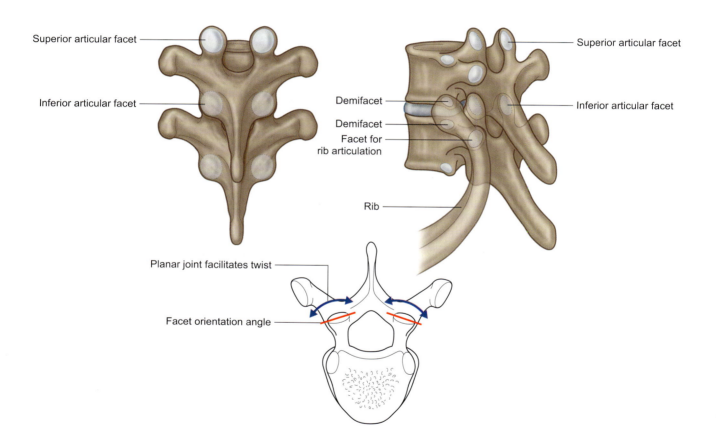

Figure 5.7. Thoracic facet joints.

THE SPINE | CHAPTER 4

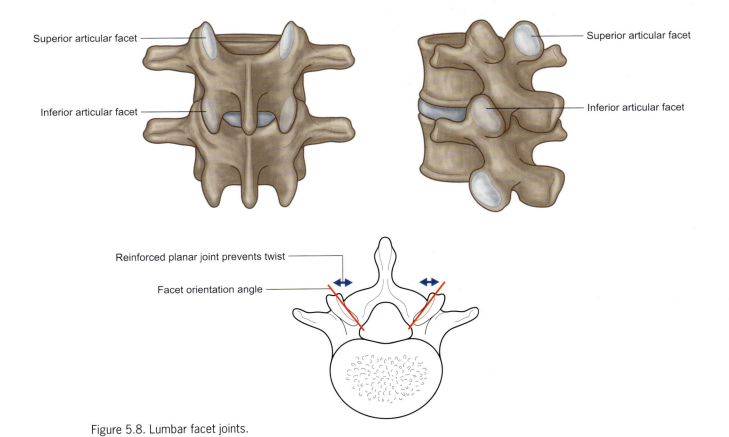

Figure 5.8. Lumbar facet joints.

Spinal rotation quick summary

What moves?	The thoracic facet joints glide over each other to *allow* the spinal twist. These are planar joints.
	The lumbar facet joints meet each other to *block* rotation. These are reinforced planar joints.
	Figures 5.7 and 5.8 show the difference between the thoracic and lumbar facet joints. For more information, refer to "The Anatomy of Twists," chapter 15.
What works?	**Spinal rotators** (fig. 5.9) internal and external obliques, multifidus, rotatores brevis/longus, on side approached
What stretches, opposes, or relaxes?	Contralateral muscles (same muscles on the opposite, lateral side of body)

PART TWO | THE BODY

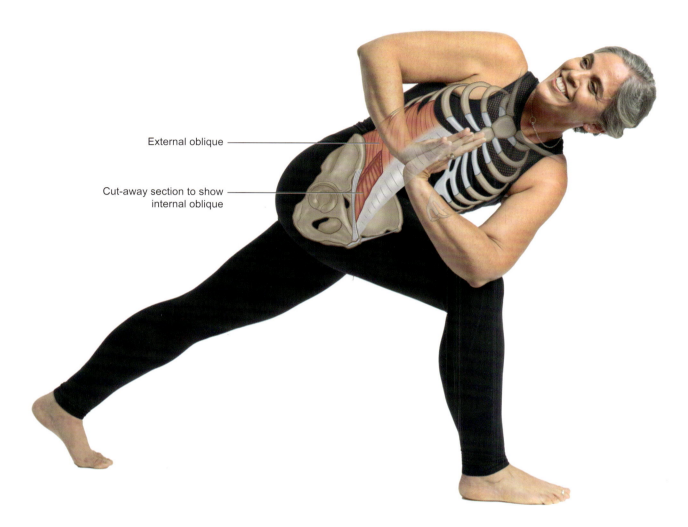

Figure 5.9. Primary muscles of spinal rotation in Crescent Twist.

Spinal Axial Extension

Axial extension is unlike other anatomical motions of the spine because it doesn't involve the same types of joint articulation. Rather, all vertebrae are moving farther away from each other, decreasing both the primary and secondary curves, lengthening the spine overall. It happens when we simply stand taller without backward bending or forward rounding (fig. 5.10).

THE SPINE | CHAPTER 4

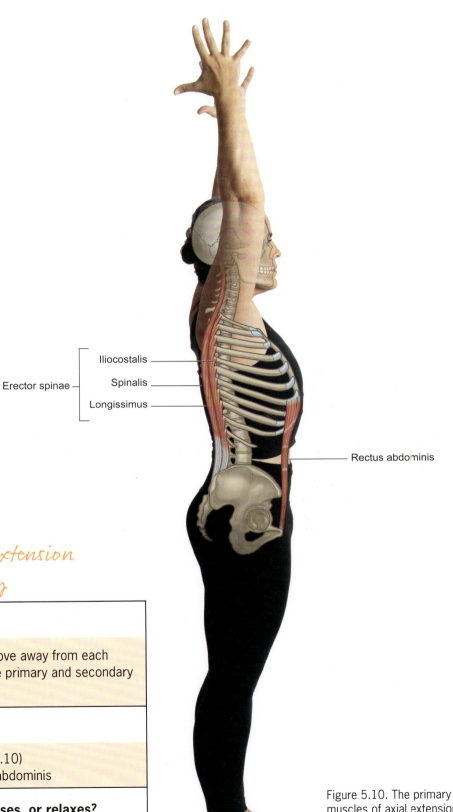

Spinal axial extension quick summary

What moves?
The vertebral bodies move away from each other, reducing both the primary and secondary spinal curves.

What works?
Axial extensors (fig. 5.10) erector spinae, rectus abdominis

What stretches, opposes, or relaxes?
All trunk muscles

Figure 5.10. The primary muscles of axial extension in Mountain pose.

PART TWO | THE BODY

Common Injuries

As we look at common injuries, keep in mind that I've chosen to include those injuries I encounter most in my classes. Like reducing the body into parts to study functional movement, reducing an injury down to a single, isolated issue is also problematic. The body is one interconnected unit; injuries which emerge in one location are often part of a larger imbalance. *Imbalance is at the root of all musculoskeletal pain and injury.*

> *Consider...*
>
> The musculoskeletal body balances under the principle of tensional integrity.[9] Imagine a tall, flexible tower supported by surrounding cables tethered to the ground on all sides. If one cable became overly tight or overly loose, the structure would be pulled off its center. This is precisely what happens in the body; muscles become too tight or too lax, and our structure (the skeleton and surrounding tissues) can be pulled off balance. This imbalance leads to degradation, pain, and chronic injury.

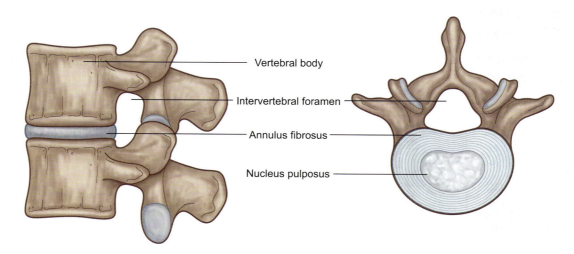

Figure 5.11. Normal intervertebral disc.

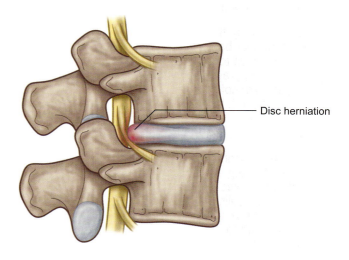

Figure 5.12. Lumbar disc herniation.

THE SPINE | CHAPTER 4

Intervertebral Disc Injury

The **intervertebral discs** (fig. 5.11) are shock absorbers supporting the skeletal spine's movement. The tougher, outer disc material is the **annulus fibrosus**, and the softer, inner material is the **nucleus pulposus**.

Over time, repetitive movement patterns and imbalanced weight bearing can cause the annulus fibrosus to weaken, resulting in a bulge or releasing nucleus pulposus material into the surrounding area (fig. 5.12).[10] Often caused by years of sitting in a flexed, rounded-forward position, this weakening usually occurs on the back side of the disc.[11]

This bulge or released material may come into contact with spinal cord nerves, causing traveling nerve pain or **neuropathy**. Disc injury most commonly happens in the lumbar spine. It also frequently takes place in the cervical spine. The bulge or inflammation usually occurs posteriorly, either to the left or to the right. This often affects the sciatic nerve (fig. 5.13), creating the symptom of sciatica which is typically felt as radiating pain originating from the lumbar spine, traveling down the hip and/or leg. Sciatica can present on either or both legs. Although sciatica is often a symptom of lumbar disc injury, it can also result from **piriformis syndrome**, when the piriformis muscle (fig. 5.13) compresses the sciatic nerve.[12] *Lumbar disc herniation and piriformis syndrome can occur independently or simultaneously.*

It is important to remember that pain is not always felt with injury. Furthermore, pain is subjective, so sometimes it is not the best indicator of an injury's severity.

Consider...

I personally had several lumbar disc herniations when I was young. I was scheduled for surgery, and miraculously the surgeon decided not to do it at the last minute. I was only 18. I suffered off and on for many years with debilitating pain before I began yoga. I also found the book, *Cure Back Pain with Yoga*, by Loren Fishman, MD, and Carol Ardman. Their teachings confirmed my own experience of healing and pain relief from backbends. To this day, backbending postures are my therapy, along with a full, balanced practice. I can't go long without doing them.

I'm not saying that backbends are good for every person with disc injury. I'm also not claiming that backbends were the only thing that healed me. We can't ever reduce healing down to one element. I was also doing many other things, including breathwork, meditation, prayer, and nutritional therapy. And yes, absolutely, sometimes surgery is needed. I'm not claiming to understand your injury, nor am I telling you what you need to do about it. We can gather information from various sources: books, physicians, physiotherapists, chiropractors, friends. But no information is valid unless it has been filtered through your unique, embodied experience.

I'm simply sharing my personal experience in case it can help your own heightened understanding of your injury. If you have any kind of injury, I highly suggest you get out of the "black box" with it. Know what it looks like and exactly where it is, so you can begin feeling how your movement is affecting it. Know what happens with certain actions. Know whether or not your practice is benefiting you. The alternative is to know nothing and to simply take someone else's word for what is happening within your body. You are the ultimate authority on your body, experience, and practice.

PART TWO | THE BODY

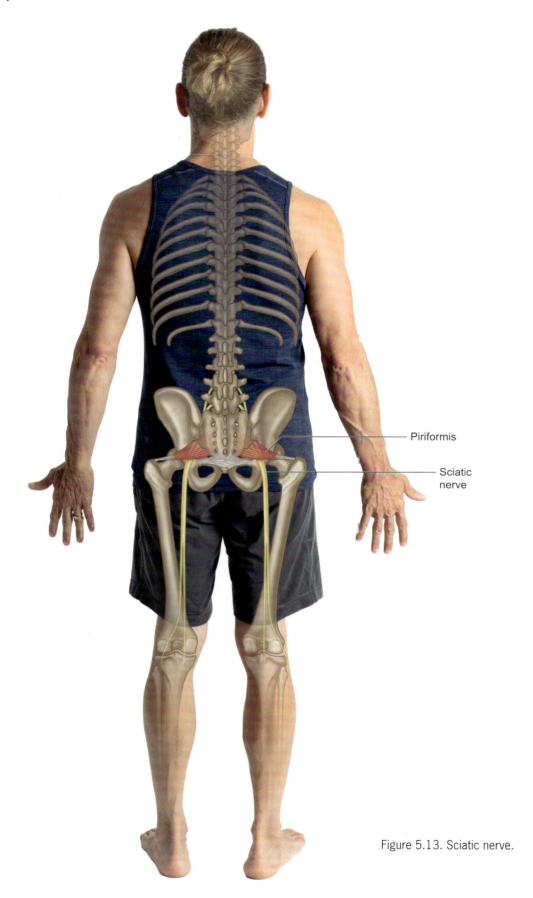

Figure 5.13. Sciatic nerve.

THE SPINE | CHAPTER 4

Posture Considerations

Always avoid yoga postures that cause lasting or residual pain.

Pain is a very tricky thing to discuss, partly because it is subjective. Also, there are different types of pain. Sometimes when you are working through an injury, a therapeutic movement can cause slight pain or discomfort. In the moment you feel discomfort, yet afterwards it feels better. This type of therapeutic "pain" lessens over time. Other times movements are alarmingly painful as the body tells you without a doubt that you shouldn't proceed. Again, this is the importance of embodiment. As the practitioner, only you can ultimately decide what is working and what is not.

If you have intervertebral disc issues, be cautious with any postures that involve a forward-flexed (rounded) lumbar spine. A disc bulge tends to push back toward the spinal cord, and this is where the pain or sensation starts.[13] Forward rounding would encourage the disc to continue pushing toward the spinal cord, possibly exacerbating the problem. Either avoid forward folding entirely, or approach it carefully with bent knees. Bending your knees will release some back-body tightness and will help you keep a longer spine rather than a rounded one.

Slowly work toward spinal extension/backward bending as you are able. Spinal extension is the one movement that encourages the disc to move away from the spinal cord and the point of aggravation. Approach the simplest of backward bends first. Sitting tall in a chair while arching into a slight backbend or lying on the floor for Sphinx pose is a good start. Many people think that backward bends should be avoided entirely with an intervertebral disc injury; this is simply not true. Each person and injury is unique. Only the affected individual can determine if and when backbending could be beneficial.

Revamp your sitting style. See "The Anatomy of Backbending," chapter 18, for more on the biomechanics of sitting.

Usually, the soft tissues surrounding any injured area will be reactive, tight, and imbalanced. Practice gentle stretches for the tight body parts. Often postures that open the outer hip compartment and release the hamstrings bring relief.

Use your doctor and physiotherapist's instructions to design a new practice that works for you along your path of healing.

PART TWO | THE BODY

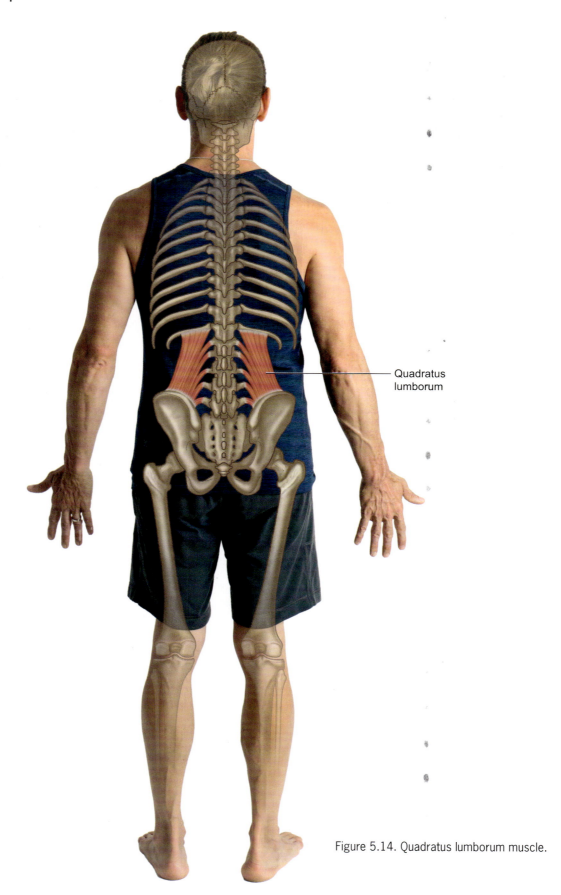

Figure 5.14. Quadratus lumborum muscle.

THE SPINE | CHAPTER 4

Lumbar Muscle Strain

Just as tensional integrity loss can degrade the intervertebral disc structure over time, it can also affect the spine's muscles, tendons, and ligaments. These conditions may occur simultaneously. When sitting is a predominant part of someone's lifestyle, their back muscles tend to get overstretched, weak, and tense. We typically think of tightness and tension only in shortened muscles, yet it also occurs in overstretched muscles. Muscle tension can create unevenly distributed forces, often leading to tears. This sometimes happens during strong effort, like lifting something heavy or moving quickly in an unusual way.

Tension, tightness, and strain can happen in any muscle. In the back, the quadratus lumborum muscle (QL) that runs from the iliac crest to the twelfth thoracic vertebrae is a very common place of strain (fig. 5.14). This muscle is responsible for stabilizing the low back while upright and for aiding in side bending. Technically, it is considered a deep abdominal muscle.

Pain with muscle strain is typically localized and does not radiate or travel like nerve pain associated with disc inflammation.

Posture Considerations

Always avoid postures that cause lasting or residual pain.

Give the injury some time to rest before practicing.

Strong backbends may put too much pressure and restriction on the QL.

Standing lateral bends toward the injured side might be too much until the injury is healed. The QL is one of the prime mover muscles in this action.

Supported spinal mobility as in Cat/Cow can be beneficial once the pain is reduced.

Seated lateral-side stretching can be beneficial once the pain is reduced. An example of this is the lateral-stretch variation of Full Pigeon (fig. 19.12).

People with this injury often find relief in supported forward folds like Child's (fig. 13.1).

Use your doctor and physiotherapist's instructions to design a new practice that works for you along your path of healing.

PART TWO | THE BODY

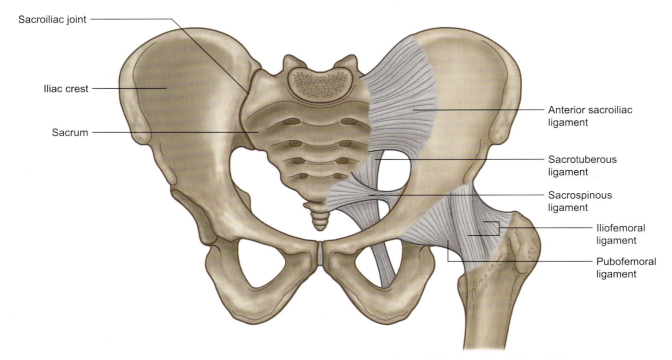

Figure 5.15. Sacroiliac joint with ligaments.

Sacroiliac Joint Dysfunction

The sacroiliac joint (SI) connects the sacrum, the triangular wedge of fused vertebrae at the bottom of the spine, with the pelvis (fig. 5.15). The part of the pelvis that meets the sacrum on either side is the ilium. This joint is where the forces of the spinal actions transfer into the pelvis and legs. By nature, it is strong and stable with very little movement. You have an SI joint on either side of your pelvis. If you reach or look back, you can feel or see two dimple-like indentions within your bony structure. These are your SI joints.

SI dysfunction occurs when the joint is misaligned.[14] Because the joint is bilateral, if one side is misaligned, the other probably is as well, at least somewhat. Frequently, SI joint pain travels from one side to the other. As with all joint misalignment, the culprit is often tensional integrity imbalance within the surrounding soft tissues. In "The Anatomy of Backward Bending," chapter 18, I discuss how an imbalance occurs between tight hip flexors and lax posterior glute muscles. Usually the imbalance is not only from the front to back sides of the hip, but from the left to right sides as well. This imbalanced tension can strain the SI joints, leading to misalignment. A typical injury pattern is imbalanced tension from postural patterns, followed by a jarring or forced action, such as stepping off a curb unknowingly or pushing too hard in a yoga pose.

THE SPINE | CHAPTER 4

Posture Considerations

Always avoid postures that cause lasting or residual pain. Every single posture can be modified. Feel what is happening within your own body. Change the pose accordingly, or skip it altogether.

Consider overall tensional integrity. Approach all your physical practices with the intention of balance. You probably need to strengthen your posterior hip muscles to bring balance back to your hip joints if you sit much of the day. Simple lunges and squats can be very beneficial. Seek out yoga poses in which you can activate the glutes more, as well as non-yoga actions that help increase posterior strength. Any time the hip is extending, take advantage of firing the glutes. You can do this in backward-bending poses or in poses in which the back leg is extended, such as Crescent Lunge.

Maintain balance in your hip joints by stretching and strengthening all three hip compartments. See "The Anatomy of Hip Opening," chapter 19. Include exercises that work the deep hip stabilizers, such as abduction work and one-leg balancing postures.

Avoid poses that create torquing tension between the spine and the pelvis. An example of this is Warrior I. The pelvis is slightly angled to the side while the aim is often squaring the front of the hips or the torso forward. When this aim to square is forced, the spine rotates away from the pelvis, landing strained tension in the SI joint. Simply allow the pelvis to angle slightly to the side, or do Crescent Lunge instead. Backward-bending poses can also sometimes place too much stress on unstable SI joints.

In all poses, keep the pelvis as stable as possible. Avoid combining forced or leveraged twists with holding the pelvis square. Read more about this in "The Anatomy of Twists," chapter 15.

Use your doctor and physiotherapist's instructions to design a new practice that works for you along your path of healing.

PART TWO | THE BODY

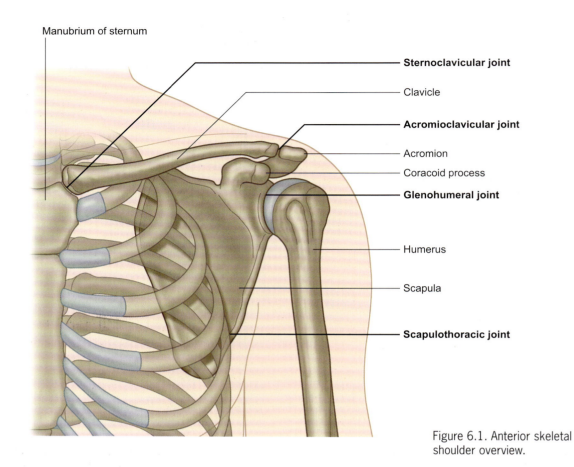

Figure 6.1. Anterior skeletal shoulder overview.

Chapter 6
The Shoulder

The shoulder is among the most complex and mobile joints of the body. While this joint's wide range of movement helps facilitate the hand's many unique actions, the shoulder's extreme complexity and mobility also make it somewhat unstable.

The shoulder consists of these four separate joints:

1. acromioclavicular—where the acromion and clavicle join,
2. sternoclavicular—where the sternum and clavicle join,
3. scapulothoracic—where the scapula and thorax join, and
4. glenohumeral—where the humerus and scapula (glenoid fossa) join.

We will focus on the glenohumeral joint and the scapulothoracic joint.

Three bones make up the glenohumeral joint: the humerus, the scapula, and the clavicle. The glenohumeral joint is designed to flex, to extend, to rotate medially, to rotate laterally, to abduct, and to adduct (fig. 6.1).

THE SHOULDER | CHAPTER 6

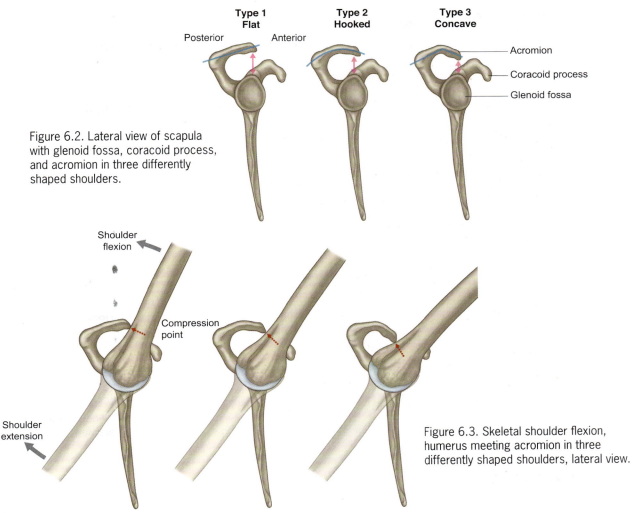

Figure 6.2. Lateral view of scapula with glenoid fossa, coracoid process, and acromion in three differently shaped shoulders.

Figure 6.3. Skeletal shoulder flexion, humerus meeting acromion in three differently shaped shoulders, lateral view.

Shoulder Flexion

This action can be seen in Warrior I (fig. 14.7) and in any other pose in which the arms are lifted above shoulder level.

Flexion occurs when the humerus moves upward to meet the acromion process, the part of the scapula that extends over the top of the humerus. Shoulder flexion is the opposite of shoulder extension. The size, shape, and orientation of the glenoid fossa, the acromion, and the head of the humerus determine how these bones articulate together. See the comparison in figure 6.2 of three unique shoulder skeletal complexes. These are all normal shoulders, but the acromions are shaped very differently.[15]

Now notice how the acromions' unique shapes affect flexion (fig. 6.3). Flexion will look and feel different in each shoulder because of these distinctions.

It is important to remember that the acromion is part of the scapula. If and when the humerus meets the acromion, the scapula and clavicle will both lift with the arm. The scapula and clavicle are connected at the acromioclavicular joint, so they always move as one unit; consequently, it is never proper to cue taking the shoulders away from the ears when the arms are lifted above parallel to the floor.

PART TWO | THE BODY

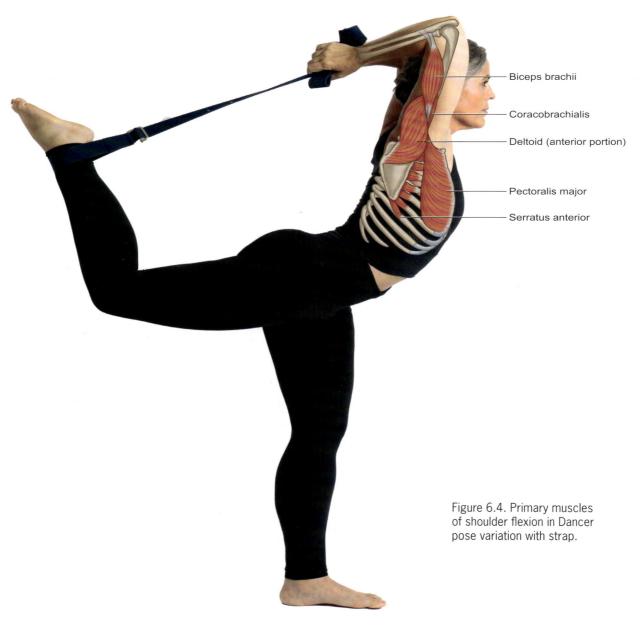

Figure 6.4. Primary muscles of shoulder flexion in Dancer pose variation with strap.

Shoulder flexion quick summary

What moves?	The humerus closes toward the acromion process. Remember, the clavicle and scapula move as one unit. They will lift together if and when the humerus meets the acromion because the acromion is part of the scapula. (See fig. 6.3.)
What works?	**Shoulder flexors** (fig. 6.4) anterior deltoid, pectoralis major, biceps brachii, coracobrachialis, serratus anterior
What stretches, opposes, or relaxes?	**Shoulder extensors** (fig. 6.5) triceps brachii, latissimus dorsi, posterior deltoid, teres major

THE SHOULDER | CHAPTER 6

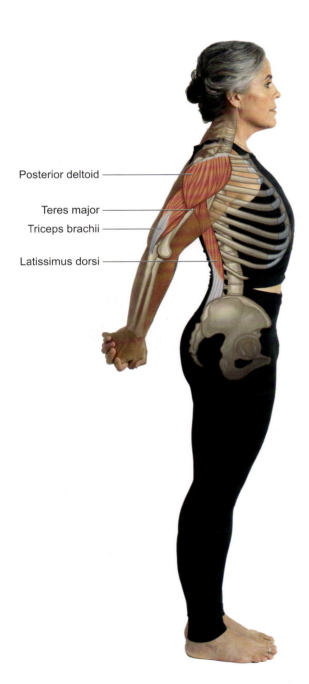

Figure 6.5. Primary muscles of shoulder extension in Mountain pose with hands clasped.

Shoulder Extension

Shoulder extension happens when we move the arms down and back (fig. 6.5). The humerus bone is moving away from the acromion, opening the front of the joint. This is the opposite of shoulder flexion (fig. 6.4).

Shoulder extension quick summary

What moves?
The humerus moves away from the front edge of the acromion process.
What works?
Shoulder extensors (fig. 6.5) triceps brachii, latissimus dorsi, posterior deltoid, teres major
What stretches, opposes, or relaxes?
Shoulder flexors (fig. 6.4) anterior deltoid, pectoralis major, biceps brachii, coracobrachialis, serratus anterior

PART TWO | THE BODY

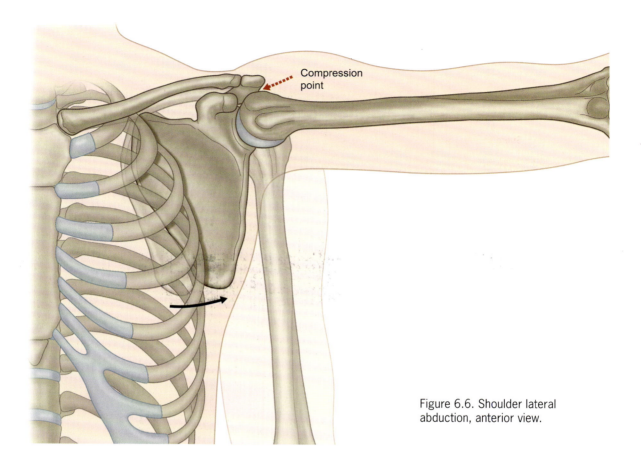

Figure 6.6. Shoulder lateral abduction, anterior view.

Shoulder Lateral Abduction

As we look at shoulder **abduction** and **adduction**, remember these actions occur in two different planes: the horizontal plane and the lateral plane. I am focusing on abduction in the lateral plane and adduction in the horizontal plane.

Lateral abduction takes place when the arms are moved away from the body's centerline as in Warrior II (fig. 6.7). As the arms reach out laterally away from the body, the head of the humerus rotates within the glenoid fossa, moving the humerus toward the acromion process. If and when the humerus meets the lateral edge of the acromion, the clavicle and scapula will tilt laterally as one unit (fig. 6.6). The deltoid and supraspinatus muscles are the primary muscles that laterally abduct the shoulder (fig. 6.7). Abduction is the opposite of adduction.

THE SHOULDER | CHAPTER 6

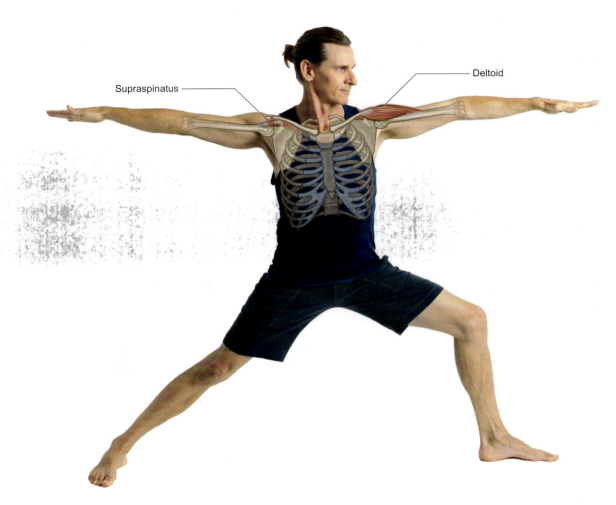

Figure 6.7. Primary muscles of shoulder lateral abduction in Warrior II.

Shoulder lateral abduction quick summary

What moves?	The humerus moves away from the body's midline. When the humerus is laterally abducted, as in Warrior II, the head of the humerus is rotationally closing into the acromion and into the subacromial space. (Fig. 6.16 shows the subacromial space.)
What works?	**Shoulder lateral abductors** (fig. 6.7) deltoid, supraspinatus
What stretches, opposes, or relaxes?	**Shoulder lateral adductors** latissimus dorsi, pectoralis major, teres major, triceps, coracobrachialis

PART TWO | THE BODY

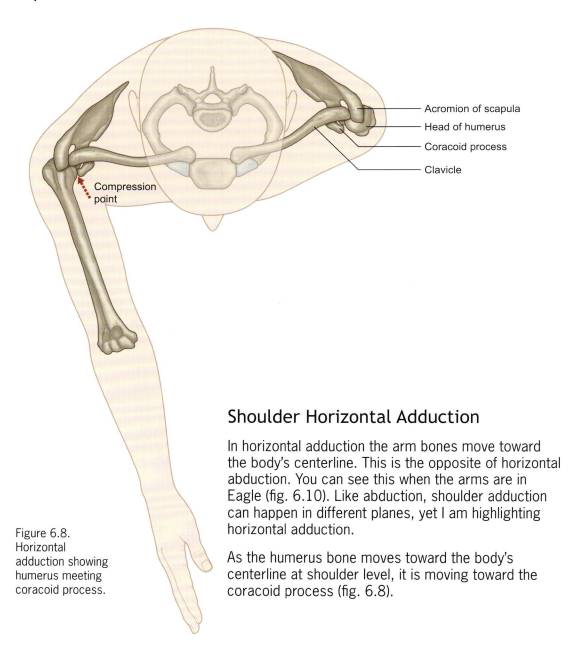

Figure 6.8. Horizontal adduction showing humerus meeting coracoid process.

Shoulder Horizontal Adduction

In horizontal adduction the arm bones move toward the body's centerline. This is the opposite of horizontal abduction. You can see this when the arms are in Eagle (fig. 6.10). Like abduction, shoulder adduction can happen in different planes, yet I am highlighting horizontal adduction.

As the humerus bone moves toward the body's centerline at shoulder level, it is moving toward the coracoid process (fig. 6.8).

Shoulder horizontal adduction quick summary

What moves?	The humerus moves toward the midline of the body. When the humerus is at shoulder level, the humerus can move toward or to the coracoid process.
What works?	**Shoulder horizontal adductors** (fig. 6.9) pectoralis major, deltoid (anterior head), coracobrachialis
What stretches, opposes, or relaxes?	**Shoulder horizontal abductors** deltoid (posterior head)

THE SHOULDER | CHAPTER 6

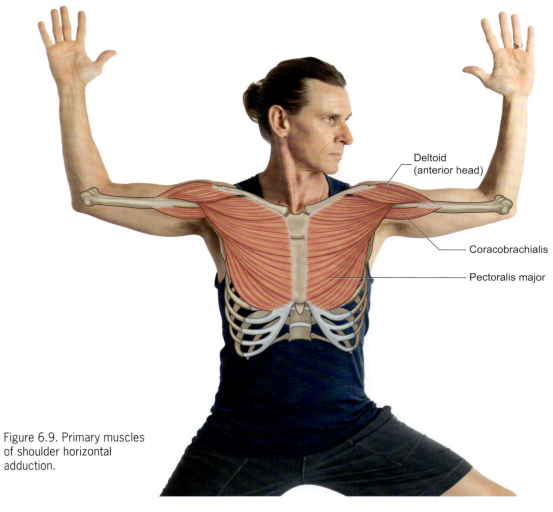

Figure 6.9. Primary muscles of shoulder horizontal adduction.

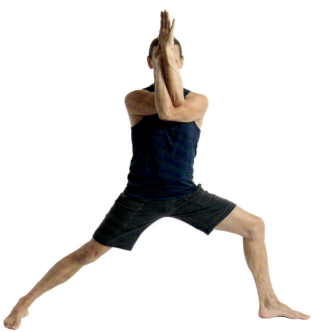

Figure 6.10. Warrior II with Eagle arm variation showing shoulder adduction.

PART TWO | THE BODY

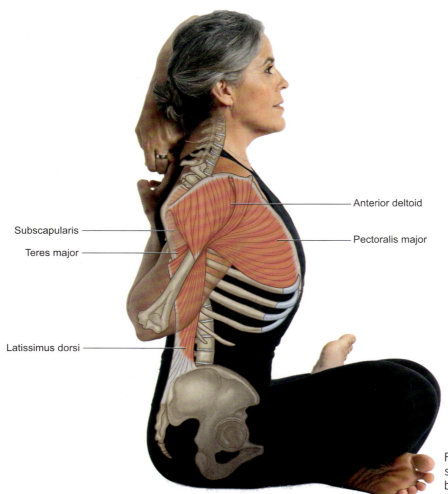

Figure 6.11. Primary muscles of shoulder medial rotation in arm bind with Full Pigeon.

Shoulder Medial Rotation

Medial, or internal rotation, is not taught as a specific alignment in yoga posture, but it does show up in some arm binds (fig. 6.11).

We always want to move in ways that encourage and maintain range of motion. *Safe movement prohibits bearing weight with an internally rotated shoulder or applying force to it; this can put too much pressure on the soft tissues associated with the front of the shoulder* (fig. 6.13). Figure 6.12 shows a very common misalignment with Dancer pose hand positioning. Medial rotation and/or extension are combined with added force or tension, putting excessive strain on the vulnerable soft tissues of the anterior shoulder complex. This also takes place in other arm binds for some people. An example is the bottom arm in Side Angle, full-bind variation. The humerus rotates toward the body's midline during medial rotation.

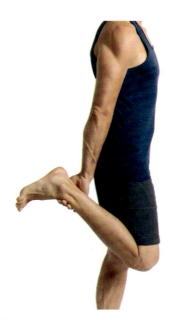

Figure 6.12. Incorrect Dancer grip with medial rotation.

48

THE SHOULDER | CHAPTER 6

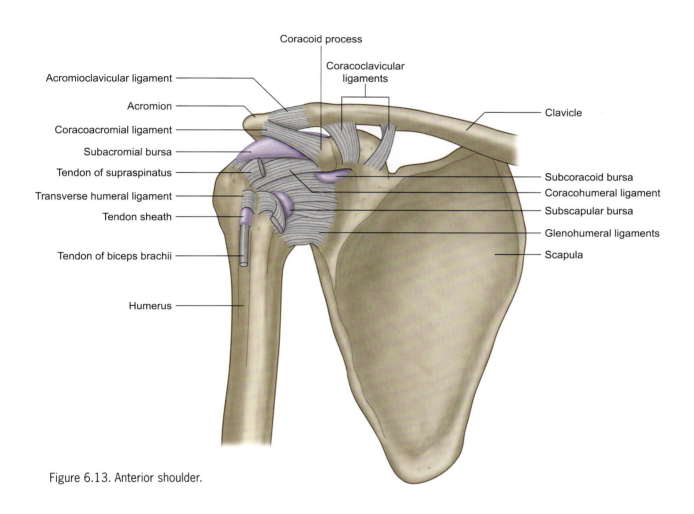

Figure 6.13. Anterior shoulder.

Shoulder medial rotation quick summary

What moves?	The head of the humerus rotates toward the coracoid process.
What works?	**Shoulder medial rotators** (fig. 6.11) pectoralis major, anterior deltoid, subscapularis, teres major, latissimus dorsi
What stretches, opposes, or relaxes?	**Shoulder lateral rotators** (fig. 6.14) posterior deltoid, infraspinatus, teres minor

49

PART TWO | **THE BODY**

Shoulder Lateral Rotation

Lateral rotation moves the palm of the hand from medial facing, or facing the body, to facing front as in Mountain. When the arms are outstretched, and the palms roll up and open in Warrior II, this is also lateral rotation. Chair is another example when the arms reach up and the pinkies rotate toward each other. These are all the same motions; they just look a little different when the arms are in different positions.

An externally rotated glenohumeral joint is often the most sound position for avoiding anterior soft tissue vulnerabilities. This also opens the often-closed fronts of the shoulders and the chest. If you visualize someone slouching while working long hours at a computer, their shoulder joints are typically internally rotated and dropped forward. Sitting up tall and opening the chest would require a lateral or external rotation of the glenohumeral joint (fig. 6.14).

The humerus rotates away from the midline with external or lateral rotation. The posterior deltoid, infraspinatus, and teres minor are the major movers of this action.

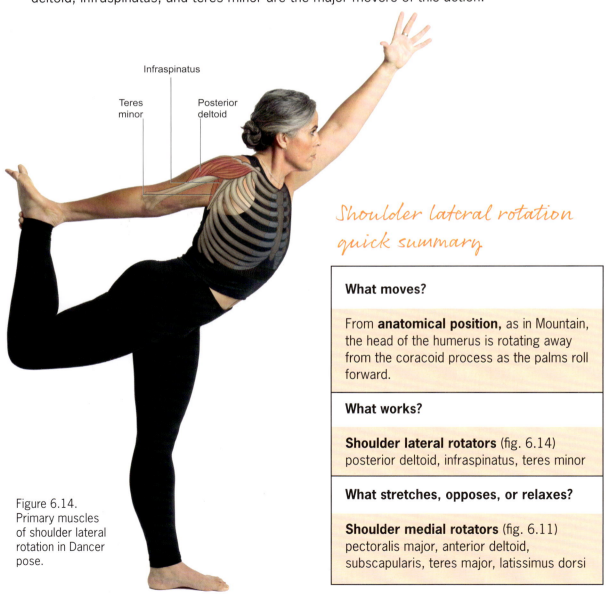

Figure 6.14. Primary muscles of shoulder lateral rotation in Dancer pose.

Shoulder lateral rotation quick summary

What moves?
From **anatomical position,** as in Mountain, the head of the humerus is rotating away from the coracoid process as the palms roll forward.
What works?
Shoulder lateral rotators (fig. 6.14) posterior deltoid, infraspinatus, teres minor
What stretches, opposes, or relaxes?
Shoulder medial rotators (fig. 6.11) pectoralis major, anterior deltoid, subscapularis, teres major, latissimus dorsi

THE SHOULDER | CHAPTER 6

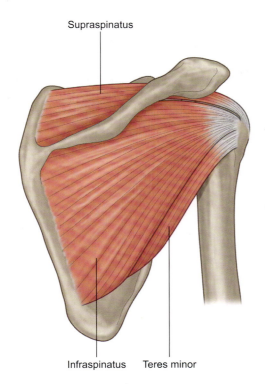
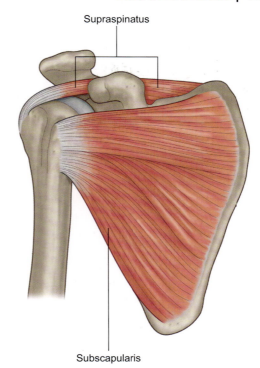

Figure 6.15. Posterior and anterior view, muscles of the rotator cuff.

Common Shoulder Injuries

Rotator Cuff Injury

The rotator cuff is made up of the four muscles and their tendons that create a supportive cuff around the glenohumeral joint. These four muscles are the supraspinatus, the infraspinatus, the teres minor, and the subscapularis (fig. 6.15). Acting collectively to stabilize the head of the humerus in its shallow shoulder socket (the glenoid fossa), these muscles also perform the work needed to move the arm bone within the socket.

Although traumatic blows to the joint can damage the rotator cuff, injuries often result from unstable structure combined with repetitive movement.[16]

Notice that the acromion process and the head of the humerus are very close. As you've seen in figure 6.3, the shape of the acromion determines just how close they are. Within this subacromial space (the space below the acromion), there is a bursa for cushioning, as well as ligaments, tendons, and muscles that extend toward their attachments on the head of the humerus. Visualize for a moment the movement of the arm in the shoulder socket. Can see how wear and tear could occur? Imagine if bone spurs were on the acromion's underside; damage of nearby soft tissues would be accelerated with movement. Unfortunately, this is very common.

Since bones can be shaped quite differently from body to body, and even on the left and right sides of the same person, some people will have less subacromial space than others. Smaller or tighter subacromial space may leave them more prone to deterioration, depending on their daily, repetitive movement. Poor posture may cause slumping forward that takes the shoulders away from ideal placement and biomechanics, inducing further wear and tear with specific, repetitive arm movement.

PART TWO | THE BODY

Descriptions of the most common rotator cuff injuries follow:

1. **Impingement**—compression caused when two or more separate bones of a joint articulate, capturing soft tissues between them
2. **Bursitis**— inflammation of the synovial bursa sac within a joint
3. **Tendinopathy**— inflammation and/or degradation of a tendon

These are not exclusively separate conditions since impingement can lead to bursitis and tendinopathy. All three can exist together.

Pain with a rotator cuff injury usually occurs when the arm is lifted above parallel to the ground. At this angle the humerus closes into the subacromial space. This is also where scapulothoracic movement (movement of the shoulder blade) joins glenohumeral movement (movement in the shoulder socket joint).

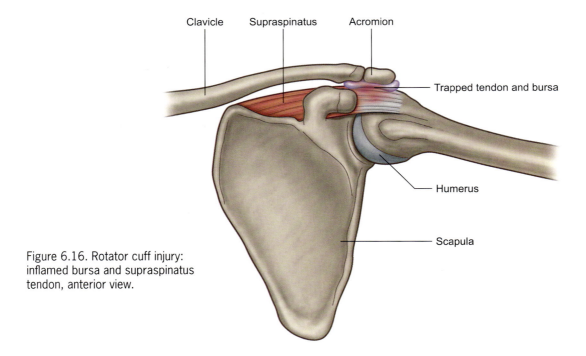

Figure 6.16. Rotator cuff injury: inflamed bursa and supraspinatus tendon, anterior view.

Proximal Biceps Tendinopathy

The long head of the biceps' tendon runs from the biceps muscle through a notched-out groove on the front of the humerus head (fig. 6.13). Then it attaches on the labrum within the shoulder socket/glenoid fossa.

Tendonitis here can result from overstretching or overstressing this tendon through poor everyday posture, compromising alignment in yoga posture, or a combination of both.

THE SHOULDER | CHAPTER 6

Damage increases when the overstretched position is combined with weight bearing, as during Low Push-Up with improper form. For more information, see "Low Plank" chapter 13. With biceps tendinopathy the fronts of the shoulders often hurt both during physical activity and when at rest; however, the pain diminishes quickly when Low Plank form is corrected.

Posture Considerations

Always avoid postures or movements that cause pain.

Keep your hands in Prayer position rather than lifting your arms.

Be cautious with weight bearing in the shoulder joints.

Be cautious with movements of your arm above shoulder level in any pose.

If it doesn't cause pain, practice engaging the muscles of scapular protraction in Dolphin pose (fig. 13.10) by strongly pressing the elbows down into the floor. This movement helps train the muscles supporting healthy positioning of the shoulder girdle while rotator cuff tears are healing. This pose has been very therapeutic for some of my students suffering from rotator cuff instability.

Use your doctor or physiotherapist's instructions to devise a practice to support your healing.

Shoulder Stability and Scapular Movements

In yoga, shoulder stability not only depends on what you are doing, but it also is influenced by where your body is spatially. For example, the most stable shoulder position in Warrior II will be very different from the most stable position in Plank because the shoulders have completely different jobs in these two poses.

The most stable shoulder position is always the one in which the arm bones are most securely integrated with the ribs or thorax. This depends on the body's action and its position. The scapula or shoulder blade is the main link between of the upper-arm bone and the ribs. It can be used to strongly bring them together. Remember that the glenoid fossa, the socket that holds the upper-arm bone, is part of the scapula (fig. 6.2). The glenoid fossa is on the front side of the scapula. As you move your body through different postures shifting your relationship with gravity, the demand on your shoulders is constantly changing. As the body moves, the scapula needs to move to accommodate the position of the humerus, or upper-arm bone, in the shoulder socket. You can increase shoulder stability in varying postures with scapular action.

The scapula moves at the scapulothoracic joint (fig. 6.1), where the scapula interacts with the ribs/thorax. The thorax is the part of the body between the neck and the abdomen. The

PART TWO | THE BODY

scapulae move in the following ways: protraction/retraction (fig. 6.17), depression/elevation (fig. 6.18), and upward (lateral) rotation/downward (medial) rotation (fig. 6.19). The muscles used for each action follow:

protraction — serratus anterior, pectoralis minor

retraction — rhomboids, trapezius

elevation — levator scapulae, trapezius (upper part)

depression — pectoralis minor, trapezius (lower part), latissimus dorsi

lateral rotation — serratus, trapezius

medial rotation — rhomboid, levator scapulae, pectoralis minor

In Plank pose, the hands, arms, and shoulders are bearing weight. As the hands and arms push into the ground, the scapulae will need to slide laterally on the ribs (protract) to strongly meet the arm bones.

As the body moves into Low Push-Up, the scapulae must move with the arm bones. They will naturally retract or move back toward the midline of the body. While some "winging" will naturally occur due to the body's spatial position and the weight bearing in the shoulders, the

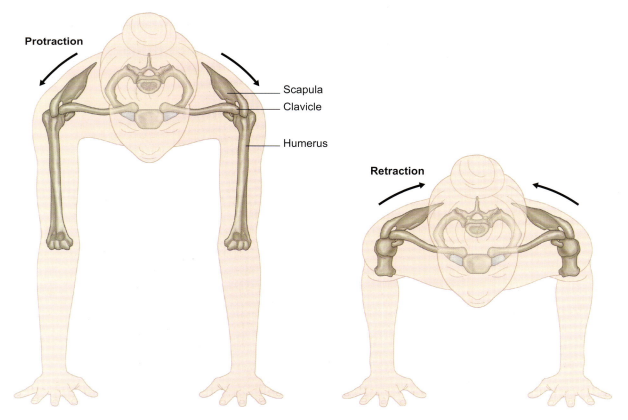

Figure 6.17. Scapular protraction in Plank. Scapular retraction in Low Plank.

THE SHOULDER | CHAPTER 6

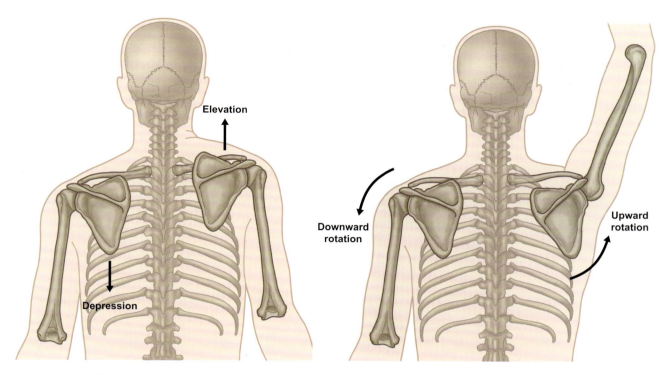

Figure 6.18. Scapular depression and elevation.

Figure 6.19. Scapular downward and upward rotation.

aim here is to keep the scapulae engaged with the thorax. Slightly depressing the scapulae, or moving them down the back, will minimize their "winging" away from the body and will engage the lower trapezius and latissimus, creating more stability for the shoulder joint and spine. This will also encourage the shoulder complex and thorax to lower together rather than letting the chest dip as the shoulder complex stays higher and winged.

In Side Plank pose, weight rests in the bottom shoulder. Protracting the scapula of the supporting arm along with trying to "hollow out" the armpit will activate the serratus muscle, providing the stability needed to hold the body's weight. See the serratus in figure 6.4 showing shoulder flexion.

When the arms are lifted above parallel to the ground in any pose, the scapulae and clavicles will move with the arms. When the arms are lifted forward and up, as in Warrior I, the scapulae will need to elevate and upwardly rotate. This is the shoulder's natural movement. It is never necessary nor biomechanically correct to take the shoulders down away from the ears when the arms are lifted. As the arms lift, allow the shoulders to go with them.

In poses like Warrior II where the arms are parallel to the ground, the shoulders will be most stable when the scapulae integrate with the thorax through slight depression and retraction. Be careful not to overdo this action. It is also important to avoid simply pulling the shoulder blades together (retraction) as this can cause dis-integration, pulling the scapulae away from the thorax. Combining retraction with depression (hugging the shoulder blades down toward the back pockets) is the key to maintaining integration.

PART TWO | THE BODY

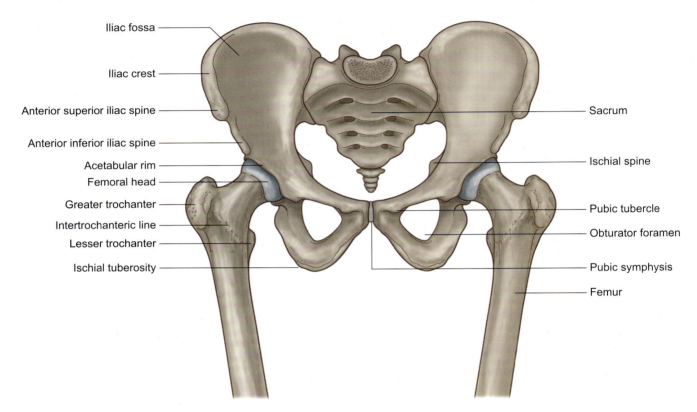

Figure 7.1. Anterior overview of the skeletal hip.

Chapter 7

The Hip

The head of the femur joins its socket, the acetabulum, to create the femoroacetabular joint. Located on each side of the pelvis, the two femoroacetabular joints are much sturdier than the shoulders due to their deeper sockets and vast muscularity. These joints sit at the center of your architecture where the movements of the trunk and the legs merge. If you are lucky, these joints will successfully bear much of your body's weight for many years. To stay mobile and active as you age, femoroacetabular joint wellness is imperative.

The femoroacetabular joint can flex, extend, rotate medially and laterally, as well as adduct and abduct. Any of these movements can also be combined for other anatomical actions.

Hip joint structure can vary from body to body and even from left to right on the same person. Factors that contribute to skeletal variability include 1) the size, shape, and orientation of the **acetabulum**, or hip socket, and 2) the length and angle of the femoral neck.[17]

THE HIP | CHAPTER 7

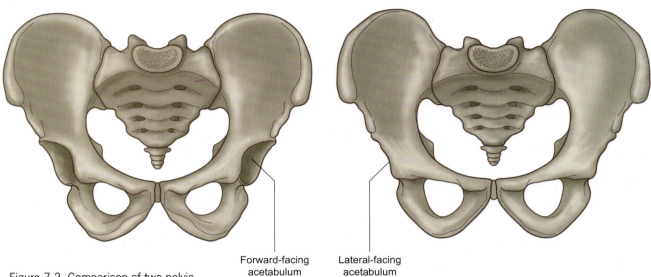

Figure 7.2. Comparison of two pelvic structures with different acetabulum orientations.

Forward-facing acetabulum

Lateral-facing acetabulum

Notice the variation between these two pelvises.[18] As you can imagine, these two bodies would have different ranges of motion in the hips. In one, the acetabulums are forward facing, and in the other, they are lateral facing (fig. 7.2).

In figure 7.3 you can see two femurs with very different shapes. One femur neck is longer and more angled while the other is shorter and straighter.[19]

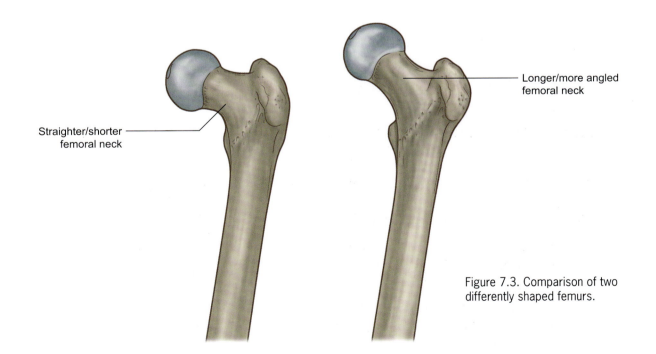

Straighter/shorter femoral neck

Longer/more angled femoral neck

Figure 7.3. Comparison of two differently shaped femurs.

57

PART TWO | THE BODY

A person's unique acetabulum shape and orientation, along with the shape, angle, and size of the femoral head and neck, determine when compression occurs. Compression restricts skeletal range of motion. Compression between the femur and the acetabulum's rim is possible in any direction; furthermore, the femur and the anterior superior iliac spine can also compress in hip flexion (fig. 7.1). See chapter 12, "Navigating the Posture," to determine if compression is affecting your range of motion.

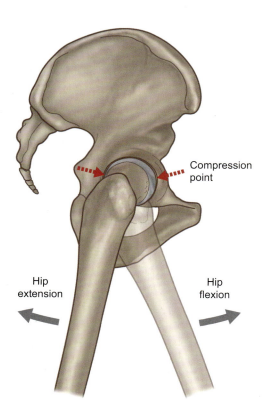

Figure 7.4. Skeletal hip flexion and extension, lateral view.

Hip Flexion

Hip flexion decreases the angle on the front of the hip as the pelvis tilts toward the legs or as the leg is lifted toward the pelvis (fig. 7.4). Hip flexion is the opposite of hip extension. The muscles of hip flexion are shown in Halfway Lift (fig. 7.5).

THE HIP | CHAPTER 7

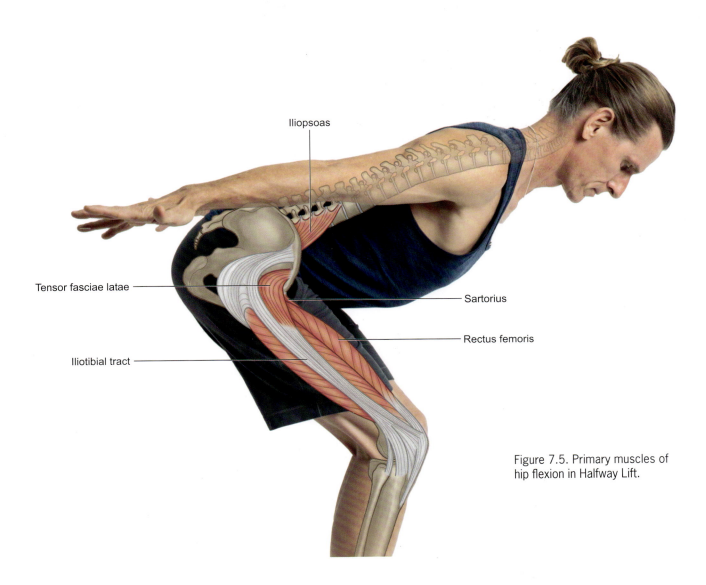

Figure 7.5. Primary muscles of hip flexion in Halfway Lift.

Hip flexion quick summary

What moves?	The femur moves toward the front rim of the acetabulum and the anterior superior iliac spine.
What works?	**Hip flexors** (fig. 7.5) iliopsoas, rectus femoris, sartorius, tensor fasciae latae
What stretches, opposes, or relaxes?	**Hip extensors** (fig. 7.6) gluteus maximus, hamstrings (biceps femoris, semitendinosus, semimembranosus), adductor magnus

PART TWO | THE BODY

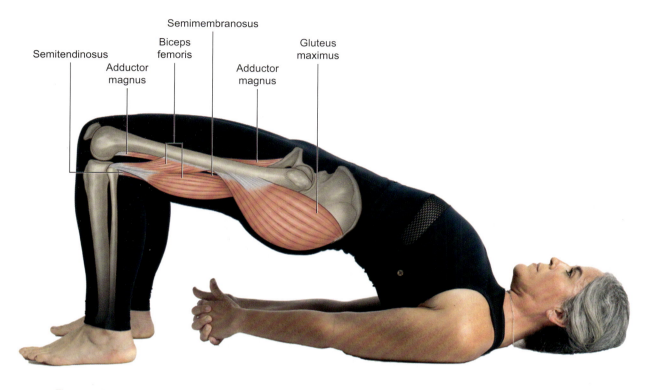

Figure 7.6. Primary muscles of hip extension in Bridge pose.

Hip Extension

Hip extension is opening the front of the hip joint, increasing the angle of the joint (fig. 7.4). It is the opposite of hip flexion. Hip extension is visible in all backward bends, including Bridge pose (fig. 7.6).

Hip extension quick summary

What moves?	The femur moves away from the anterior rim of the acetabulum and toward the posterior rim and ischium.
What works?	**Hip extensors** (fig. 7.6) gluteus maximus, hamstrings (biceps femoris, semitendinosus, semimembranosus), adductor magnus
What stretches, opposes, or relaxes?	**Hip flexors** (fig. 7.5) iliopsoas, rectus femoris, sartorius, tensor fasciae latae

THE HIP | CHAPTER 7

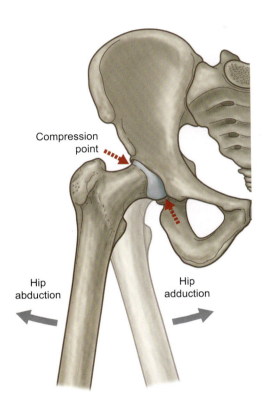

Figure 7.7. Anterior view of skeletal hip adduction and abduction.

Hip Adduction

Hip adduction happens when the thigh moves toward or beyond the body's midline (fig. 7.7), as in Eagle (fig. 7.8). Adduction is the opposite of abduction.

Hip Abduction

Hip abduction happens when the thigh moves away from the body's midline (fig. 7.7), as in Tree (fig. 7.9). Abduction is the opposite of adduction.

PART TWO | **THE BODY**

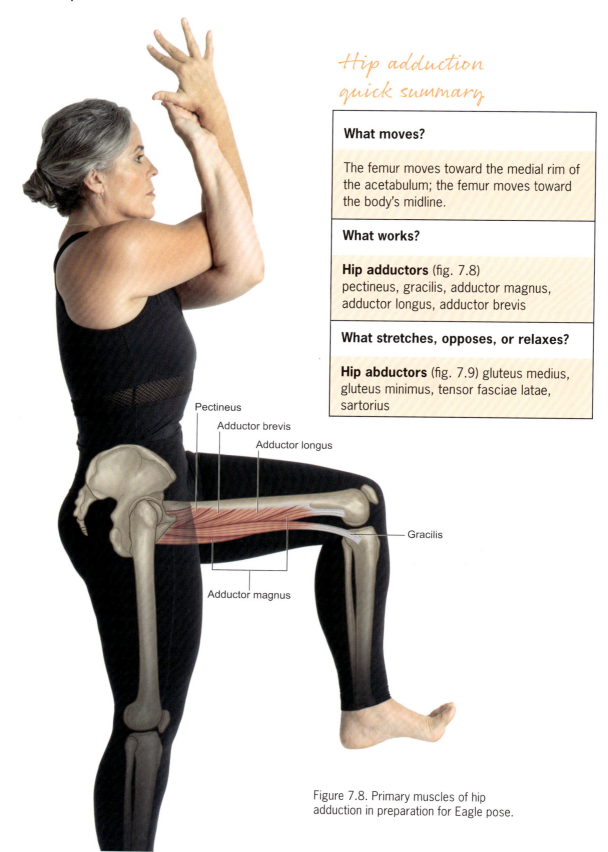

Hip adduction quick summary

What moves?	
The femur moves toward the medial rim of the acetabulum; the femur moves toward the body's midline.	
What works?	
Hip adductors (fig. 7.8) pectineus, gracilis, adductor magnus, adductor longus, adductor brevis	
What stretches, opposes, or relaxes?	
Hip abductors (fig. 7.9) gluteus medius, gluteus minimus, tensor fasciae latae, sartorius	

Figure 7.8. Primary muscles of hip adduction in preparation for Eagle pose.

THE HIP | CHAPTER 7

Hip abduction quick summary

What moves?
The femur moves toward the lateral rim of the acetabulum; the femur moves away from the body's midline.
What works?
Hip abductors (fig. 7.9) gluteus medius, gluteus minimus, tensor fasciae latae, sartorius
What stretches, opposes, or relaxes?
Hip adductors (fig. 7.8) pectineus, gracilis, adductor magnus, adductor longus, adductor brevis

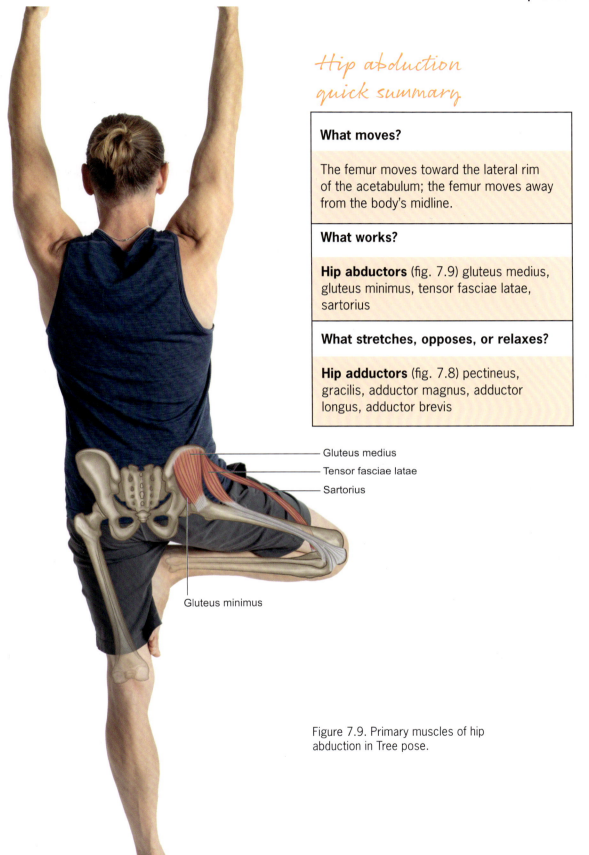

Figure 7.9. Primary muscles of hip abduction in Tree pose.

PART TWO | THE BODY

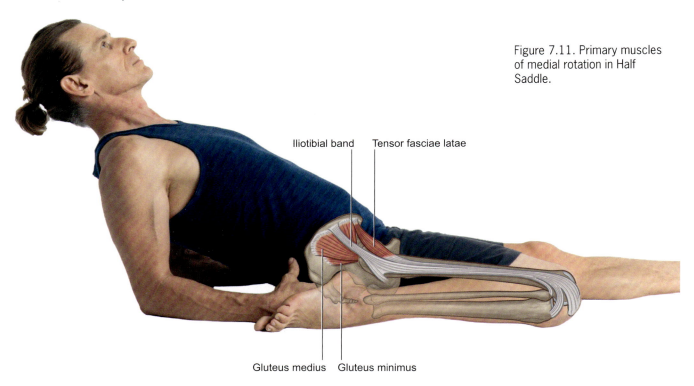

Figure 7.11. Primary muscles of medial rotation in Half Saddle.

Hip Medial Rotation

Medial (internal) rotation of the hip happens when the femur rotates toward the body's midline (fig. 7.10). Medial rotation is the opposite of lateral rotation. You can see it in Half Saddle (fig. 7.11).

Hip medial rotation quick summary

What moves?
The femur rotates toward the medial rim of the acetabulum; the femur rotates toward the body's midline.

What works?
Hip medial rotators (fig. 7.11) gluteus minimus, gluteus medius, tensor fasciae latae

What stretches, opposes, or relaxes?
Hip lateral rotators (fig. 7.12) piriformis, superior gemellus, obturator internus, inferior gemellus, quadratus femoris, obturator externus, (gluteus maximus lower fibers), sartorius

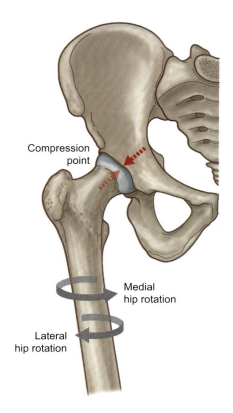

Figure 7.10. Anterior view of skeletal hip medial and lateral rotation.

THE HIP | CHAPTER 7

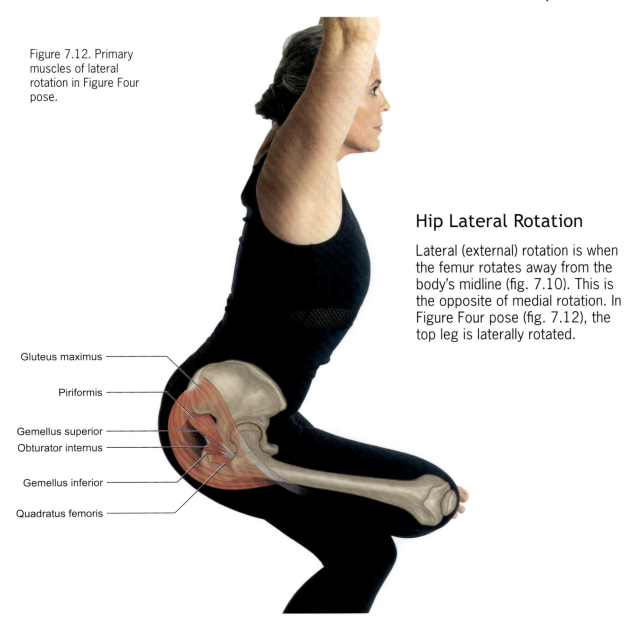

Figure 7.12. Primary muscles of lateral rotation in Figure Four pose.

- Gluteus maximus
- Piriformis
- Gemellus superior
- Obturator internus
- Gemellus inferior
- Quadratus femoris

Hip Lateral Rotation

Lateral (external) rotation is when the femur rotates away from the body's midline (fig. 7.10). This is the opposite of medial rotation. In Figure Four pose (fig. 7.12), the top leg is laterally rotated.

Hip lateral rotation quick summary

What moves?	The femur rotates toward the lateral rim of the acetabulum; the femur rotates away from the body's midline.
What works?	**Hip lateral rotators** (fig. 7.12) piriformis, superior gemellus, obturator internus, inferior gemellus, quadratus femoris, obturator externus, (gluteus maximus lower fibers), sartorius
What stretches, opposes, or relaxes?	**Hip medial rotators** (fig. 7.11) gluteus minimus, gluteus medius, tensor fasciae latae

PART TWO | THE BODY

Common Hip Injuries

Femoroacetabular Impingement (FAI)

FAI occurs when imbalanced articulation between the femur head and the acetabulum damages cartilage. The damage can be on the labrum (the acetabulum's cartilage lining), on the cartilage surface of the femur head, or on both.

Torn Labrum

A tear in the **labrum** (fig. 7.13) often accompanies FAI. Repeatedly pushing to extreme ranges of motion may result in these types of injuries. Apparently certain hip structures are much more prone to injury than others.[20] This is true with all joint structures.

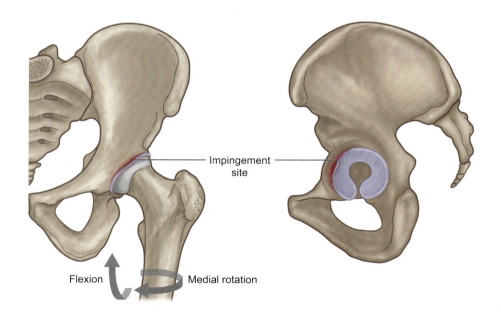

Figure 7.13. Anterior and lateral view of torn labrum in left hip.

THE HIP | CHAPTER 7

Posture Considerations

Always avoid postures that cause lasting or residual pain. *Remember, pain is not always felt with injury. Furthermore, pain is subjective, so it is not always the best indicator of an injury's severity.*

Yoga is commonly misunderstood as a practice aimed predominantly at increasing flexibility and achieving extreme ranges of motion. As I said before, the hip injuries mentioned above often result when a uniquely shaped skeletal hip complex is repetitively pushed through extreme ranges of motion. If life-long, functional, musculoskeletal wellness is your aim, approach your practice pursuing balanced strength and flexibility. I am not saying, "Never approach extreme ranges of motion." Every body is unique, so the results of certain repetitive actions will differ from person to person. The key is to approach your practice as a practice of *embodiment*. Learn to tune in and to feel. Honor the wellness of your unique structure, and be choosy about the postures you repetitively practice day after day. The truth is, only you can know what is right for your body. Listen to what others have to say. Then filter it all through your own experience. Remember to ask yourself the question, "What is my goal?"

Notice if your practice is balancing the musculature surrounding your hip joints. Your practice should include not only balanced hip opening, but also balanced hip strengthening. Typical practices include lots of hip flexion and extension work; be sure you are also including poses that strengthen the abductors, the adductors, and the medial and lateral rotators.

If you are injured, this is the perfect time to practice compassion and self-love. Be present in your body's new sensations. Use your doctor and physiotherapist's instructions to create a new practice. You will still be able to do many things; you may just need to do them a little differently. Enjoy this fresh perspective and the opportunity to move in other ways. Along your path of healing, your vision of your body and of practicing yoga will broaden tremendously.

Hamstring Tendinopathy

Hamstring tendinopathy is inflammation or tissue damage at the tendinous attachment on either end of one of the three hamstring muscles (fig. 7.14). What I see in yoga students most often is proximal tendinopathy, typically described as a "pain in the butt," because the attachments affected are at the ischial tuberosity, or sitting bone.[21] Damage usually results from overuse with movements like jumping and running, or from overstretching or pushing end ranges of motion too forcefully, too quickly, or too repetitively over time. Yoga practices including lots of repetitive folding can provoke this injury if the quality and quantity of hamstring stretch are not properly managed.

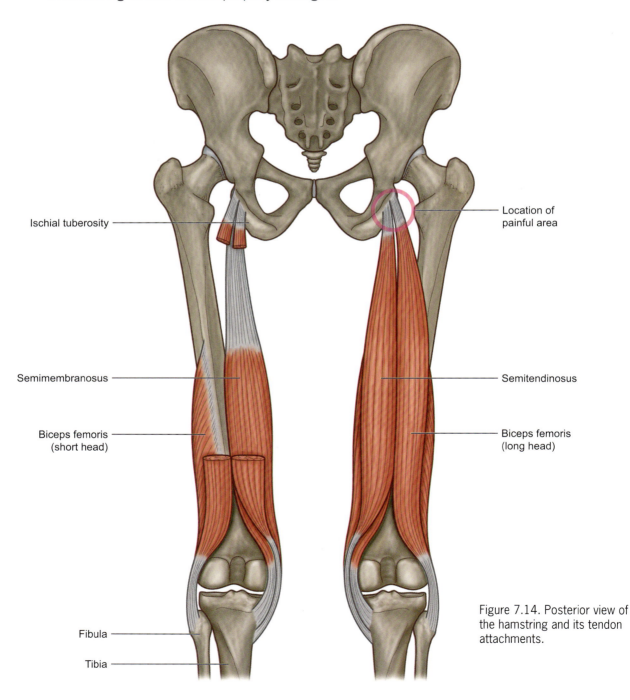

Figure 7.14. Posterior view of the hamstring and its tendon attachments.

THE HIP | CHAPTER 7

Distal hamstring tendinopathy is often confused with knee injury because the attachments are near the knee joint.

Posture Considerations

Avoid postures that cause lasting or residual pain.

If your practice involves a Sun Salutation warm-up, take five minutes to lie on your back with a strap gently stretching your hamstrings. This position is very stable since the pelvis is anchored to the floor. Proceed slowly, aiming for more stretch sensation in the muscle centers than at their distal ends. Take long, slow, deep breaths. This will better prepare the muscles and tendons for the repetitive Sun Salutation folding. *(This is a precautionary suggestion.)*

If you already have this injury, avoid full hip flexion. Depending on your injury's severity, you can either eliminate or minimize all folds. Placing two tall blocks under your hands can be helpful during these poses. Work on maintaining a nice, long spine and some openness in the fronts of the hip creases. This applies to any posture that entails hip flexion; there are many.

Teachers often tell students simply to bend their knees if they have hamstring tightness or injury. Bent knees typically allow more anterior tilt of the pelvis and more hip flexion. This can be a problem with hamstring tendinopathy because it puts even more strain at the attachment points, further exacerbating the injury. While slightly bent knees will help reduce tightness in the entire back body, this will be most effective when combined with less hip flexion.

The only way to avoid this common injury is to tune in and notice how your poses feel within your body. Pushing beyond your range of motion in any pose is not beneficial musculoskeletally. Repetitively putting undue strain on these tendinous attachments will inevitably damage them. Consider a pose like Standing Split. Often the aim is getting the lifted leg higher and higher. This goal is frequently linked with instruction to keep the hips square. For many people, these combined actions excessively strain the ischial tuberosity attachments of the standing leg (fig. 7.14).

Once again, remember that everyone is different. Some people will be able to go much farther in this pose with their natural range of motion. You can't always judge what is happening on the inside from what is happening on the outside. I prefer to teach Standing Split in a way that encourages functional strength. Rather than having students maximize their leg lift, I have them keep the lifted leg close to parallel to the floor with square hips (fig. 7.15). From here, the focus moves away from excessive hamstring stretch and switches to leg, hip, and trunk strengthening.

PART TWO | **THE BODY**

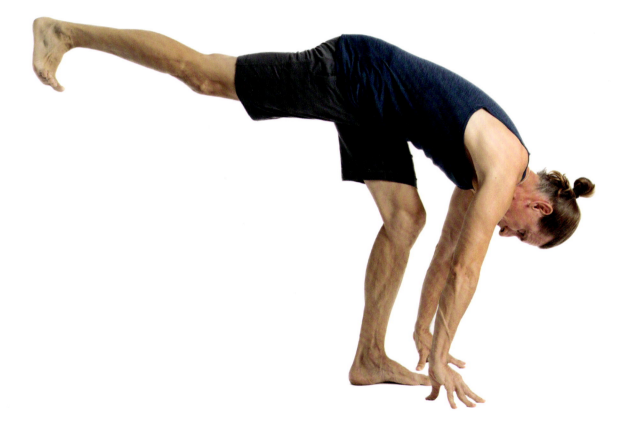

Fig. 7.15 Standing Split variation.

THE HIP | CHAPTER 7

Imperfections are not inadequacies; they are reminders that we're all in this together.

—Brené Brown

PART TWO | THE BODY

Chapter 8
The Knee

The knee is the largest and most complex joint of the body. This joint is vital to our daily movements, bearing much of our body's weight while enabling the upper leg to work with the lower leg and foot. It can extend and flex as well as rotate minimally both medially and laterally. Made up of the femur, the tibia, and the kneecap (or patella), the knee is also referred to as the tibiofemoral joint (fig. 8.1).

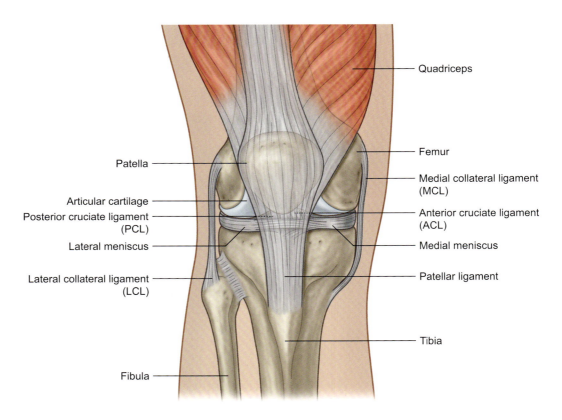

Figure 8.1. Anterior view of right knee.

THE KNEE | CHAPTER 8

Knee Extension

Extension occurs when the leg straightens, and the angle on the back side of the knee joint opens. The back of the tibia angles farther away from the back of the femur. In Triangle both knees are in extension (fig. 8.2). Extension is the opposite of flexion.

Knee extension quick summary

What moves?	The posterior angle between the tibia and the femur opens as the two bones move toward alignment.
What works?	**Knee extensors** (fig. 8.2) quadriceps (rectus femoris, vastus medialis, vastus lateralis, vastus intermedius)
What stretches, opposes, or relaxes?	**Knee flexors** (fig. 8.3) hamstring (biceps femoris, semitendinosus, semimembranosus), gracilis, sartorius, popliteus, gastrocnemius

Knee Flexion

Flexion happens when the leg bends, and the angle on the back side of the knee joint gets smaller. The back of the tibia moves closer to the back of the femur. The bent leg in Headstand variation (fig. 8.3) is in flexion. This is the opposite of extension (fig. 8.2)

Knee flexion quick summary

What moves?	The posterior or back-side angle between the tibia and femur closes as the two bones move closer together.
What works?	**Knee flexors** (fig. 8.3) hamstring (biceps femoris, semitendinosus, semimembranosus), gracilis, sartorius, popliteus, gastrocnemius
What stretches, opposes, or relaxes?	**Knee extensors** (fig. 8.2) quadriceps (rectus femoris, vastus medialis, vastus lateralis, vastus intermedius)

PART TWO | THE BODY

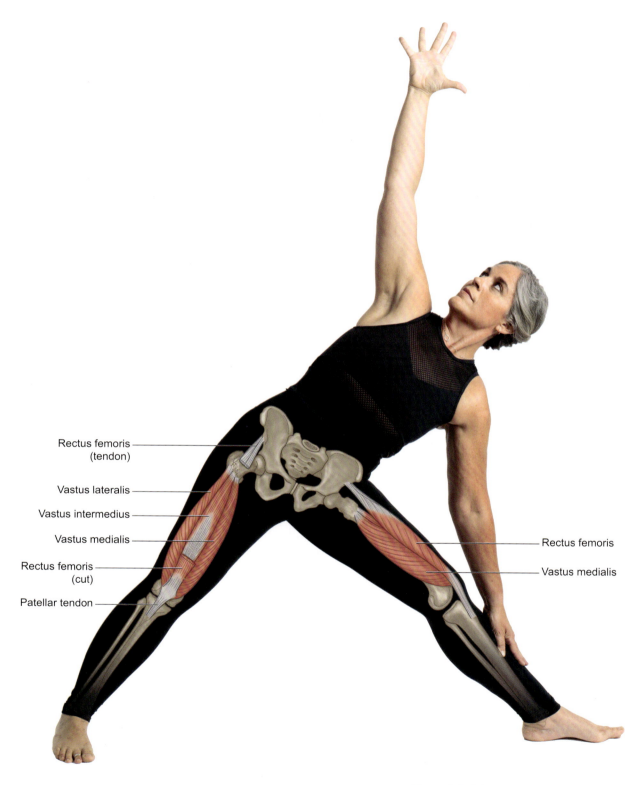

Figure 8.2. Primary muscles of knee extension in Triangle pose.

THE KNEE | CHAPTER 8

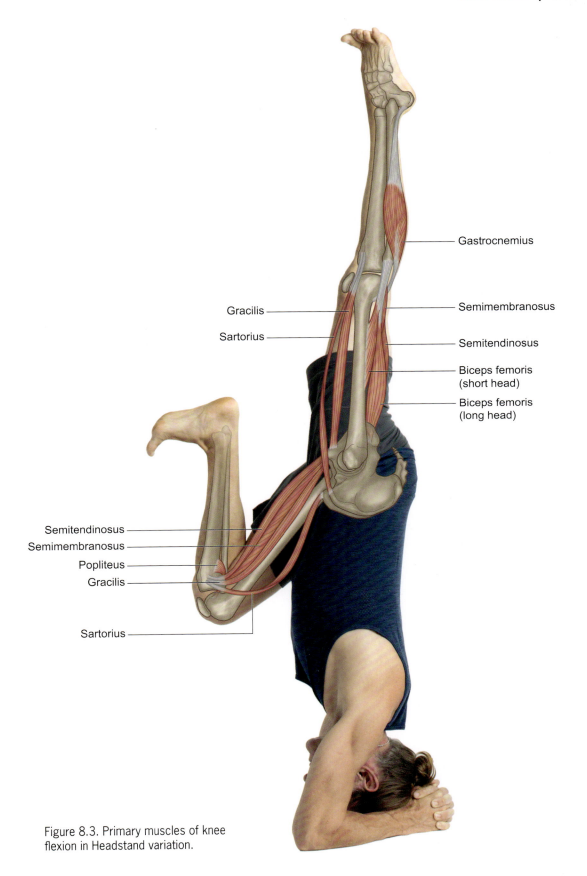

Figure 8.3. Primary muscles of knee flexion in Headstand variation.

75

Knee Medial Rotation

Knee rotation is minimal and only happens when the knee is in flexion, or bent. When the knee is locked in extension, no rotation is possible. Knee rotation is natural, healthy movement; however, it is best to practice this action conservatively in yoga. Rotation situates the body in a way that places pressure on the lateral knee ligaments. Regularly moving your body through its natural ranges of motion supports joint health, but forcing your body to go too far is unsafe. This is another reminder of the importance of embodying your posture. Drop in, and feel what is happening. Once you can visualize the knee's structure and its supportive ligaments, you will feel your body from within more easily.

Medial rotation at the knee happens when the tibia rotates toward the body's midline. In seated Hero's pose the knee is in medial rotation (fig. 8.4). Note that the hip joint is also in medial rotation. You can see how a person's unique skeletal joint complex greatly affects their ability to do a posture like Hero's. As always, the bones' shape, size, and orientation primarily determine range of motion. The joint capsule and the surrounding soft tissues are also influential.

Knee medial rotation quick summary

What moves?	
The tibia rotationally glides at its knee joint connection to the femur as it moves toward the body's midline.	
What works?	
Knee medial rotators (fig. 8.4) sartorius, gracilis, semimembranosus, semitendinosus, popliteus	
What stretches, opposes, or relaxes?	
Knee lateral rotators (fig. 8.5) biceps femoris — short head, biceps femoris — long head	

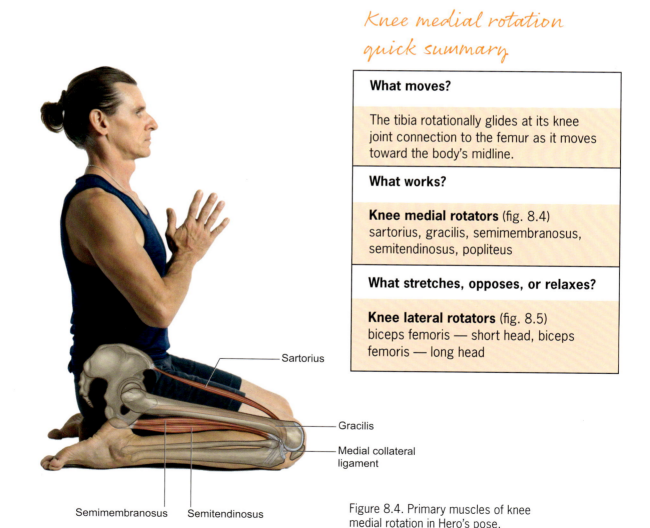

Figure 8.4. Primary muscles of knee medial rotation in Hero's pose.

THE KNEE | CHAPTER 8

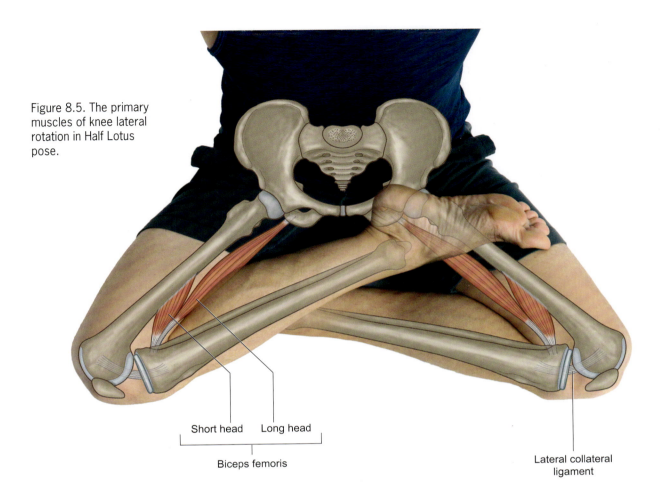

Figure 8.5. The primary muscles of knee lateral rotation in Half Lotus pose.

Knee Lateral Rotation

Lateral rotation happens when the tibia rotates away from the body's midline. In Half Lotus (fig. 8.5), the knee must laterally rotate for placing the foot on the opposite thigh.

Knee lateral rotation quick summary

What moves?	The tibia rotationally glides at its knee joint connection to the femur as it moves away from the body's midline.
What works?	**Knee lateral rotators** (fig. 8.5) biceps femoris — short head, biceps femoris — long head
What stretches, opposes, or relaxes?	**Knee medial rotators** (fig. 8.4) sartorius, gracilis, semimembranosus, semitendinosus, popliteus

77

PART TWO | THE BODY

Common Knee Injuries

Many different types of knee injuries can occur. Ligament or meniscus damage are most common. Instead of looking at injuries individually, it will be more beneficial to zoom out and consider how and why injury might happen. In figure 8.1, note the many ligaments supporting the overall structure. These ligaments are designed to protect and maintain healthy ranges of motion. When the knee is forced beyond its natural ranges of extension, flexion, medial rotation, or lateral rotation, the ligaments can be injured. Injury can result from traumatic force or from repetitive actions that cause stress in any direction. A sprain is an overstretched or torn ligament in any joint.

Injured ligament	Direction of force
ACL (anterior cruciate ligament)	Hyperextension, possibly from a sudden move, stop, or change of direction[22]
PCL (posterior cruciate ligament)	Blow to the front of knee while it is bent, hyperflexion, or hyperextension[23]
LCL (lateral collateral ligament)	Blow from medial side of knee[24]
MCL (medial collateral ligament)	Force from severe lateral twist[25]

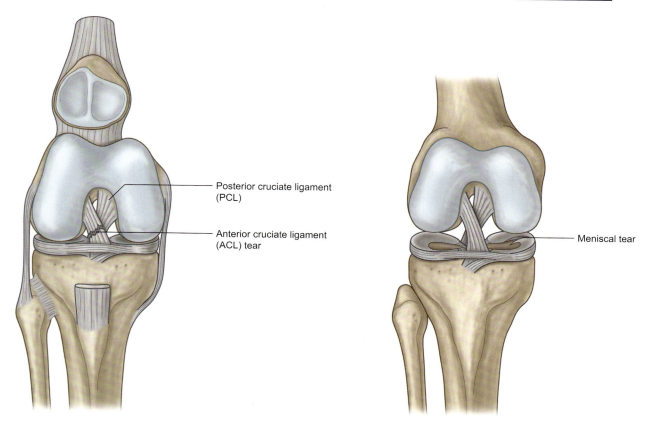

Figure 8.6. Anterior cruciate ligament tear, anterior view of right knee with patella lifted.

Figure 8.7. Anterior view of right knee meniscal tear.

THE KNEE | CHAPTER 8

As the meniscus provides shock absorption and cushion, it can also be damaged from traumatic force or from repetitive wear and tear caused by imbalanced articulation (fig. 8.7). Imbalanced articulation can result from excess weight or pressure, biomechanics, arthritis, or deformation from other causes.[26] Remember, the distinct parts of the body work in an interconnected way. When one part is injured, another imbalance probably occurs farther up or down the chain of connectivity. For example, a hip injury may lead to knee imbalance or injury, or vice-versa.

Remember that the ligaments, cartilage, and menisci are designed to withstand pressure; that is actually part of their job. Consider knee placement in a pose like Half Pigeon. Pressure is definitely put on the soft tissues. Some pressure can be healthy. Injurious pressure occurs when the unique knee joint is pushed beyond its safe range or when a pre-existing injury is aggravated.

This is another example of the importance of posture embodiment. Only you can feel what's happening inside your body. Learn to distinguish between the sensations of healthy poking and prodding and the type of pain or sensation associated with degradation. While we can't always know what is happening within our bodies, we can turn up our inner listening.

Posture Considerations

Never do poses that cause lasting, residual, or increased pain.

Develop an understanding of the knee's structure and its stabilizing ligaments. Respect your personal ranges of motion; this will require feeling from within.

Maintain strength in your hip stabilizers by practicing one-leg balancing postures.

Regularly take your knees through their natural ranges of motion to maintain joint health and mobility.

If your knee is injured, depending on the injury, you may have limited range of motion, most commonly with flexion. You will need to modify poses with this action, decreasing the knee bend or practicing different postures instead.

Avoid postures that put pressure or strain near the injured area. Poses requiring knee flexion with weight bearing, like Half Pigeon, Child's, and Hero's, will need to be avoided or modified.

If you have a knee injury, use your doctor and physiotherapist's orders to create a new practice that supports healing.

PART TWO | THE BODY

Chapter 9
The Ankle

The ankle is intricate and complex, composed of numerous bones and joints. Here we will discuss only the ankle's primary joint, the **tibiotalar joint**. This hinge joint is where the leg's tibia articulates with the foot's talus bone. Its strength and mobility allow us to comfortably navigate movement and to balance between the foot and the **proximal** joints of the knee and hip. The primary movements of this joint are dorsiflexion and plantar flexion (fig. 9.2). The anatomical movements of inversion, eversion, pronation, and supination all involve additional ankle joints.

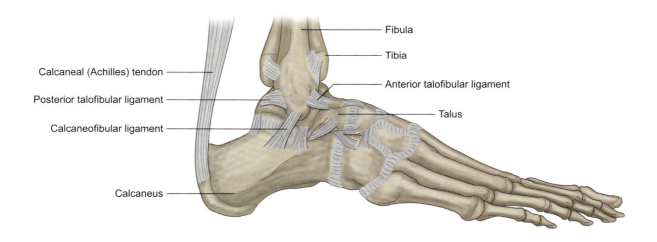

Figure 9.1. Lateral view of the ankle.

THE ANKLE | CHAPTER 9

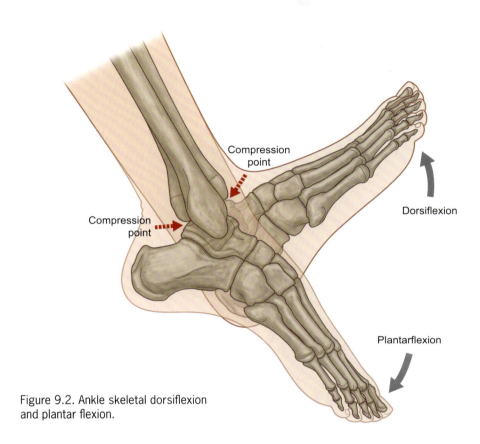

Figure 9.2. Ankle skeletal dorsiflexion and plantar flexion.

Ankle Dorsiflexion

Dorsiflexion is most commonly referred to as "flexed feet." It occurs when the foot draws toward the front of the leg, decreasing the angle in the ankle front (fig. 9.2). The front of the tibia approaches the talus, or the talus moves toward the tibia as the foot flexes. The top foot in Half Moon is often in dorsiflexion (fig. 9.3).

The dynamic action of dorsiflexion can be quite different depending on how we are holding our bodies and what actions we are performing. For example, consider the difference between dorsiflexing in Low Lunge versus dorsiflexing the lifted foot in a pose like Half Moon. The lunge dorsiflexion depends mainly on the body's weight and gravity, while in Half Moon the lifted leg must work the dorsiflexors to flex the foot. Possible skeletal limitation would only show up in a lunge-like pose. Can you see how limited dorsiflexion could impact your ability to get your heels to the ground in a Yogi Squat (fig. 19.18)?

PART TWO | THE BODY

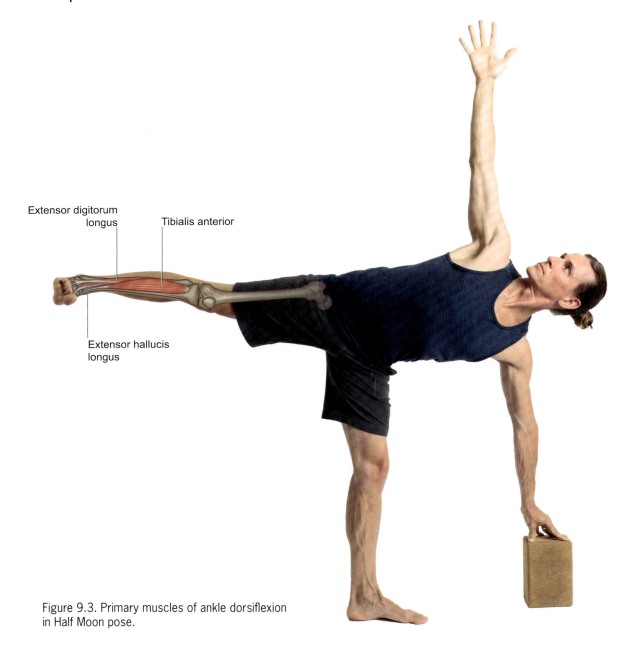

Figure 9.3. Primary muscles of ankle dorsiflexion in Half Moon pose.

Ankle dorsiflexion quick summary

What moves?	The tibia and anterior talus hinge toward each other.
What works?	**Ankle dorsiflexors** (fig. 9.3) extensor hallucis longus, extensor digitorum longus, tibialis anterior
What stretches, opposes, or relaxes?	**Ankle plantar flexors** (fig. 9.4) flexor hallucis longus, flexor digitorum longus, tibialis posterior, soleus, gastrocnemius, plantaris

THE ANKLE | CHAPTER 9

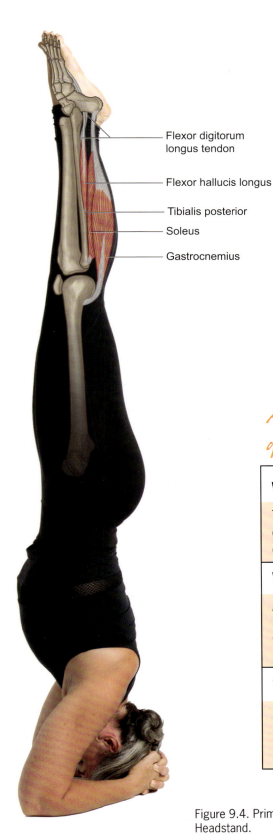

Ankle plantar flexion quick summary

What moves?
The tibia and posterior talus hinge toward each other. The posterior talus and calcaneus hinge toward each other.
What works?
Ankle plantar flexors (fig. 9.4) flexor hallucis longus, flexor digitorum longus, tibialis posterior, soleus, gastrocnemius, plantaris
What stretches, opposes, or relaxes?
Ankle dorsiflexors (fig. 9.3) extensor hallucis longus, extensor digitorum longus, tibialis anterior

Figure 9.4. Primary muscles of ankle plantar flexion in Headstand.

Ankle Plantar Flexion

Plantar flexion occurs with pointed toes or feet as the foot moves away from the front of the leg, opening the angle in the ankle front. The back of the tibia closes toward the talus, or the talus hinges toward the back of the tibia (fig. 9.2). Also referred to as pointing the foot, plantar flexion is seen in the ankles in figure 9.4, Headstand variation.

The shape, size, and orientation of the ankle-complex bones will help determine the range of motion in dorsiflexion or plantar flexion (fig. 9.2). Some people will have more skeletal range of motion than others. To better understand how to feel and distinguish between your skeleton stopping you versus soft tissue limitation, read chapter 12, "Navigating the Posture."

Common Ankle Injury

Sprained Ankle

Ligaments are the bands of dense connective tissues that maintain structural support around all joints. When excessive force in any direction is placed on the joint, a ligament can be overstretched or torn. This is called a **sprain**. In an ankle sprain, the lower lateral ligaments are most commonly affected.[27] These include the anterior talofibular ligament, the calcaneofibular ligament, and the posterior talofibular ligament (fig. 9.1). Damage to these ligaments typically results from rolling the ankle, tripping, or mis-stepping.

Ankle Impingement

Impingement in any joint results when two or more bones of the joint come together. Exaggerating or maxing out ranges of motion typically causes this. Nearby soft tissues are often "trapped" or "pinched" between the bones. Ankle impingement can happen on the front or back of the tibiotalar joint (fig. 9.1).[28] Anterior (front-side) impingement happens with dorsiflexion (fig. 9.2), and posterior (back-side) impingement happens with plantar flexion (fig. 9.2). As always, weight bearing or force in extreme ranges of motion will further add to degradation. Keep in mind that everyone is shaped differently. When, how, and where one meets a maxed-out range of motion will depend on their structure and will be unique from person to person. Consequently, as a practitioner of yoga, it is your responsibility to feel from within. One place you might meet tibiotalar compression is in a pose like Triangle (fig. 14.20). If your stance is so wide that you feel pressure or pain in the back of the ankle of your front leg, compression is likely.

THE ANKLE | CHAPTER 9

Posture Considerations

Heightening your awareness is the best way to avoid injury in yoga or other physical disciplines. Avoid going beyond your natural, sturdy range of motion. Your body is always talking to you; learn to listen. Learn to distinguish between the strong sensations of gaining strength and the sometimes-subtle warning signals that something isn't right.

With a new injury, it is crucial to give it time to heal before bearing weight and/or pressure.

Your doctor or physiotherapist might recommend using a brace to support the ankle in the early stages of weight bearing.

Depending on the location and nature of your injury, you may be limited with weight bearing in certain positions. Be patient, and change or skip poses as needed.

Once healing progresses, bear weight in varying positions to restore strength. It will also be important to regain range of motion with simple movements.

Direct more attention toward overall body balance. Be aware of how your weight is distributed through your feet, and use your entire body to increase equanimity.

As with any injury, use your doctor and physiotherapist's orders to devise a practice that works for you. You never have to abandon your mat time altogether.

PART TWO | **THE BODY**

Chapter 10

The Elbow

Connecting the upper and lower arm, the elbow helps enable versatile, agile movements of the human hand. This joint bears substantial weight in postures like Plank (fig. 13.18) and Downward Dog (fig. 13.9). Located where the humerus, ulna, and radius meet, the humeroulnar joint is the actual elbow joint (fig. 10.1). Here the humerus and ulna articulate together in a synovial hinge joint. Although supination and pronation of the forearm don't technically result from the hinge joint moving, these actions occur between the ulna and radius, so they are also included.

THE ELBOW | CHAPTER 10

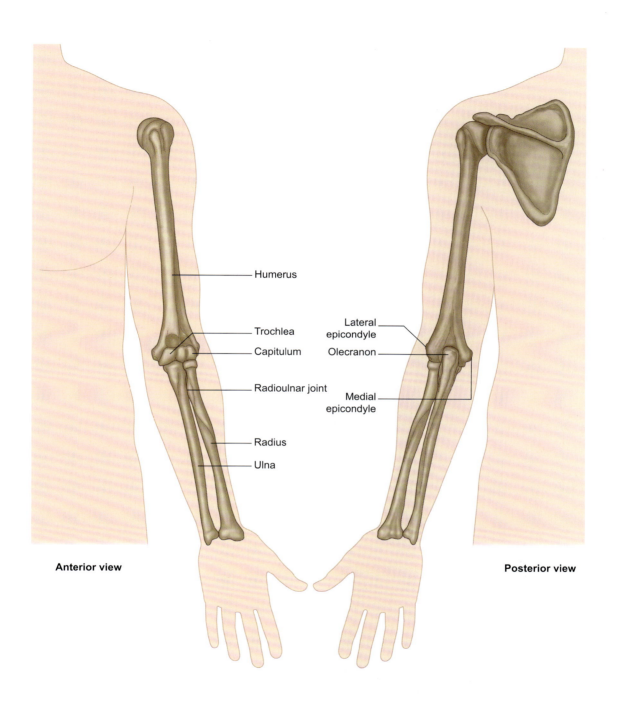

Figure 10.1. Overview of the elbow.

PART TWO | **THE BODY**

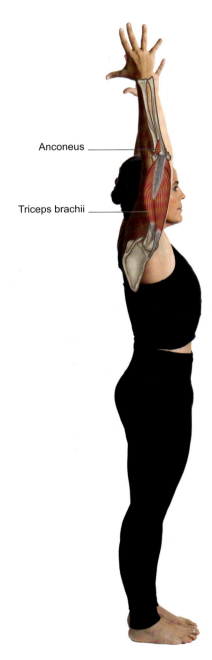

Elbow Extension

Elbow extension happens when the arm straightens. With extension, the elbow crease angle (palm side of arm) gets larger. This is the opposite of elbow flexion. Both elbows are in extension in Extended Mountain (fig. 10.2).

Figure 10.2. Primary muscles of elbow extension in Extended Mountain pose.

Elbow extension quick summary

What moves?	The olecranon process of the ulna moves toward compression with the posterior humerus or olecranon fossa.
What works?	**Elbow extensors** (fig. 10.2) anconeus, triceps brachii
What stretches, opposes, or relaxes?	**Elbow flexors** (fig. 10.3) brachialis, biceps brachii (short and long heads), brachioradialis

THE ELBOW | CHAPTER 10

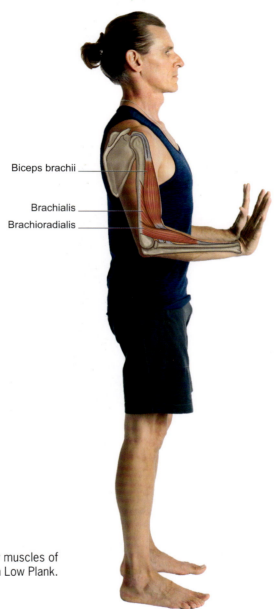

Elbow Flexion

With elbow flexion, the elbow crease gets smaller. This is the opposite of elbow extension. In Low Plank, both elbows are in flexion (fig. 10.3).

Figure 10.3. Primary muscles of elbow flexion in Low Plank.

Elbow flexion quick summary

What moves?	The radius and ulna move toward the humerus, decreasing or closing the anterior angle of the elbow.
What works?	**Elbow flexors** (fig. 10.3) brachioradialis, biceps brachii (short and long heads), brachialis
What stretches, opposes, or relaxes?	**Elbow extensors** (fig. 10.2) anconeus, triceps brachii

89

PART TWO | THE BODY

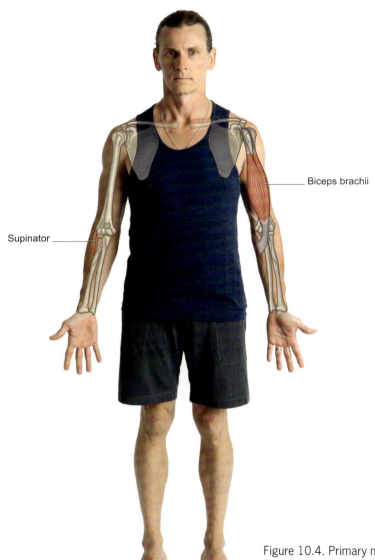

Forearm Supination

The forearm's radius and ulna interact at the radioulnar joints. Movement at this joint turns the palm. Supination occurs when the palm is turned to face up. As the palm rolls face up (supination), the radius rolls over and away from compression with the ulna. This is the opposite of pronation. In Mountain pose with palms facing forward, the forearms are supinated (fig. 10.4).

Figure 10.4. Primary muscles of forearm supination in Mountain.

Forearm supination quick summary

What moves?	From a palm-down position, the radius rolls over laterally, away from compression with the ulna.
What works?	**Forearm supinators** (fig. 10.4) supinator, biceps brachii
What stretches, opposes, or relaxes?	**Forearm pronators** (fig. 10.5) pronator teres, pronator quadratus

THE ELBOW | CHAPTER 10

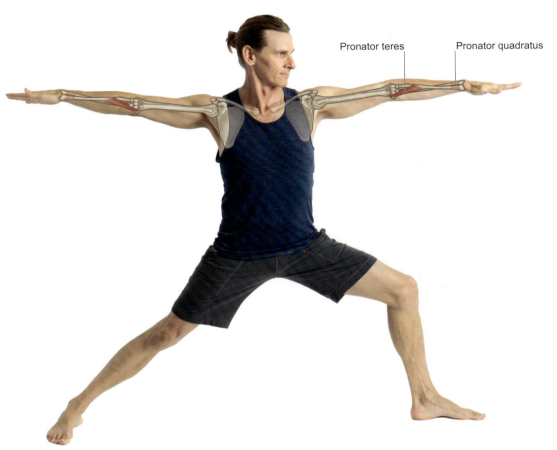

Figure 10.5. Primary muscles of forearm pronation in Warrior II.

Forearm Pronation

Pronation happens when the palms are turned face down. As the palms roll face down, the radius rolls over and closes in toward compression with the ulna. This is the opposite of supination. With palms face down in Warrior II, the forearms are pronated (fig. 10.5).

Forearm pronation quick summary

What moves?	From a palm-up position, the radius rolls over medially, toward compression with the ulna.
What works?	**Forearm pronators** (fig. 10.5) pronator teres, pronator quadratus
What stretches, opposes, or relaxes?	**Forearm supinators** (fig. 10.4) supinator, biceps brachii

Common Elbow Injuries

Ligaments are like strong pieces of tape supporting the bones at the joint intersections. They are designed both to allow and to limit movement simultaneously. When a traumatic blow or repetitive misalignment places excessive strain or force on the joint, degradation results. In yoga, misalignment combined with excessive weight bearing in the joint can cause ligament sprain. Sprain often occurs in people with hypermobile elbow joints.[29] Hypermobility is not necessarily a problem; it is simply the consequence of their unique bone shapes. Hypermobility combined with weight bearing is the concern. For example, if someone with hypermobile arms straightens them to the point of hyperextension in Warrior II, it won't have the same effect as holding Side Plank with a hyperextended elbow. When weight is placed on a hyperextended joint, the ligaments take the brunt of the force; this can lead to ligament sprain.

Posture Considerations

Be cautious about locking out your elbow joints when they are bearing weight if you have hypermobility. Keep a slight bend in the elbow, and focus on using the muscles around the joint for stability.

Strengthen the muscles around the hypermobile joint with elbow extension and flexion work.

Any hypermobile joint can be made more stable with strengthening.

If you are injured, the joint will need rest. Modify your practice to avoid bearing weight with your arms while healing.

THE ELBOW | CHAPTER 10

Inviting our thoughts and feelings into awareness allows us to learn from them rather than be driven by them.

—Daniel J. Siegel

PART TWO | **THE BODY**

Chapter 11
The Wrist

The critical junction between the forearm and the hand, the wrist is essential for our complex hand movements. This joint must not be ignored in yoga, especially in poses requiring the hands to bear weight. An extremely complex joint, it is actually made up of many smaller radiocarpal joints. Consisting of the radius and ulna of the arm along with the carpals of the hand, the wrist can flex, extend, adduct, and abduct; however, we will not review wrist adduction and abduction since they are not common in yoga posture instruction.

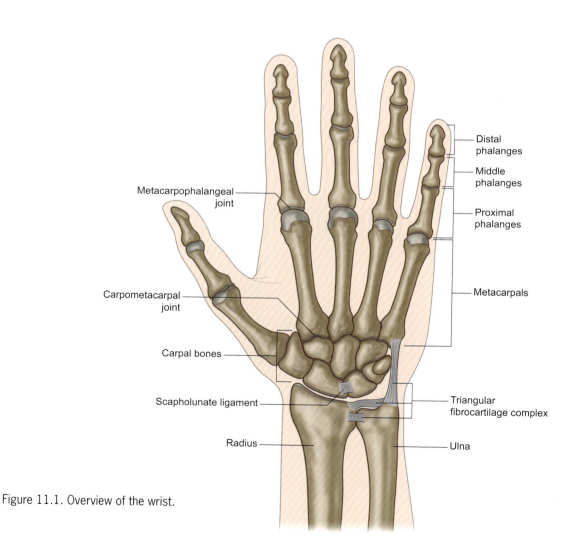

Figure 11.1. Overview of the wrist.

THE WRIST | CHAPTER 11

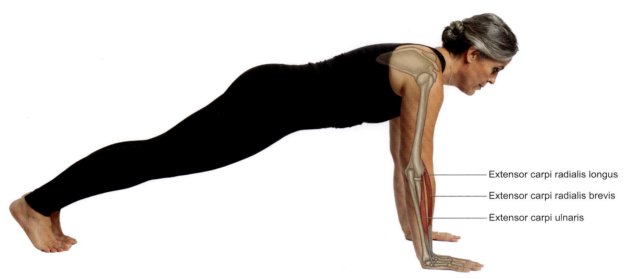

Figure 11.2. Primary muscles of wrist extension in Plank pose.

Wrist Extension

Many weight-bearing yoga postures involve wrist extension; Plank (fig. 11.2) and Low Plank are two examples. Wrist extension is the opposite of wrist flexion, so it is an effective counter stretch for the wrist flexor muscles that get tight from typing or other repetitive work with the hands and fingers. Extension occurs when the angle on the top side of the wrist decreases; the wrist angle on the palm side increases.

In postures where body weight is held in your hands, do not let excessive weight collapse into your wrists, and do not hyperextend your wrist joints, going farther into extension than your natural range.

Wrist extension quick summary

What moves?	The radius and ulna hinge toward the carpal bones on the dorsal (top) side of the wrist, closing this side of the joint.
What works?	**Wrist extensors** (fig. 11.2) extensor carpi radialis brevis, extensor carpi radialis longus, extensor carpi ulnaris
What stretches, opposes, or relaxes?	**Wrist flexors** (11.3) flexor carpi radialis, flexor carpi ulnaris, palmaris longus, flexor digitorum superficialis

PART TWO | THE BODY

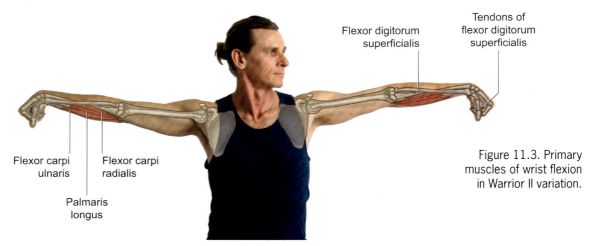

Figure 11.3. Primary muscles of wrist flexion in Warrior II variation.

Wrist Flexion

Wrist flexion occurs when the angle on the palm side of the wrist gets smaller (fig. 11.3). It is the opposite of wrist extension; therefore, flexion is an effective counter stretch for all the postures in which the wrists are extended.

Wrist flexion quick summary

What moves?	The radius and ulna move toward the carpals on the palmar side as the joint angle lessens.
What works?	**Wrist flexors** (fig. 11.3) flexor carpi radialis, flexor carpi ulnaris, palmaris longus, flexor digitorum superficialis
What stretches, opposes, or relaxes?	**Wrist extensors** (fig. 11.2) extensor carpi ulnaris, extensor carpi radialis brevis, extensor carpi radialis longus

Consider...

In every yoga pose, weight is landing somewhere. Our feet, legs, and hips usually bear weight since we are an upright species. When we stand on one leg, weight shifts; this pattern of holding our body weight isn't quite as natural as standing on two feet. In one-leg standing postures you need to be aware of how you are holding your weight in the foot and ankle, the knee, and the standing hip. Stacking your joints in a sound, stable, balanced way is key, along with activating up and out of your joints, engaging, and connecting with the rest of the body. Think of lifting up and away from the floor rather than letting the floor hold you. Your body's connectivity with the floor can always be a point of activation.

Bearing weight in your hands takes lots of practice because we don't typically walk on our hands; consequently, our brains and bodies must develop a new relationship with gravity. Poses like Downward-Facing Dog, Crow, Plank, Low Plank, Handstand, and Side Plank require focusing on how we hold weight in our hands, wrists, and shoulders. These joints are all more mobile and less stable than the standing joints of the ankles, knees, and hips. Activating your legs and core to help hold your body weight distributes the force more evenly, giving the hands, wrists, and shoulders some relief. Using the floor as a point of activation, pushing the floor away is also vital. Lastly, Cylindrical Core engagement is what pulls everything together when bearing weight in the hands. Learn more about Cylindrical Core under Halfway Lift, chapter 13 and figure 13.17.

THE WRIST | CHAPTER 11

Common Wrist Injuries

Carpal Tunnel Syndrome

The median nerve runs through the carpal tunnel (fig. 11.4), literally a small tunnel-like space in the wrist. This nerve controls sensation and movement in all the fingers except the pinky. Swelling in and around the carpal tunnel presses on the median nerve resulting in numbness, tingling, weakness, and/or pain.[30] This swelling can be caused by illness, repetitive motions, excessive weight bearing, or repeated, extreme ranges of motion.

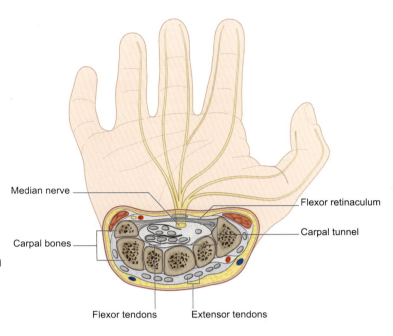

Figure 11.4. Carpal tunnel with median nerve.

Wrist Sprain

The wrist contains numerous ligaments, but I have only included the most commonly injured ligaments in figure 11.1. These are the scapholunate and the triangular fibrocartilage complex (TFCC).[31] The TFCC stabilizes the wrist on the pinky side and consists of several ligaments and other cartilaginous structures. A sprain is damage to a ligament. As in every other joint, the ligaments are like strong pieces of super tape connecting the bones. Ligaments allow, protect, and maintain natural ranges of motion. Injury occurs when ligaments overstretch, tear slightly, or tear completely due to a fall or blow or due to repetitive force beyond their natural ranges of motion.

Posture Considerations

Do not overextend the wrist (fig. 13.23), especially with force or weight bearing. When your hand is placed flat on the floor, do not let your forearm go beyond vertical.

Use the rest of your body strength to lift weight out of your hands and wrists instead of letting weight dump into your wrist joints.

If your wrist is injured, you might need to avoid postures requiring weight bearing in the hands altogether for a while. Another option is going to your forearms in poses like Plank and Downward Dog.

While healing from injury, maintain mobility by doing gentle wrist stretches. Wrist injuries typically need time and rest to heal. Remember, you can do an entire practice without ever bearing weight in your hands.

Use your doctor and physiotherapist's instructions to design a new practice that works for you along your path of healing.

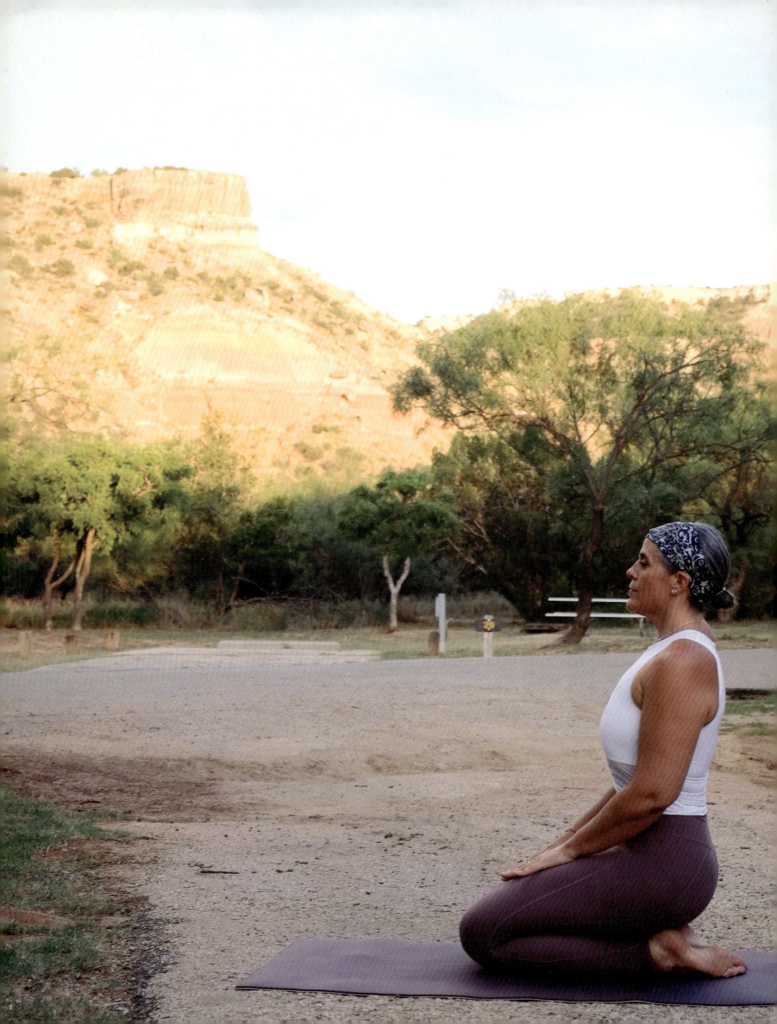

PART THREE
The Posture

Willingness

In the willingness to feel,
there is healing. In the
choice not to closet, cast
aside or deny experience,
energy is freed, and I
dive deeper into life.

There may be maturity in
choosing not to act, but
there are no rewards for
suppression and denial.

To be fully alive is saying
yes to the wide array of
human feelings. When I
soften, release and breathe,
I discover I am more than
what I think, feel, reason,
or believe.

Danna Faulds
Go In and In

Chapter 12

Navigating the Posture

Whether we are adopting a nutrition plan, an exercise routine, or a yoga alignment method, most of us want to be told exactly what to do. Following someone else's rules seems easier than trying to figure things out for ourselves. Although information gathered from others is valuable, our individual genetic blueprints, life histories, and current situations make us unique, each with very distinct needs. When I attended nutritional therapy school, my biggest takeaway was this: we are bio-individuals, so one plan can never fit everyone. What works well for someone else may not work well for you.

Foundational principles guide nutrition, but the best approach relies on personal experience. Together, the nutritional therapist and the client gather information to develop an action plan. They begin a trial-and-error journey. The client tries something and then waits to feel how the body and mind respond. One of the hallmarks of a successful nutritional therapy plan is the client's increased body awareness, or learning to listen to signals from within to make adjustments along the way. Connecting how the body feels with food choices, sleep quality, and life circumstances is incredibly beneficial. In fact, recognizing cause-and-effect relationships is crucial to transforming any aspect of our lives. This increased awareness is often what helps us make new choices that, in turn, profoundly affect our overall health and well-being.

Teaching yoga is much like being a nutritional therapist in that my main aim is to awaken students' awareness, so they can move, breathe, and be in a way that supports all aspects of wellness. As a teacher, I use my personal practice experience, along with my understanding

PART THREE | THE POSTURES

of the body in posture and yoga philosophy, to guide students toward finding their own ways. Like nutritional therapy, yoga alignment is guided by sound principles. General anatomical and biomechanical theories apply, but students gain the most complete information through their individual experiences. I can never truly know anyone else's experience of the pose as felt from within; only they can know that.

Using EPM, you can learn to feel and align your poses from within. Don't dismiss knowledge gleaned from your teachers. Rather, honor and respect all information gathered from others, and then live within your own experience. This requires paying attention while opening up, being curious and willing to experiment, expanding your capacity to trust yourself. *To find your own authentic practice, you must awaken to your inner experience of the postures.*

Be patient while you develop the skill of interoceptive awareness, feeling what's happening on the inside. If this is new to you, it may take some time. Here are a few guiding principles to help you find your way back into your own body.

Getting to Know Your Muscles

Getting to know your muscles can be tricky and intimidating, but it also can be highly rewarding as you pursue embodiment. EPM requires a fine-tuned awareness and the willingness to focus on feelings you might normally dismiss. The way you approach your study can significantly impact your understanding and retention of this information.

For me, thinking of the muscles as groups rather than individuals helps me feel their actions within my body more easily. For instance, I can immediately feel my spinal extensors engaging when I bend backward, but feeling my longissimus muscle working is very challenging. Furthermore, if you are a teacher, using muscle groups rather than individual muscle names can accelerate your students' understanding of the muscles working within their bodies. As you move into the posture descriptions, you will find the primary anatomical actions required for each pose, along with which muscle groups are working, stretching, releasing, or opposing.

I say this several times in various ways throughout this book: *your body does not work in parts and pieces, so no action occurs in isolation.* Looking at the joint actions only gives us partial information; however, this is a great place to start investigating the body's movements. What is happening at one joint is highly influenced by what is taking place at the body's other joints. Some muscles cross two joints; in this case, what occurs in one muscle depends on the unique, combined actions at both joints. Additional forces may increase demand on muscular actions. Perhaps another body part is being held in a way that adds force to the nearby joint action. Hip flexion in Standing Forward Fold, for example, is very different from hip flexion in Supported Leg Raise, in which the weight of the leg must be supported. Gravity is another force that shifts muscular demand around the joint. For instance, holding the shoulders in extension in Low Push-Up is drastically different from holding the shoulders in extension with an arm bind in Mountain pose.

Still, while many factors should be considered, in my opinion, studying the individual joint actions is the best way to begin understanding how muscles work. As you study the joint actions and muscle groups, keep actively investigating what you are experiencing within your body. Notice how your muscles feel, not only when they are working and strengthening, but when they are releasing and stretching as well. Feel how your muscles move your joints, and be curious about

NAVIGATING THE POSTURE | CHAPTER 12

the different sensations within the unique body-action combinations from pose to pose.

Remember, the joint actions listed for each pose are those needed to move into it. Once you are there, whether you hold the pose or not and how long you hold it will change the demand on your muscles. Muscles can work three ways: (1) **isometrically** or statically, such as the triceps while holding Plank, (2) **eccentrically** while lengthening, such as the triceps while lowering to Low Push-Up, or (3) **concentrically** while shortening, such as the triceps while pressing from Low Plank to High Plank. Yoga provides many opportunities for your muscles to work in all three ways as you come in and out of poses. Any time you hold still in a pose, your muscles are working isometrically. Within the pose descriptions, I do not label every action as either isometric, concentric, or eccentric; however, I give you several examples of each action.

These are some additional factors determining how muscles work: (1) how you get into the pose, (2) how long you are in the pose, (3) the angles of your joints or how deep you are in the pose, (4) your body proportions, and (5) how your body is held in space. In this book, I assume you aren't trying to learn to calculate joint forces and muscle activations, but rather you are attempting to enhance your personal experience in yoga posture. Many other books are much better resources for learning kinesiology and biomechanics. Here I am sharing basic information about the muscular joint actions, hoping to increase your awareness on the mat.

Distinguishing Between Compression and Tension

While moving your body into various yoga postures, unless you are Gumby, you will encounter barriers, a sense that something is stopping you. Pay attention to this useful information your body is giving you. To navigate alignment most effectively, you need to notice what is limiting your pose. *Honoring your own natural ranges of motion on the mat is a primary step toward cultivating awareness and self-compassion for all aspects of your life.* This requires acute self-observation which you will also need for a life-long, sustainable practice supporting structural wellness.

Compression occurs when two objects meet, and no further movement is possible. The belly or chest meeting the thighs in a forward fold is an example. In yoga, the most commonly occurring type of compression is skeletal compression at joints. Joints are the places where two or more bones articulate and where we access skeletal movement. Joints have end ranges of motion; if they didn't, we'd be so dangerously mobile that we would be unable even to sit upright. The end of **range of motion** can be thought of as a stopping point where the bones meet, the barrier you cannot pass. Your unique bone shapes and how they fit together will determine your skeletal ranges of motion. And poses and actions will look and feel different from body to body because everyone has different ranges of motion. In part 2, "The Body," you can see examples of skeletal variations. Within each anatomical joint action, I answer the question, "What moves?" so you can further investigate how you are feeling your own skeleton move with certain actions, possibly finding your compression limits.

This concept is helpful only if you know what compression feels like in your body. It literally feels like two objects are meeting. Some describe it as pinching, pressure, or "stuckness."

PART THREE | THE POSTURES

Some say they can feel that they just don't go any farther. I will never forget many years ago when I was teaching one of my regular classes, and I called Full Pigeon pose. I looked around to see one of my students frustrated. I asked her what was wrong, and she replied, "I can't stand this pose." She went on to say she never felt a stretch in her hips like everyone else, and she felt stuck. I asked her to show me where she felt stuck, and she pointed to her front hip creases. She said, "I can't go anywhere." I suggested that she try taking her knees wider. When she did, she was able to hinge farther forward in the pose. She looked up at me with her eyes wide and laughed. After practicing for nearly ten years, this was the first time she had ever felt an outer-hip stretch in Full Pigeon. She had been meeting compression in her hip fronts with flexion. When she moved her knees wider, she was able to avoid compression enough to move into the stretch. *When two bones meet, something is often caught or impinged between them, like cartilage, tendon, ligament, or muscle. This will sometimes cause pain, but not always.*

Although our skeletal shape plays a key role in how we access movement, our bones don't solely determine joint range of motion. As you more closely observe movement in your body, remember that bones, muscles, and connective tissue are involved, too. Joints contain all these components. Most human body joints, including all the joints discussed in this book, are synovial joints. (An example of non-synovial joints are the sutures of the skull.) **Synovial joints** have a capsule, or sleeve, of cartilaginous material that surrounds the articulating bones providing support, protection, and a well-lubricated environment for movement. The outer part of the capsule is tough and fibrous and sometimes incorporates ligaments and tendons. The inner part of the capsule is a synovial membrane that produces lubricating synovial fluid. When you move through postures and meet limitation, joint capsule tightness may be limiting your movement. Once again, this is beneficial since the joint is supposed to provide support and protection. Respect your natural range of motion.

Tension results from tightness in soft tissues, including fascia, tendons, ligaments, and muscles. These tissues shorten and tighten for many different reasons. Depending on your genetic constitution, you may have naturally tighter or looser soft tissues. We also create set points in our soft tissues through our daily, repetitive actions. Physical activities such as running or cycling will tend to over-strengthen certain muscles while not demanding much from others. Tension arises in our bodies for many reasons and is typically easier than compression to identify since it feels "tense" or "tight." Some describe it as a pulling, or "rubber band" feeling. Learning to distinguish between tension and compression in your body will be very helpful. Besides recognizing the characteristic sensations of pinching, pressure, tenseness, or tightness, the location of a sensation can tell us a lot. With practice, deciphering these feelings will become very natural.

Compression happens in the direction of motion. For example, when forward folding (like my student in Full Pigeon), the pelvis moves toward the femur(s). Compression in this action will be felt in the front hip crease, the direction of motion. I provide examples of direction of motion and compression points in part 2, "The Body."

Tension happens behind the direction of motion, or on the joint's other side. In the forward-folding example, tension will be felt in the back of the hip (like my student when she finally felt the outer-hip stretch in Full Pigeon).

NAVIGATING THE POSTURE | CHAPTER 12

For each anatomical action in "The Body," I answer the question, "What stretches, opposes, or relaxes?" I also specifically identify places of possible compression or tension within each individual pose description in the "What am I feeling?" tables (see "Using the Posture Descriptions" below). This helpful information can guide you as your inner awareness increases. Once you determine whether you are feeling tension or compression, you will want to know how to handle it. *Teachers, you can profoundly change your students' experiences once you understand this concept well.*

Navigating Tension

If your aim is to increase or maintain musculoskeletal wellness, you only want to stretch enough to return to natural flexibility, or that state in which you are free of excess tightness and tension. *Stretching beyond where your body returns to balance can eventually degrade your structure and cause weakness and/or injury.* If you feel that tension is stopping you in your pose, first decide if you indeed have excess tightness, or if you have met the edge of your natural flexibility. In other words, do you really need further stretch? If you do, finding a healthy level of stretch is key. First off, you don't want strong, localized sensation at a focused point. Make sure the stretch isn't landing predominantly in an attachment point or where the muscle meets tendon. You will feel this as a strong tug or sharp pull near a bone. Aim to spread out the stretch sensation as much as possible by making minor shifts in your position and activation.

Consider taking advantage of **reciprocal inhibition**, the principle that muscles work in pairs; as a result, when we activate muscles on one side of a joint, muscles on the other side release. For instance, if you want to stretch your hip flexors on the front of the hip, try engaging the muscles of hip extension at the same time. Remember, a little stretch goes a long way. Once you have an evenly distributed, manageable stretch sensation, use your breath as your guide. Take long, deep, steady breaths. Tap into what you are feeling.

Navigating Compression

If you notice skeletal compression within a joint in a certain pose, play with the angles of your bones a bit. Basically, move things around. By slightly changing your body placement, you may be able to navigate around the compression somewhat or completely. A very basic example of this can be seen in Downward-Facing Dog (fig. 13.9). Certain body types will have skeletal compression with shoulder flexion in this pose (fig. 6.3). By taking the hands wider and angling them differently, compression can possibly be shifted or avoided.

Realizing Proportions Matter

You may have wondered why certain poses come easier than others. Or you may wonder why certain poses are always awkward, no matter how you approach them, or how long you have practiced them. One reason could be your body proportions.

PART THREE | THE POSTURES

In yoga postures, we can't avoid the laws of matter, motion, energy, and force that govern the rest of the world. Your structure largely determines which poses come easily and which seem impossible. It will also determine the pose's appearance. Some people have long torsos and short legs. Some carry more weight in their lower bodies, while others are bulkier in their upper torso and arms. I have a student who has a short torso and long arms, and she finds arm balancing incredibly easy. Her body shape provides a center of gravity that makes balancing weight in her hands very manageable.

Can you see how Crow (fig. 20.3) will look very different from body to body depending on body proportions? For some, it is simple to get the knees to the backs of the arms, yet for others, the knees can only be placed on the outside of the arms. Even alignment such as the optimal bottom-hand placement in Triangle is determined in part by body proportions. As mentioned under the "Special Considerations" for Headstand (fig. 20.7), the humeri (upper-arm bones) need to be long enough to clear the head to provide a stable forearm base. If they aren't, the pose can't be done without compressing the cervical spine.

We will each be able to do certain poses much more easily than others purely because of the way we are shaped. This is not bad news or good news; it is just more information. I'm certainly not saying you should avoid challenging postures—unless they are harming your body, of course. The more we know about our bodies, the more we can navigate our experiences on the mat with relevancy and authenticity. Instead of feeling frustrated with poses that don't work for your body, learn to approach these poses with curiosity and allowance, while allocating your energy differently.

Playing Your Edge with Strength

Growth requires stretching into the unknown. It demands that we courageously step out of comfort and familiarity. Many yoga poses provide beautiful opportunities to expand our strength. Even if a pose is challenging, it can be approached with a sense of grounding, ease, and steadiness. Our breath can reveal our attitude, not only in our yoga poses but in all of life. As we grow stronger, we encounter new sensations in our bodies as well as new experiences for our brain. Yoga invites us to find strength while maintaining a sense of calm. It is a dichotomy that teaches us to be in the center of the storm while still seeing clearly, encouraging us to face our fears with compassion and awareness. This calm and clarity can initially result from the intentional practice and use of breath; then, eventually the ease can become automatic. While challenging your strength on the mat, if you pay close attention, you will know when you have gone too far. Feel what is happening in your attitude and breath; pay close attention to your body. With mindful awareness you will find the perfect amount of effort. Allow your breath to be your guide.

NAVIGATING THE POSTURE | CHAPTER 12

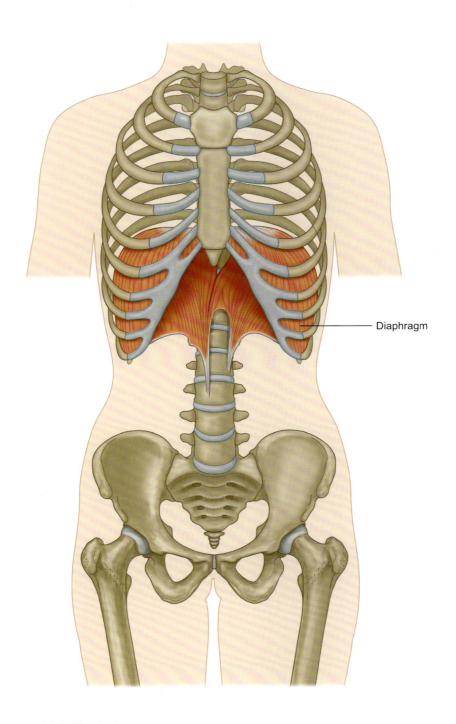

Figure 12.1. The diaphragm.

PART THREE | THE POSTURES

Using Breath and Gaze

Health care providers and wellness practitioners often prescribe breathing exercises as stress-lowering tools because how we breathe profoundly affects our autonomic nervous system. Stress reduction and autonomic balance are fundamental aspects of yoga. Longer, slower, deeper breathing correlates with vagus nerve stimulation and **parasympathetic** response (p. 8).[32] The breath is often described as the doorway to the autonomic nervous system since it is the one function that can happen either autonomically or voluntarily.[33] The sensory experience of breath is a principal tool for landing in the present moment. Your breath can also be an intelligent guide through your practice on the mat. Let's look at how normal breathing occurs.

The **diaphragm** and the external intercostals (the muscles between the ribs) are the main muscles of breathing. The diaphragm is an umbrella-shaped muscle separating the thoracic and abdominal cavities. Preceding an inhale, the diaphragm and the external intercostal muscles contract. The center of the diaphragm draws down into the abdominal cavity while the external intercostals expand the lower edges of the ribs upward and outward. These actions increase the volume of the thoracic cavity, reducing the pressure within the lungs to less than atmospheric pressure.[34] Air always flows from greater to lesser pressure; thus, the inhale occurs.

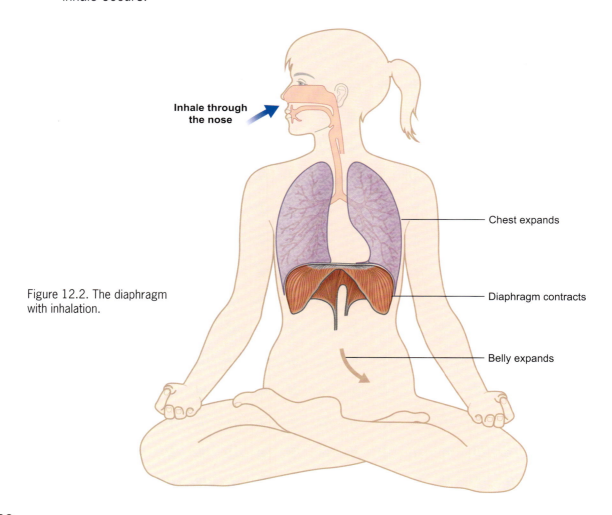

Figure 12.2. The diaphragm with inhalation.

After the lungs are full of air, the diaphragm and the external intercostals relax. The diaphragm goes back up into the thoracic cavity, and the ribs return to their original position. This relaxation reduces the thoracic cavity volume, increasing the pressure within the lungs and forcing air out with the exhale.

As inhalation and exhalation continue, this constant shape change is taking place, back and forth between the thoracic and abdominal cavities. With the inhale, the thoracic cavity volume increases while the abdominal cavity volume decreases (the belly pooches out). With the exhale, the thoracic cavity decreases while the abdominal cavity increases (the belly softens).

Place your hand on your belly for a moment. Feel your belly's tightness as it pushes into your hand when you inhale. Feel the softness as you exhale. Visualize and feel the diaphragm moving to create this dynamic shape change.

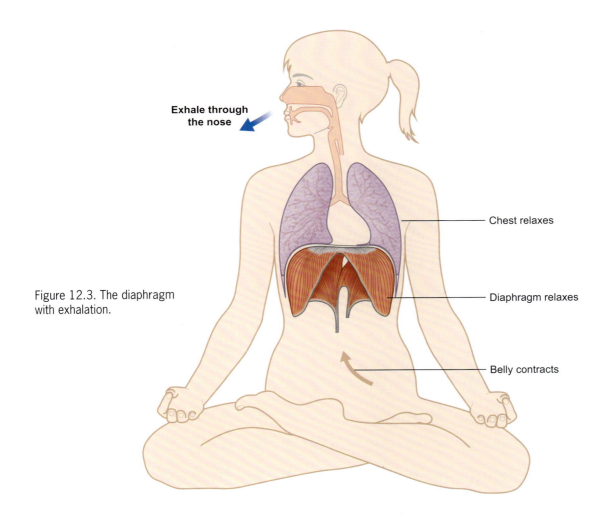

Figure 12.3. The diaphragm with exhalation.

PART THREE | THE POSTURES

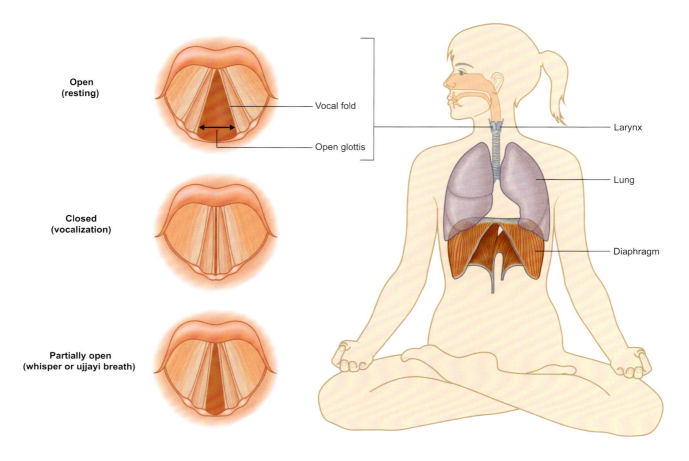

Figure 12.4. The throat space with glottis: resting, vocalization, and whisper.

> ### Consider...
> Did you know that lung capacity varies from person to person? In Vinyasa yoga, linking breath and movement is emphasized. This emphasis sometimes expands into classes in which teachers encourage group-synchronized breath. Just as our body structures vary, our vital lung capacities can also vary.[35] In addition, respiratory illnesses and cardiovascular fitness profoundly affect lung volume. Once students develop the skill of victorious breath, their breath pace will probably slow, yet it is important for teachers to understand and honor unique breath variability from mat to mat.

NAVIGATING THE POSTURE | CHAPTER 12

Ujjayi breath is sometimes referred to as "victorious breath" or "oceanic breath." It is the type of **pranayama** or breath-control exercise most used during yoga postures. Open your mouth and whisper a long "haaaaa." Now, repeat this with your mouth closed. The throat's action while whispering is similar to its action with ujjayi breath. A slight restriction, closing, or valving at the glottis restricts the air flow, creating a physical sensation of air moving on the back of the throat, as well as a subtle sound (fig. 12.4). This also results in a slower breath pace than normal. As mentioned in chapter 2, "Yoga and the Posture," purposeful, slow breath is a fundamental contributor to the stress-reducing attributes of yoga.

Along with victorious breath, using an intentional point of gaze, or **drishti**, is very helpful while practicing. Focusing the eyes can be the initial anchor for focusing the mind and body. As the gaze lands and steadies, the body and mind will follow. Within each pose, focus your gaze on a single point. Where you look can vary from pose to pose. Simply pick a point that makes the most sense with the pose.

Using the Posture Descriptions

Before you dive into the individual postures, understanding how they are grouped will be helpful. I have sorted poses by their similar anatomical actions and qualities. I find this useful when creating balanced sequences for my classes. If a pose is in a certain category, it may not exclusively belong there. For example, Child's Pose is with "Foundation Postures." Technically, it is also a forward fold. I have grouped them in a way that makes sense for this book. Each category opens with an overview of alignment elements to consider. Detailed descriptions of several poses follow. The pose categories are Foundation Postures, Standing Postures, Twists, Standing Balance Postures, Forward Folds, Backward Bends, Hip Openers, and Arm Balances and Inversions.

Each posture description begins with the pose's most common names. Typically, this will include a Sanskrit name and one or two English names. Sanskrit is an ancient Indian language used in yoga for centuries. The Sanskrit pose names may be unfamiliar. They usually end in "asana," which means "posture." None of the names are better, or "most" correct; they are merely different words used by different people.

Then, I explain the posture alignment. I am doing this like I would teach my own students. You will notice I often use the word *toward* in alignment instruction. I feel that directing an action toward something is more important than adamantly giving precise body placement. Your body variability will determine the best alignment for you. Please remember these are just some alignment ideas. How you align a pose and the actions you take depend on your aims in the pose. In my opinion, no alignment "list" could ever be complete.

Next, you will see a photo illustration of the pose with its anatomical actions labeled. Again, the photo is only an example of one body in the pose. The image is an initial reference; your pose will be different. Try to move away from needing your pose to meet an aesthetic ideal.

PART THREE | THE POSTURES

Each posture description includes a detailed table titled, "What am I feeling?" These tables provide plenty of information. Please do not get bogged down here. They are resources for investigating aspects of the pose further, as you need them.

This table has four components:

1. The "How do I get there?" column gives the construction elements, the anatomical actions that must take place to achieve the pose. You can think of these as the puzzle pieces combining to build the whole posture. For an expanded explanation of these anatomical actions, refer to part 2, "The Body." As you study an individual action of the pose, don't forget this is partial information. Anatomical actions don't happen in isolation. They happen within the interconnected web that is your body. The whole, integrated body will affect the movement, stability, range of motion, and action at a differentiated part.

2. The "What is strengthening?" column conveys which groups of muscles are the primary workers. Your structure, your pose, and your level of conditioning will determine how much you are actually strengthening. Although any of the groups of muscles listed could be places you might be getting stronger, I have highlighted the most common tendencies I see in my students.

3. The "Where could I notice tightness?" column relates which groups of muscles are the antagonists. Although you could notice tightness in any of the groups of muscles listed, I have highlighted the most common tendencies I see in my students.

4. The "Could I feel skeletal compression here?" column tells you which anatomical motions are most likely to entail skeletal compression with uniquely shaped bones.

These tables will help you investigate when something feels limited, challenging, or uncomfortable. Additionally, when you want to know what you are strengthening, stretching, and moving in any given posture, this information will be invaluable. Using these tables while referring to part 2, "The Body," will advance your understanding of what you are feeling in your body.

In "Special Considerations," I share additional perspective and understanding to further support you while using Embodied Posture Methodology in your practice and/or teaching. Next you will see "Modifications" and "Variations" of the posture. Again, this is not a complete list. I've just given a few ideas here. The last section is titled, "Exploration/Possible Cues." This is where I share some of my personal thought processes as a teacher, as well as my own curiosities and explorations in my body on the mat. If you are a teacher, you could use these in your classes. As a student, use these to inspire exploration of your unique pose.

Chapter 13
Foundation Postures

Foundation Postures Overview

Foundation postures include Mountain (fig. 13.13) and its closest relatives. The feet and legs are placed in line with the pelvis, and these are all symmetrical poses; the left side of the body mirrors the right. These poses build a foundation for equanimity within the entire body. Carry this sense of equanimity through all your non-foundational, asymmetrical postures. The Foundation Postures are perfect for establishing the embodiment of breath, body, and mind synchronicity.

PART THREE | THE POSTURES

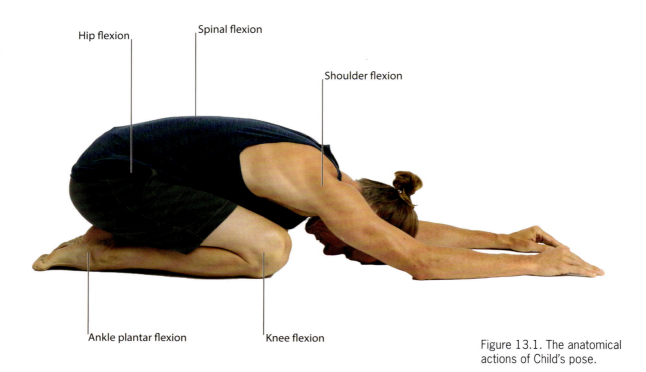

Figure 13.1. The anatomical actions of Child's pose.

Child's Pose

Child's
Pose of the Child
Balasana

Child's pose symbolizes surrender to life's physical and mental demands. Relax into this passive stretch for the back of your body at the beginning of a practice or any time you need a break.

Start on your hands and knees. Take your knees wide to the edges of your mat. Untuck your toes, laying the tops of your feet on the mat. Draw your big toes toward together. Rest your hips back toward your heels. Reach your arms forward and long, resting your forehead on the ground.

***You will notice that I often use the word *toward* in my alignment instructions. This is because I prefer to focus on an action *toward* something rather than adamantly giving precise body placement. Your body variability will determine the best alignment for you.

FOUNDATION POSTURES | CHAPTER 13

Child's. What am I feeling?

HOW DO I GET THERE?	WHAT IS STRENGTHENING?	WHERE COULD I NOTICE TIGHTNESS?	IS COMPRESSION POSSIBLE?
Spinal flexion	*Passive*	Spinal extensors, fig. 5.3	
Shoulder flexion *Can be active or passive*	Shoulder flexors, fig. 6.4	Shoulder extensors, fig. 6.5	✓ Fig. 6.3
Scapular elevation and upward rotation *Natural placement with arms lengthened forward; can be active or passive*	Elevators and upward rotators of the scapulae, p. 54	Depressors and downward rotators of the scapulae, p. 54	
Elbow extension *Can be active or passive*	Elbow extensors, fig. 10.2	Elbow flexors, fig. 10.3	
Hip flexion	*Passive*	Hip extensors, fig. 7.6	✓ Fig. 7.4
Knee flexion	*Passive*	Knee extensors, fig. 8.2	
Ankle plantar flexion	*Passive*	Ankle dorsiflexors, fig. 9.3	✓ Fig. 9.2

My discoveries:

PART THREE | THE POSTURES

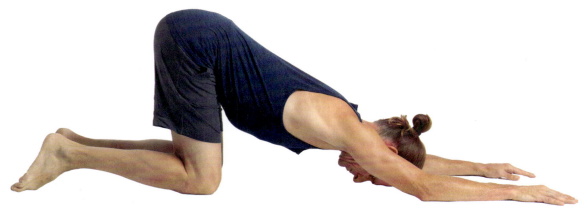

Figure 13.2. Child's pose modification with higher hips.

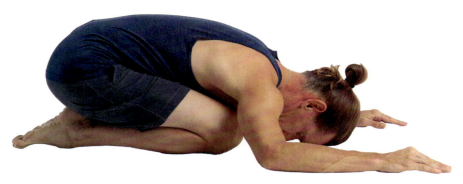

Figure 13.3. Child's pose modification with Cactus arms.

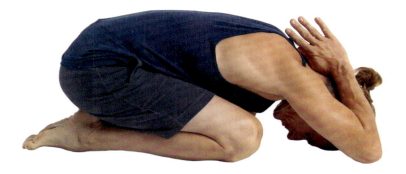

Figure 13.4. Child's pose variation with Reverse Prayer hands.

Special Considerations

Four big ranges of motion must be accessed to achieve this pose: ankle plantar flexion, knee flexion, shoulder flexion, and hip flexion. Injury or limited range of motion in any of these will limit the pose.

Bulkiness on the front of the body (breasts/abdomen) as well as ankle, knee, and/or hip injury can limit this pose.

Modifications

Tuck your back toes under if you have limited ankle range of motion, tenderness, or foot cramping.

Bend less at your knees and/or hip joints (higher hips) if the range of motion is limited in your knees or hips.

Bend your elbows, or take your arms back along your sides if your shoulder-flexion range of motion is limited, and/or you have discomfort in your shoulders.

Place a block under your forehead.

Place your forehead on your stacked fists.

If Child's pose is not working at all, replace it with Tabletop (fig. 13.5) or Downward-Facing Dog (fig. 13.9).

Variations

Stretch through your armpits and chest with Reverse Prayer hands.

Bring your knees together.

Exploration/Possible Cues

As you take your knees wide, allow your ribs and belly to soften toward the ground.

Notice your breath in this shape.

Enjoy the stretch on the back sides of your hip joints and along your spine.

Try bringing your knees closer together so that your thighs touch your ribs. Feel the difference in your back and in your breath.

Reach forward with your hands, lengthening out of your hips.

PART THREE | THE POSTURES

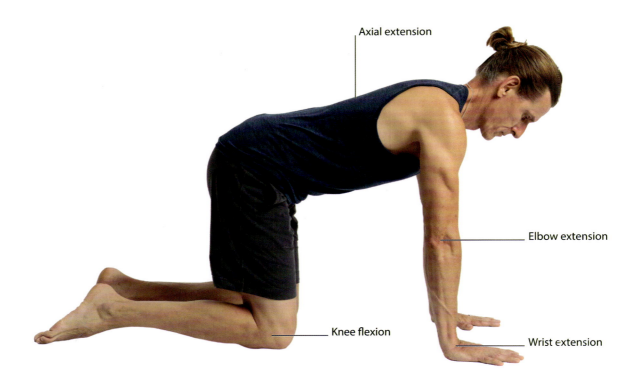

Figure 13.5. The anatomical actions of Tabletop.

Tabletop

Tabletop
All Fours
Bharmanasana

Tabletop allows for an unhurried arrival on the mat as we come into the body and breath. It is often taught early in yoga classes as a foundation for many other posture variations done from the hands and knees. This posture is simplistic yet very effective for wiring in the sensory experience of equanimity.

Place your hands directly under your shoulders and your knees directly under your hips. Keep your fingers spread wide and active. You can tuck or untuck your toes for stability. Maintain neutral in your spine. Notice your weight distribution from left to right and from front to back. Stay for several breaths while you wire in the sense of balance.

FOUNDATION POSTURES | CHAPTER 13

Tabletop. What am I feeling?

HOW DO I GET THERE?	WHAT IS STRENGTHENING?	WHERE COULD I NOTICE TIGHTNESS?	IS COMPRESSION POSSIBLE?
Axial extension	**Axial extensors, fig. 5.10**	Entire trunk	
Elbow extension	Elbow extensors, fig. 10.2	Elbow flexors, fig. 10.3	
Wrist extension	Wrist extensors, fig. 11.2	Wrist flexors, fig. 11.3	
Shoulder flexion	Shoulder flexors, fig. 6.4	Shoulder extensors, fig. 6.5	
Ankle dorsiflexion or plantar flexion	Ankle dorsiflexors, fig. 9.3 Ankle plantar flexors, fig. 9.4	Ankle plantar flexors, fig. 9.4 Ankle dorsiflexors, fig. 9.3	
Knee flexion	Knee flexors, fig. 8.3 *Passive*	Knee extensors, fig. 8.2	

My discoveries:

I have highlighted the most common tendencies I see in my students. It is possible to feel strengthening or to notice tightness in any of the muscle groups listed within their respective columns.

Special Considerations

Sometimes it is hard to sense exactly what your body is doing when you are holding postures requiring more strength. But in Tabletop you can notice how pelvic tilt feels in a less physically demanding pose. Moving through anterior and posterior tilt, as in Cat/Cow movements, can help you feel the correlation between the pelvis and the spine. Then you can replicate this articulation more successfully in standing postures.

PART THREE | THE POSTURES

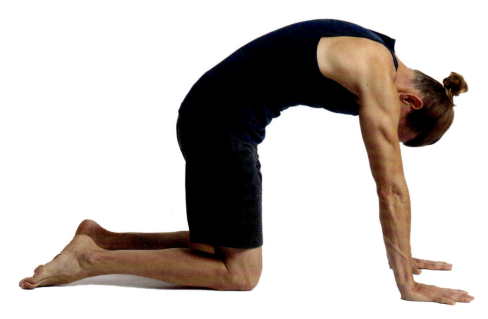

Figure 13.6. Cat pose.

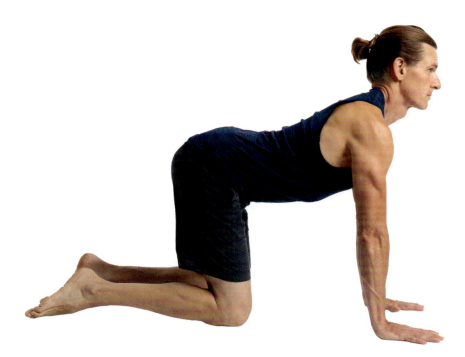

Figure 13.7. Cow pose.

FOUNDATION POSTURES | CHAPTER 13

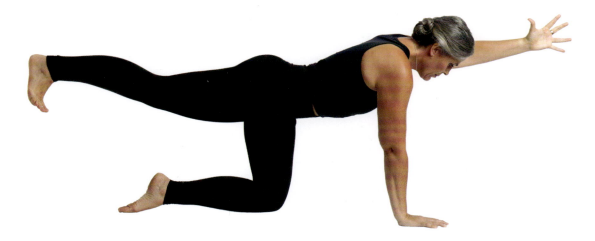

Figure 13.8. Spinal Balance.

Modifications

If you can't put pressure on your knees, try placing padding under them. If this doesn't help, Downward Dog is a good substitution.

Variations

Cat and Cow are actions typically taken from Tabletop for spinal mobility.

Spinal Balance is a balancing and strengthening Tabletop variation.

Rotate your fingertips externally and toward your knees for a nice wrist-flexor stretch here.

For a calf stretch, extend a leg back, tuck the toes under, and shift your weight back until you reach the desired stretch. Repeat on the other side.

Exploration/Possible Cues

Shift your weight in different directions to feel how your body bears weight.

Distribute your weight as evenly as possible through both hands and knees.

Use this pose to learn how neutral spine feels.

As you go into Cat, slide your shoulder blades apart.

In Cat, push the floor away.

As you go into Cow, reach the center of your chest forward.

As you go into Cat, rock your weight slightly back. As you go into Cow, rock your weight slightly forward.

PART THREE | THE POSTURES

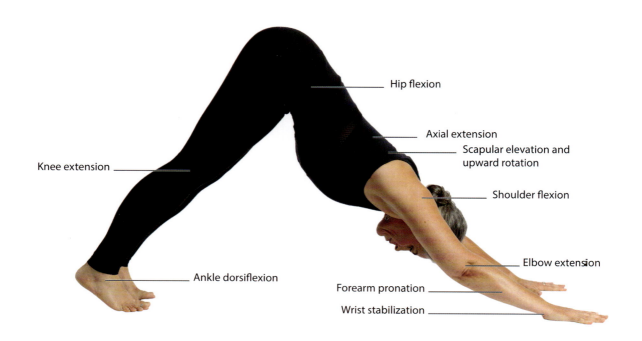

Figure 13.9. The anatomical actions of Downward-Facing Dog.

Downward-Facing Dog

Downward-Facing Dog
Adho Mukha Svanasana

This is typically the first pose that comes to mind when someone hears the word *yoga*. Considered a resting pose for seasoned practitioners, Downward-Facing Dog is often challenging for beginners. It is a full-body strengthener, an inversion, and an effective release for the back side of the body.

Begin in Tabletop position with active hands pointing straight forward, slightly wider than shoulder-width distance apart. Then slide your hands a couple of inches forward. Tuck your toes under, and lift your knees up and off the ground, creating a bold, upside-down V shape with your body. Allow your head to hang freely, and gaze back at the ground between your feet. Bend your knees enough to achieve axial extension, lengthening your spine. Draw your hips back, up, and away from your wrists, limiting weight bearing in your hands. Remain active along one bright line of energy from your hands to your seat. A slight internal rotation of your thighs might help overall stability and core activation, depending on your hip structure. Feel all four points of contact with the floor, and breathe deeply.

FOUNDATION POSTURES | CHAPTER 13

Downward-Facing Dog. What am I feeling?

HOW DO I GET THERE?	WHAT IS STRENGTHENING?	WHERE COULD I NOTICE TIGHTNESS?	IS COMPRESSION POSSIBLE?
Axial extension	**Axial extensors, fig. 5.10**	Entire trunk	
Wrist stabilization	**Wrist flexors, fig. 11.3** *The wrists are somewhat neutral, yet the flexors work isometrically to prevent collapse into extension.*		
Forearm pronation	Forearm pronators, fig. 10.5	Forearm supinators, fig. 10.4	
Shoulder flexion	**Shoulder flexors, fig. 6.4**	**Shoulder extensors, fig. 6.5**	✓ Fig. 6.3
Scapular elevation and upward rotation *Natural placement with arm positioning*	Elevators and upward rotators of the scapulae, p. 54	Depressors and downward rotators of the scapulae, p. 54	
Elbow extension	**Elbow extensors, fig. 10.2**	Elbow flexors, fig. 10.3	
Hip flexion	Hip flexors, fig. 7.5 *The degree of hip flexor activation will depend on the unique combination of hip flexion angle and knee-extension angle, along with body proportions. The amount of activation or stretch in any muscle at any joint depends on these factors, among others.*	**Hip extensors, fig. 7.6**	
Knee extension	Knee extensors, fig. 8.2	Knee flexors, fig. 8.3	
Ankle dorsiflexion	*Passive*	Ankle plantar flexors, fig. 9.4	✓ Fig. 9.2

My discoveries:

PART THREE | THE POSTURES

Special Considerations

Some instructors may teach you to have a shorter base (feet closer to hands), while others teach a longer base (feet farther away from hands). Neither is right or wrong, but each offers different benefits. A shorter base typically results in more **posterior** body stretch. A longer base is less stable but allows more spine lengthening. *As always, if you are adamant about doing anything a particular way, simply know why.*

You might be cued to work toward getting your heels to the floor in this pose. Your ability to do this will be determined by your unique skeletal ankle complex. Some bodies will easily be able to touch heels to the floor while others will never be able to, simply because of the bones' shapes. It is neither right nor wrong to get your heels to the floor in Downward Dog.

Foot, ankle, leg, hip, shoulder, and/or spine injury will limit this pose.

Various cues address shoulder placement in this pose. As I've mentioned before, no cues are inherently "bad"; they just aren't always 100% relevant. Here is an example:

> Recently I had a student in my class who asked me to help with her Downward-Facing Dog alignment. She said her shoulders were very uncomfortable in the pose, and subsequently, she was having shoulder pain. I asked her to show me the pose. As she moved into it, she strongly rotated her elbow creases forward while jamming her shoulder blades away from her ears. While I watched where the joint was flexing in her shoulder creases, I saw congestion building. As I always do, I began by asking her what she felt. She answered that she felt extreme pressure in her shoulder joints and pointed to her shoulder creases. I asked her first to take a moment to focus on what she was feeling inside, then to wiggle into what felt comfortable, disregarding what she thought was the *right* thing to do with her shoulders.
>
> I watched as she took a few breaths. She allowed her shoulder blades to move toward her ears. Then she relaxed the rotation she had been forcing in her arm bones. I watched as the congested area in her shoulder creases began to soften. She finally said, "This is what feels good." By simply unravelling the alignment directions she had been forcing, she allowed her shoulders to find their natural alignment. Obviously, she was trying to do the pose correctly by following the specific action cues she had learned. These cues may serve certain bodies at certain times, but they weren't working for her body in this pose.
>
> In chapter 6, "The Shoulder," I discuss shoulder stability and scapular movements. Any time the arms are overhead, as in Downward-Facing Dog, the scapulae naturally elevate and rotate upward. The scapulae are sliding to meet the humerus heads for natural stability. The student had felt from within to find natural, sturdy alignment. This is an excellent example of approaching the pose based on interoception, or noticing what is happening on the inside, rather than attempting to force the shape of the pose to fit an aesthetic ideal, or what it is "supposed" to look like from the outside. This is Embodied Posture.

FOUNDATION POSTURES | CHAPTER 13

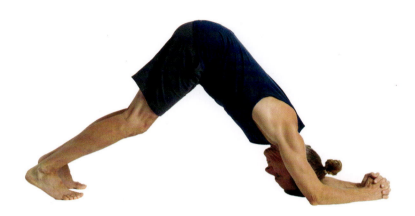

Figure 13.10. Dolphin.

Modifications

Replace Downward-Facing Dog with Tabletop if needed (fig. 13.5).

Take Child's pose for rest intermittently while you are building strength (fig. 13.1).

Placing your hands wider or angling your hands out will help if shoulder compression limits you.

If hand or wrist pain is an issue, do Dolphin instead (fig. 13.10). Or you can change the angle of your hands/wrists by placing a rolled-up mat underneath the base of your hands to lessen wrist extension.

I've seen students using fists to avoid weight bearing in extended wrists and flat hands. This modification is not stable and can lead to further pain in the fingers, hands, and wrists. If you choose to do this, minimize the time spent weight bearing in this position, and proceed with caution. Better yet, instead of making fists, try using a dumbbell or handle device that eliminates wrist extension.

If you have hand or wrist pain, remember to take weight off of them by shifting your center of gravity. To do this, pull back, up, and away through your hips. Often beginners miss this activation and end up bearing too much weight in the hands and wrists, causing pain.

PART THREE | THE POSTURES

Variations

Placing blocks under your hands changes the physics of this pose and may help you find the mobility to step or hop forward.

Three-Legged Dog adds an increased lateral stretch and a balance element.

Try Puppy pose on your knees to allow a more restorative stretch for your chest and the fronts of your shoulders.

Exploration/Possible Cues

If you feel discomfort or compression in your shoulders, try taking your hands a little wider, and/or angle your hands out slightly.

Activate your lower body to lift weight up and out of your shoulders.

Can you make your shoulder joints a little more spacious?

Bend your knees, and pull back and up from your hip creases, creating spaciousness in your entire spine.

Keep softness in the back of your neck.

Push the ground forward and away to pull your hips back and up.

Imagine your hips floating up like a balloon, diagonally lifting away from your hands.

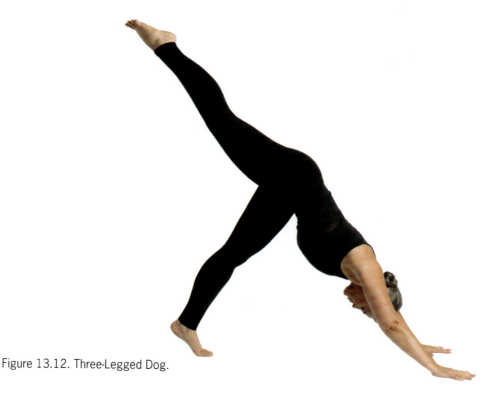

Figure 13.12. Three-Legged Dog.

FOUNDATION POSTURES | CHAPTER 13

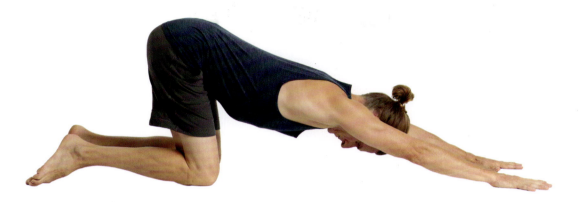

Figure 13.11. Puppy pose.

Consider...

Growth occurs in the midst of the unfamiliar. This is true for our bodies and for our brains. Consider the things you do on autopilot. Do you actually think about all the turns and lane changes on your commute to work? Probably not. Our brains create neural pathways for everything we do. For often-repeated actions, the neural pathways resemble very fast, easily accessible super highways. But when we face something unknown, we must slow down and take the back roads while we create fresh neural pathways. As we repeat the new activity, these neural pathways get stronger until they, too, become super highways, which then become habits, things we can do on autopilot. Our brains thrive on learning new things.

From a musculoskeletal perspective, repetitive actions form set patterns of range of motion and muscle use in our bodies. If we move in the same limited ways day after day, we can overuse some parts of our bodies while losing range or strength in other parts. Any time we are doing something on the mat that feels awkward or challenging, it is a moment of growth. I'm not talking about things that feel awkward because they are harming your body; I'm talking about things that are challenging because they are different and new. Our bodies thrive on movement variability. This is one reason why elite athletes place so much value on cross-training.

Approach yoga posture with healthy, ongoing curiosity. Don't think of a pose as something you will finally master; think of it as something to experience new each time you practice. Let each pose be your vehicle to practice feeling from within, being fully present as you explore it. The postures are beautiful tools for increasing our ability to be aware. Our bodies are a bit different every single day, so don't be afraid to approach your postures differently from practice to practice. Play with the physics of the pose. Change your stance—some days bigger, some days smaller. Take different arm variations. Transition differently into poses. If you always go into a particular pose from Downward Dog, try moving into it from Mountain. Make up poses and new variations of poses. Do those things that you aren't "good" at. You never know what you might discover. And take your yoga off the mat. At its heart, yoga is a practice of mindful awareness, so you can do this with anything. Incorporate walks, runs, biking, and even strength training into your yoga. Yoga is a state of mind. Don't let anyone tell you what your yoga can and can't be.

PART THREE | THE POSTURES

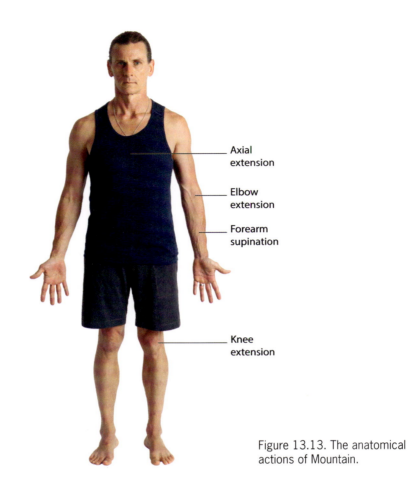

Figure 13.13. The anatomical actions of Mountain.

Mountain

Mountain
Tadasana

Mountain pose is the template for all other poses. All other postures contain foundational elements of this one.

Take an upright, sturdy, neutral stance. Place your feet hip-width distance apart or closer for stability. Distribute your weight evenly through the three corners of your feet. Actively engage your legs as you lengthen up and away through your crown. Depending on your hip structure, a slight internal rotation/activation of your thighs might help steady your core, lower body, and feet. Face your palms forward for openness across your chest. Gently integrate your shoulder blades by hugging them slightly down and together, keeping a sturdy, upright position. (Don't overdo this.) Maintain all the natural curves of your spine. Draw your sacrum toward your heels just enough to bring a slight broadening to the low-back space. Gaze forward, stand tall, and be present with the feeling of equanimity.

FOUNDATION POSTURES | CHAPTER 13

Mountain. What am I feeling?

HOW DO I GET THERE?	WHAT IS STRENGTHENING?	WHERE COULD I NOTICE TIGHTNESS?	IS COMPRESSION POSSIBLE?
Axial extension	Axial extensors, fig. 5.10	Entire trunk	
Shoulder lateral rotation	Shoulder lateral rotators, fig. 6.14	Shoulder medial rotators, fig. 6.11	
Scapular depression and downward rotation Natural, relaxed position with arms down	Depressors and downward rotators of the scapulae, p. 54	Elevators and upward rotators of the scapulae, p. 54	
Forearm supination	Forearm supinators, fig. 10.4	Forearm pronators, fig. 10.5	
Elbow extension	Elbow extensors, fig. 10.2 *Passive with gravity*	Elbow flexors, fig. 10.3	
Knee extension	Knee extensors, fig. 8.2	Knee flexors, fig. 8.3	
Hip stabilization with adduction	Hip adductors, fig. 7.8	Hip abductors, fig. 7.9	

My discoveries:

Special Considerations

Foot positioning is taught many ways. Some teachers/traditions teach feet together; some teach feet hip-width distance apart. Because we all have unique skeletal structures, you need to find what is most stable for you. Some factors determining your most stable foot placement include the width of your pelvis; the orientation and shape of your hip, knee, and ankle complexes; and the shape of your leg bones. Typically, somewhere between feet hip-width-distance apart and feet together will work best.

PART THREE | THE POSTURES

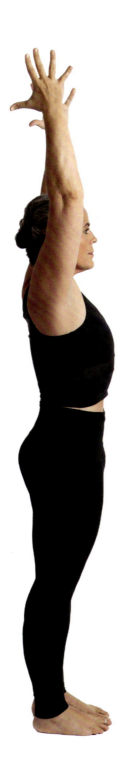

Modifications

Stand near a wall.

Use a folding chair for support. Place your hands on the back of the chair, or simply have it nearby if needed for balance.

Variations

Reach your arms up for Extended Mountain.

Exploration/Possible Cues

Use this pose to establish the feeling of equanimity in your body.

Notice balance from left to right, front to back, and top to bottom.

Shift your weight in different directions to feel changes in sensation and balance.

Imagine a string lifting your crown up and away from the ground.

Allow your breath to support the expansion of your spine.

Figure 13.14. Extended Mountain.

FOUNDATION POSTURES | CHAPTER

What I am looking for is not out there, it is in me.
—Helen Keller

THE POSTURES

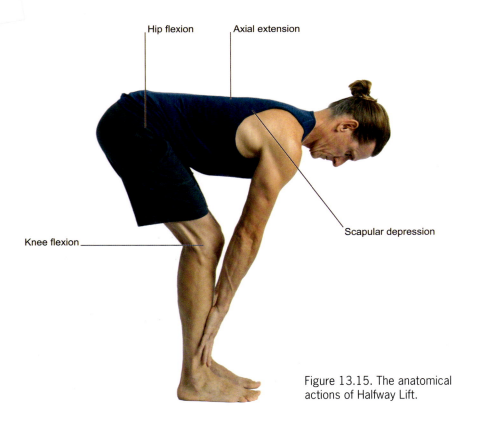

Figure 13.15. The anatomical actions of Halfway Lift.

Halfway Lift

Halfway Lift
Standing Half Forward Bend
Ardha Uttanasana

Halfway Lift is the dynamic link between Forward Fold and Mountain pose in many **vinyasa** sequences. Vinyasa is a style of yoga that emphasizes synchronization of breath and movement. In other words, pose actions are linked with an inhale or an exhale. Halfway Lift, for example, is fueled by the energy of an inhale. It is an excellent leg strengthener and spine stretch.

From a Forward Fold position, bend your knees slightly. Draw your hips back as you lift and elongate your spine. Lift high enough that you have to engage your back muscles. Place your fingertips on your shins, and reach your crown long and away from your hips. Draw your shoulder blades away from your ears, and meet the fullness of your inhalation.

FOUNDATION POSTURES | CHAPTER 13

Halfway Lift. What am I feeling?

HOW DO I GET THERE?	WHAT IS STRENGTHENING?	WHERE COULD I NOTICE TIGHTNESS?	IS COMPRESSION POSSIBLE?
Axial extension	Axial extensors, fig. 5.10	Entire trunk	
Scapular depression and retraction	Depressors and retractors of the scapulae, p. 54	Elevators and protractors of the scapulae, p. 54	
Hip flexion	Hip extensors, fig. 7.6 Extensors engage eccentrically and/or isometrically to oppose gravity toward further hip flexion during a hold.		
Knee extension	Knee extensors, fig. 8.2 Even if knees are bent, activation is isometric extension opposing gravity during a hold, eccentric on the way into the pose.	Knee flexors, fig. 8.3	

My discoveries:

Special Considerations

This posture could technically be considered a forward fold because of the hip flexion. I don't classify it as one because it emphasizes spinal elongation rather than folding.

Most yoga classes tend to be imbalanced between strengthening the pushing and pulling muscles. Strengthening the pushing muscles is usually emphasized much more. Consequently, I always aim to bring more upper-back strengthening into my classes when possible. Halfway Lift provides an opportunity for upper-back engagement if we highlight it. Doing the pose with Airplane Wings helps wire in this activation, so I like to call at least the first few Halfway Lifts with Airplane Wings to remind students to focus on the back-body muscles. This variation of the pose is also a great place to practice using Cylindrical Core (fig. 13.17).

Modifications

Place your hands on blocks or on your thighs near your knees.

Bend your knees more.

PART THREE | THE POSTURES

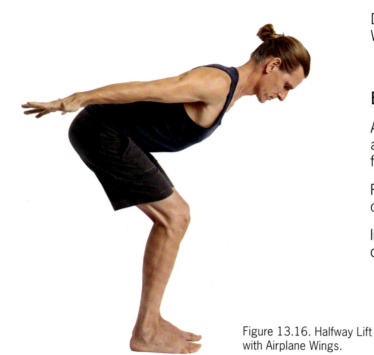

Variations

Do Halfway Lift with arms in Airplane Wings as shown at left.

Exploration/Possible Cues

Actively push your hips back as an anchoring point as you draw your crown forward.

Pull back through your belly and hip creases to telescope your spine forward.

Imagine the muscles that engage while doing pull-ups. Engage them here.

Figure 13.16. Halfway Lift with Airplane Wings.

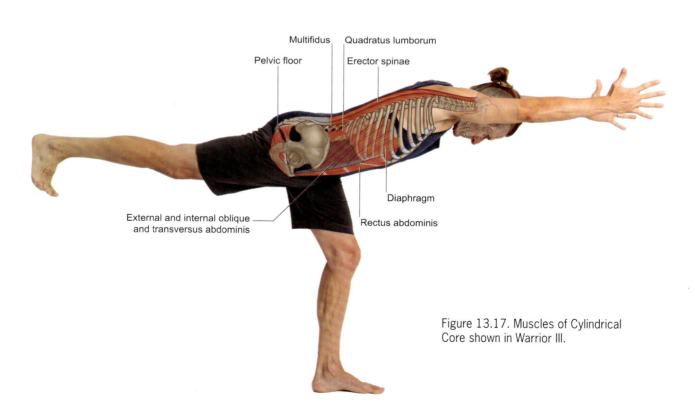

Figure 13.17. Muscles of Cylindrical Core shown in Warrior III.

FOUNDATION POSTURES | CHAPTER 13

Consider...

Tuning in to the use of Cylindrical Core (fig. 13.17) takes focused awareness. Usually when we think of core strengthening, sit-ups, leg lifts, and bicycles come to mind. Movements like these mainly strengthen and tighten the iliopsoas muscles (fig. 18.5), sometimes creating imbalance and placing unnecessary pressure on the spine. These exercises aren't necessarily bad, but they can be much more effective when combined with awareness and activation of the intrinsic muscles that support the spine. Thinking of the spine as a cylindrical container with a top, bottom, and sides is helpful. The diaphragm muscle is the top; the abdominal muscles and back muscles make up the front, sides, and back; the pelvic floor is the bottom.

In exercises done while lying on your back, like leg lifts, aim to engage the abdominis rectus and the transverse abdominis to stabilize your pelvis. An unstabilized pelvis will result in a pooched-out belly and excessive lumbar backbend. These movements can be a bit tricky if you aren't used to them; this may take a little practice. To engage the transverse abdominis, squeeze your digestive organs in closer to your spine. You should feel your belly flattening and your waist getting smaller. To engage the rectus abdominis, think of zipping up your belly from pubis to sternum, much like you would to put on your favorite pair of skinny jeans. This action also flexes the spine, so aim to just zip up without rounding your spine. These added activations of the abdominis rectus and the transverse abdominis will make your leg lifts and crunches much more effective while balancing out the iliopsoas strength that coordinates the muscles between your trunk and legs.

When we shift the body in space to poses in which the spine requires more structural support, engaging the total Cylindrical Core is vital. To determine which poses require the most spinal structural support, think of the muscular demand in a pose like High Lunge. To stand or sit upright, our trunk muscles must work to hold the spine; yet, we don't often notice this until we've been upright for a while, and our muscles get tired. Although the muscles have to work in the upright position of High Lunge, the torso's weight is stacked directly over the legs so that the lower body is bearing most of the weight. Now imagine leaning forward in High Lunge, taking your spine to a diagonal position. This creates a completely new gravitational relationship between your trunk and the ground. The spine is no longer stacked directly over the pelvis. This is an example of where activation of the Cylindrical Core is most useful.

To activate the entire cylinder, think back to the visualization of the container with a top, bottom, front, back, and sides. Start by activating the rectus abdominis and the transverse abdominis with the zipping up and hugging in actions. From there, feel your abdominals wrapping around your sides connecting to your back; then add pelvic floor engagement. Engage your pelvic floor by lifting the center of the musculature as if you really "needed to go." The last step in Cylindrical Core activation is to keep the lid on the container with deep, strong breaths. Feel the powerful action of the diaphragm (fig. 12.1) as it pushes down toward your abdominals with the inhalation.

PART THREE | THE POSTURES

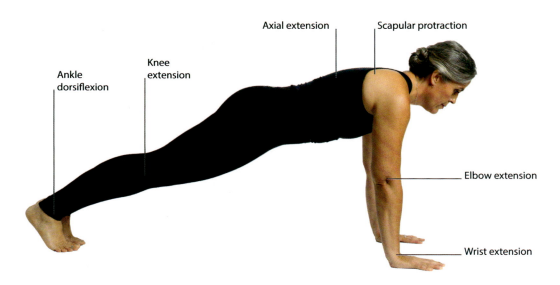

Figure 13.18. The anatomical motions of Plank.

Plank

Plank
High Push-Up
Kumbhakasana

Fiery, strong, and empowering, this pose builds overall strength and confidence. It is basically Mountain pose shifted horizontally in space.

Begin in Tabletop. Lift your knees off the floor by extending one leg back and then the other. Tuck your toes under strongly, and press back through your heels as if you were standing firmly on the ground. Activate and engage both legs. Draw your sacrum down toward your heels while hugging your front lower ribs into your belly. This will help you avoid dropping into a backbend and hammocking toward the ground. Fire up your Cylindrical Core (fig. 13.17), and push into your hands and arms making them two strong pillars. Stabilize your shoulders with scapular protraction (fig. 6.17). Remain lifted and spacious through your shoulder joints.

FOUNDATION POSTURES | CHAPTER 13

Plank. What am I feeling?

HOW DO I GET THERE?	WHAT IS STRENGTHENING?	WHERE COULD I NOTICE TIGHTNESS?	IS COMPRESSION POSSIBLE?
Scapular protraction	**Protractors of the scapulae, p. 54**	Retractors of the scapulae, p. 54	
Shoulder flexion	**Shoulder flexors, fig. 6.4**	Shoulder extensors, fig. 6.5	
Elbow extension	Elbow extensors, fig. 10.2	Elbow flexors, fig. 10.3	
Wrist extension	Wrist extensors, fig. 11.2	**Wrist flexors, fig. 11.3**	
Forearm pronation	Forearm pronators, fig. 10.5	Forearm supinators, fig. 10.4	
Ankle dorsiflexion	Ankle dorsiflexors, fig. 9.3	**Ankle plantar flexors, fig. 9.4**	
Cylindrical Core activation	**Cylindrical Core, fig. 13.17**		
Knee extension	**Knee extensors, fig. 8.2**	Knee flexors, fig. 8.3	
Hip stabilization	**Hip flexors, fig. 7.5** Hip flexors work isometrically to prevent the hips from sagging into extension.		

My discoveries:

Special Considerations

Hand, wrist, shoulder, or back injury will limit this pose.

The shoulder socket is on the front side of the scapula, part of the same bony structure (fig. 6.2). Remember that stable shoulder positioning changes depending on how you are supporting your body in space (p. 54.) Shoulder stability while standing in Warrior II looks very different from stability in Plank. As the pillars of your arm bones support your body weight, sliding the scapulae/shoulder sockets out a bit to meet them (protraction, fig. 6.17) will provide the most support. Don't overdo the protraction and collapse around your chest.

If your elbows hyperextend, keep them slightly bent here.

Modifications

Take your knees to the ground as needed while building strength.

Forearm Plank is an option if you have hand or wrist injuries. The alignment is the same except for arm placement.

Variations

For added strength and balance work, try lifting an arm or leg.

Exploration/Possible Cues

As you come into Plank, imagine connecting all your strength from your feet, legs, core, and hands.

Keep the back of your neck nice and long. Pick a point of gaze on the floor slightly in front of your hands.

Your hands should be brightly energetic with fingers spread wide; keep them active.

Draw the pit of your belly up into your low spine.

Hold your body like one solid wood Plank.

Lift the space between your shoulder blades.

Slightly dome your upper back.

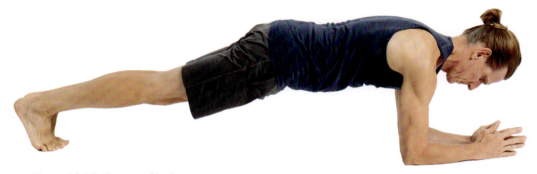

Figure 13.19. Forearm Plank.

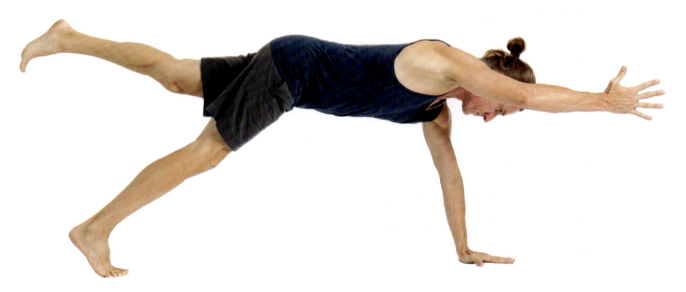

Figure 13.20. Plank variation with leg and arm reach.

PART THREE | THE POSTURES

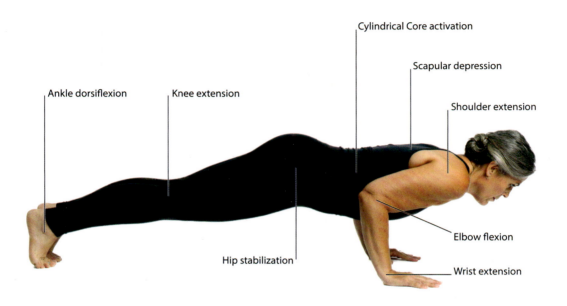

Figure 13.21. The anatomical actions of Low Plank.

Low Plank

Low Plank
Low Push-Up
Chaturanga Dandasana

A full-body strengthener, Low Plank is an integral part of any flow class. Refining the alignment of this often-repetitive pose is crucial.

From Plank alignment, shift your heels forward, taking your chest forward a few inches. Keep your hands planted in Plank alignment. Fire up the engagement of your Cylindrical Core (fig. 13.17) and legs so that your upper body is not working alone. Maintaining the Plank-like structure of your body, lower toward a 90-degree bend in the elbows or higher, but no lower. Keep your elbows near over your wrists as you lower. As always, use your breath for strength, and honor where you are.

FOUNDATION POSTURES | CHAPTER 13

Low Plank. What am I feeling?

HOW DO I GET THERE?	WHAT IS STRENGTHENING?	WHERE COULD I NOTICE TIGHTNESS?	IS COMPRESSION POSSIBLE?
Cylindrical Core activation	**Cylindrical Core, fig. 13.17**		
Shoulder extension *When moving from Plank to Low Plank*	**Shoulder flexors, fig. 6.4** *Shoulder flexors work eccentrically and/or isometrically to oppose further collapse into extension with gravity.*		
Scapular depression	**Depressors of the scapulae, p. 54**	Elevators of the scapulae, p. 54	
Elbow flexion	**Elbow extensors, fig. 10.2** *Elbow extensors work eccentrically while lowering, and isometrically while holding to oppose gravity.*		
Wrist extension	Wrist extensors, fig. 11.2	**Wrist flexors, fig. 11.3**	
Ankle dorsiflexion	Ankle dorsiflexors, fig. 9.3	Ankle plantar flexors, fig. 9.4	
Knee extension	**Knee extensors, fig. 8.2**	Knee flexors, fig. 8.3	
Hip stabilization	**Hip flexors, fig. 7.5** *Hip flexors work isometrically to prevent the hips from sagging into extension.*		

My discoveries:

PART THREE | THE POSTURES

Special Considerations

Shoulder, wrist, or back injury will limit this pose.

Lower only to where you still have stability. It is often more effective not to lower all the way to 90 degrees.

Lowering beyond 90 degrees excessively strains the soft tissues in the front of the shoulder, specifically the long head of the biceps tendon (fig. 6.13).

Scapular retraction (fig. 6.17) is a natural movement of the scapulae when moving from Plank to Low Plank. To keep the scapulae from winging away from the thorax, activate scapular depression, or snug your shoulder blades toward your back pockets as you lower.

Often practitioners unknowingly place repetitive strain on their shoulders in Low Plank. A tell-tale sign is tenderness or pain in the fronts of both shoulders. If you have this, you should work on refining your alignment in this pose. Read about proximal biceps tendinopathy in chapter 6, "The Shoulder."

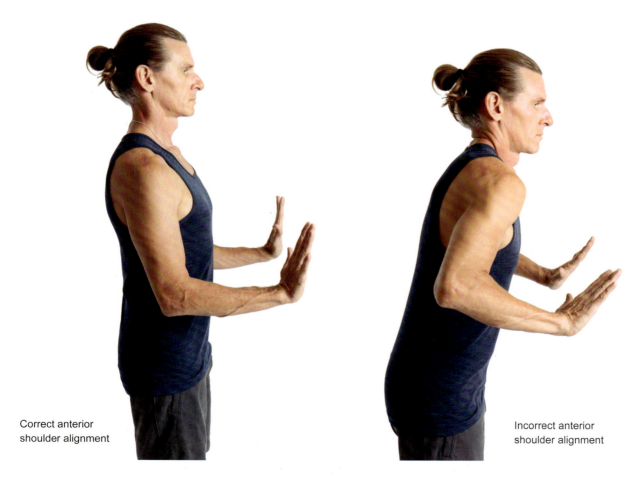

Correct anterior shoulder alignment

Incorrect anterior shoulder alignment

Figure 13.22. Correct vs. incorrect anterior shoulder alignment Low Plank.

FOUNDATION POSTURES | **CHAPTER 13**

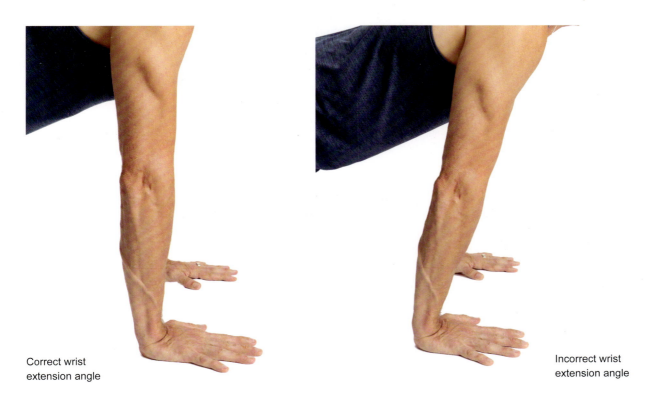

Correct wrist extension angle

Incorrect wrist extension angle

Figure 13.23. Correct vs. incorrect wrist extension angle in Low Plank.

Avoid overextending the wrists. This happens when your forearms move too far forward, decreasing the angle between the forearms and the hands.

This pose can also be done safely without shifting your weight forward prior to lowering. The elbows would not stack over the wrists, but instead they would stay slightly back. This especially helps keep excess weight and tension off the wrists and shoulders.

Modifications

Place your knees on the ground while building your strength.

Lowering the knees, then thighs, then belly, and lastly chest is another way to modify this pose. I prefer this for beginners as it helps them maintain good form while guiding their elbows straight back with control. Always emphasize *controlled lowering*.

PART THREE | THE POSTURES

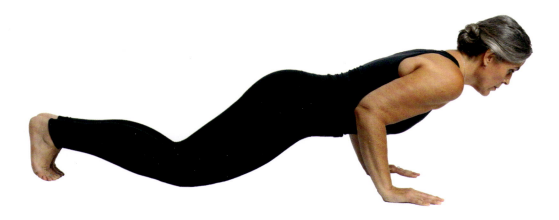

Figure 13.24. Low Plank modification with knees down.

Variations

It's best to stick with the base pose here. Low Plank requires such full-body strength integration that variations like lifting a leg or arm put the supporting joints at too much risk.

Exploration/Possible Cues

Don't forget to engage your legs and core so your arms aren't doing all the work.

Strongly engage your quadriceps to straighten your knees as you lower all the way down.

If you feel steady in Plank pose, begin moving toward Low Plank, and tap your knees down the moment you reach instability. This will help increase your strength little by little.

Keep your chest open as you lower.

Keep your head in line with your body as you lower.

Lower your belly and hips at the same time as your shoulders.

Your entire body should lower as a solid Plank.

FOUNDATION POSTURES | **CHAPTER 13**

There is a voice that doesn't use words. Listen.
—Rumi

PART THREE | THE POSTURES

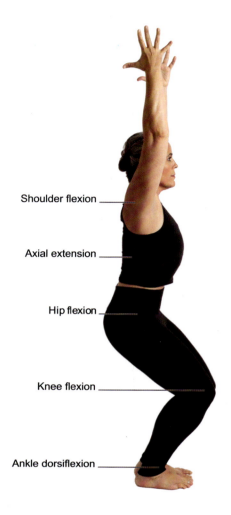

Figure 13.25. The anatomical actions of Chair.

Chair

Chair
Utkatasana
Awkward Pose
Fierce Pose

Chair embodies strength and equanimity. It helps build overall strength and stamina while providing an expansive upper-body stretch.

Begin in Mountain pose alignment (fig. 13.13). Bend your knees much like sitting in a chair. Allow your hips to lower back behind you. You can keep your feet together or apart for stability. Ground into the three corners of both feet evenly. Keep your chest upright while maintaining all the curvatures of your spine. Draw your sacrum (fig. 5.15) down toward the floor to slightly broaden the lumbar spine space while drawing the front lower ribs into the belly. Reach up actively all the way through the tips of your fingers, and gaze straight ahead.

FOUNDATION POSTURES | CHAPTER 13

Chair. What am I feeling?

HOW DO I GET THERE?	WHAT IS STRENGTHENING?	WHERE COULD I NOTICE TIGHTNESS?	IS COMPRESSION POSSIBLE?
Axial extension	**Axial extensors, fig. 5.10**	Entire trunk	
Shoulder flexion	**Shoulder flexors, fig. 6.4**	**Shoulder extensors, fig. 6.5**	✓ Fig. 6.3
Scapular elevation and upward rotation *Natural placement with arms lifted*	Elevators and upward rotators of the scapulae, p. 54	Depressors and downward rotators of the scapulae, p. 54	
Elbow extension	**Elbow extensors, fig. 10.2**	Elbow flexors, fig. 10.3	
Hip flexion	**Hip extensors, fig. 7.6** *While lowering into Chair, hip extensors work eccentrically to oppose gravity. While holding, they work isometrically.*	*Remember, when you see an eccentric contraction, those muscles are also lengthening.*	
Hip adduction *Stabilizing action*	**Hip adductors, fig. 7.8**	Hip abductors, fig. 7.9	
Knee flexion	**Knee extensors, fig. 8.2** *While lowering into Chair, knee extensors work eccentrically to oppose gravity. While holding, they work isometrically.*		
Ankle dorsiflexion	Ankle dorsiflexors, fig. 9.3	Ankle plantar flexors, fig. 9.4	✓ Fig. 9.2

My discoveries:

PART THREE | THE POSTURES

Special Considerations

As you sink deeper into Chair, counterbalance occurs. As the hips go back and down, something must counter that weight forward, typically the knees. If you are limited in ankle flexion range of motion (fig. 9.2), your knees will not be able to go forward, and you will have trouble going low without leaning your torso forward to balance. Taking your arms forward can give a nice counterweight so that your torso doesn't have to lean forward.

The best foot positioning will depend on your unique hip complex. Place your feet in a way that supports your pelvis. You will know you have the right placement when you feel stable and strong from hips to feet.

Foot, ankle, leg, hip, shoulder, or spine injury will limit this pose.

Modifications

Take your arms down.

Try varying arm positions to help with balance or any shoulder-flexion compression.

Don't sit as low if you lack strength and stamina here.

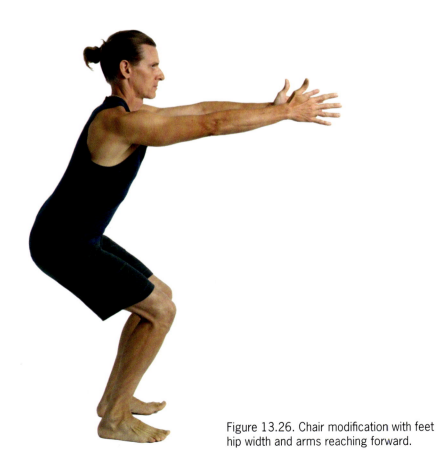

Figure 13.26. Chair modification with feet hip width and arms reaching forward.

FOUNDATION POSTURES | CHAPTER 13

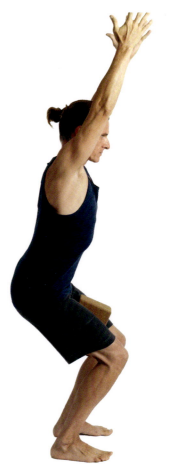

Figure 13.27. Chair variation with block squeeze.

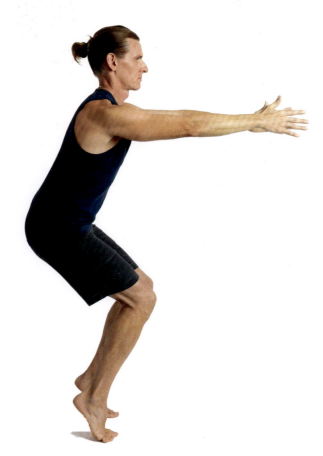

Figure 13.28. Chair with heels up and arms forward.

Variations

Place a block between your thighs to activate hip adductors (fig. 7.8) and lower-body stability.

Lift your heels up, and move your arms forward to generate added strength and balance.

Exploration/Possible Cues

Create more length from your crown to your tail without going into backward bend.

Drop your lowest ribs back into your belly.

Anchor your sitting bones down toward the floor to broaden across your low back.

Use your inhale to bring more space between your vertebrae.

Use your exhale to ground through your feet.

PART THREE | THE POSTURES

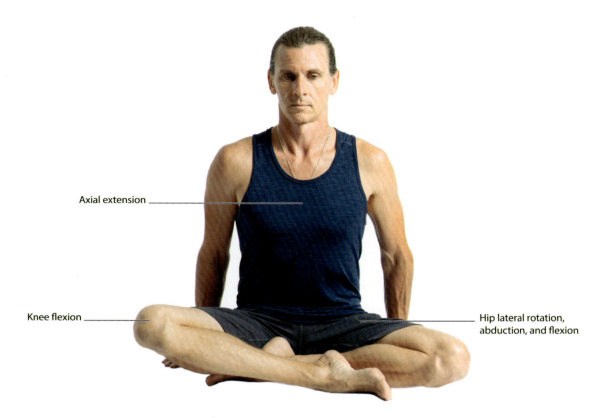

Figure 13.29. The anatomical actions of Easy pose.

Easy Pose

Seated Meditation Pose

Easy Pose

Sukhasana

When I lead trainings and retreats, mindfulness meditation and breathwork are part of the daily regime. For those who aren't used to sitting on the floor, training the trunk muscles to hold the spine upright for more than a couple of minutes can be challenging. We are used to sitting in chairs with backs, and even then, our tendency is to slump forward. In this slumped-forward position, the trunk muscles don't have to work to hold the spine as it collapses forward onto itself. Consequently, the Easy Pose is not so easy after all. But it is worth the effort since it is a tremendous back strengthener, and it helps us maintain mobility in our lower-body joints.

Sit on the floor, and cross your legs while allowing your thighs to lie out to the sides. Shift your sitting bones back, and maintain all the natural curves of your spine. Sit nice and tall. Place your hands gently on your thighs. Close your eyes, and visualize your spine. Feel your muscles holding it. Engage your muscles just enough to support your spine; don't overdo it. Stay, and breathe. Begin with a couple of minutes. Then aim to increase your time until you can sit comfortably for 30 minutes.

FOUNDATION POSTURES | **CHAPTER 13**

Easy Pose. What am I feeling?

HOW DO I GET THERE?	WHAT IS STRENGTHENING?	WHERE COULD I NOTICE TIGHTNESS?	IS COMPRESSION POSSIBLE?
Axial extension	**Axial extensors, fig. 5.10**	Entire trunk	
Hip lateral rotation	Passive	**Hip medial rotators, Fig. 7.11**	✓ Fig. 7.10
Hip abduction	Passive	**Hip adductors, fig. 7.8**	✓ Fig. 7.7
Hip flexion	Passive	Hip extensors, fig. 7.6	✓ Fig. 7.4
Knee flexion	Passive	Knee extensors, fig. 8.2	

My discoveries:

Special Considerations

This is one of the best poses for countering the biomechanics of modern-day sitting.

If you have severe back weakness or injury, begin your sitting practice in a chair.

If you have any lower-body injury or limitation, sitting in a chair is a good option.

Back, hip, or knee injury will limit this pose.

Modifications

A cushion or block will help lift your hips higher than your legs, preventing your feet from falling asleep in Easy Pose. It can also provide a more stable position for the pelvis.

Variations

Many differently shaped cushions and benches are available to help you if you have trouble sitting directly on the floor.

Hero's pose is an option if this pose doesn't work for you.

PART THREE | THE POSTURES

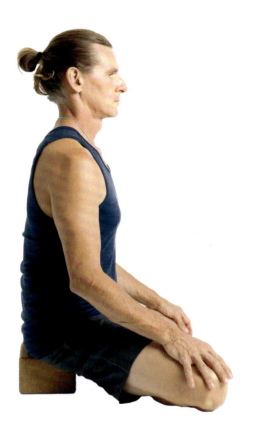

Figure 13.30. Easy Pose on block.

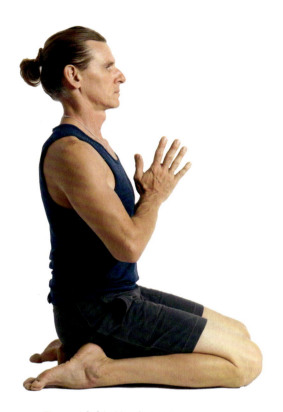

Figure 13.31. Hero's pose.

Exploration/Possible Cues

Lift the entire line of your spine up through the crown of your head.

Imagine your breath supporting the strength of your body.

Keep a subtle back-and-down engagement around your shoulder blades.

Align your pelvis first with a slight anterior tilt (fig. 14.6). This should take you to neutral. Then allow the rest of your spine to stack naturally from there.

Imagine that you have a long tail and that you don't want to sit on it. Take it behind you.

Let your head be like a helium balloon rising up, while the muscles of your neck soften.

Be careful not to go into backbend when you draw your arm bones back.

FOUNDATION POSTURES | **CHAPTER 13**

In prayer, it is better to have a heart without words than words without a heart.
—Mahatma Gandhi

PART THREE | THE POSTURES

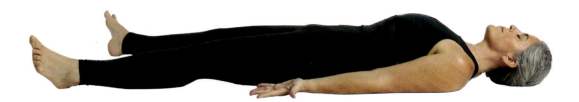

Figure 13.32. Final Rest.

Final Rest

Final Rest
Corpse Pose
Savasana

Near the beginning of practice, we arrive in Mountain's strong equanimity (fig. 13.13). The end of our practice is always sealed with a surrender to the fully supported equanimity of Final Rest. This pose embodies an invitation to our **autonomic nervous system** (p. 8) for nourishing, healing rest. Fully resting while wide awake is rare. This is the time to allow it.

Simply lie down in your most comfortable position, and scan your body from top to bottom for any effort you can release. Let the floor hold your body's weight. Let go of any effort with your breath. Drop in.

Special Considerations

If you have any low-back discomfort, being flat on your back might not work. See Modifications.

Modifications

Placing blocks or a bolster under your knees will create slack in the posterior body, typically relieving any discomfort.

If this doesn't work, lie on your side.

FOUNDATION POSTURES | CHAPTER 13

Final Rest. What am I feeling?

HOW DO I GET THERE?	WHAT IS STRENGTHENING?	WHERE COULD I NOTICE TIGHTNESS?	IS COMPRESSION POSSIBLE?
Total body surrender		In this neutral position, notice any sensations of stretch or tightness. This is good information on any muscular imbalances you might have.	

My discoveries:

Variations

Any restful position can work here. Occasionally I like teaching a supported option with a block under the head and one under the heart.

Exploration/Possible Cues

Find your most relaxed, comfortable position.

Scan your body from top to bottom. Invite it to surrender.

Allow your breath to return to its autonomic or natural state.

Feel the softness in your breath.

Feel your body move with your breath.

Invite your mind to stay right here where your body has landed.

Embody openness, surrender, and release.

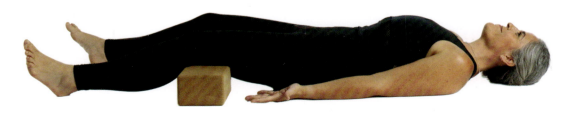

Figure 13.33. Final Rest modification with blocks under knees.

PART THREE | THE POSTURES

Chapter 14
Standing Postures

Standing Postures Overview

In these postures both feet are on the ground but placed asymmetrically. They differ from the foundation postures in which the feet are evenly aligned with the pelvis. These poses are not backbends, forward bends, or twists. I have broken down this category into two sub-groups: open-hip standing postures and closed-hip standing postures.

STANDING POSTURES | CHAPTER 14

Open-Hip Standing Postures

These poses require hip **abduction** (fig. 7.9), or an open relationship between the femurs and pelvis. These are the poses practiced with hips facing to the side. This shape can be achieved by moving the pelvis in relation to the femur, as in moving from Warrior I to Warrior II or by moving the femur in relation to the pelvis, as in drawing the front thigh toward the pinky toe in Warrior II.

- Warrior II
- Reverse Warrior
- Triangle
- Extended Side Angle

Closed-Hip Standing Postures

Closed-hip postures are those in which we keep the thigh bones somewhat neutral with the pelvis. In other words, there is a closed relationship between the thighs and pelvis. We can think of these as the poses in which the hips are facing forward.

- High Lunge
- Pyramid

The big idea regarding open-hip and closed-hip postures is that they require unique articulation in the hip complex or the femoroacetabular joint (fig. 7.1). Because everyone's bones and soft tissues are shaped differently, students' experiences will differ from mat to mat. Some people have more front-facing hip sockets while others are more side oriented. Also, femur heads vary in size and shape. Therefore, thinking of skeletal structure alone, we'll see many alternatives. Additionally, when we consider soft tissues, we realize a vast range of postural possibilities exists. All poses will not look alike due to factors such as whether students' hips truly face the side or the front, and how they need to place their feet for their hips. If we try to force "textbook alignment," we are completely dismissing the uniqueness of our bodies and ignoring the transformative practice of feeling each pose from within.

Although Warrior I is often taught as a closed-hip posture, I prefer to teach it as a blend of open and closed. This helps to avoid unnecessary leveraged tension in the pelvis and knee that can result from forcing the hips into a forward-facing, closed position.

PART THREE | THE POSTURES

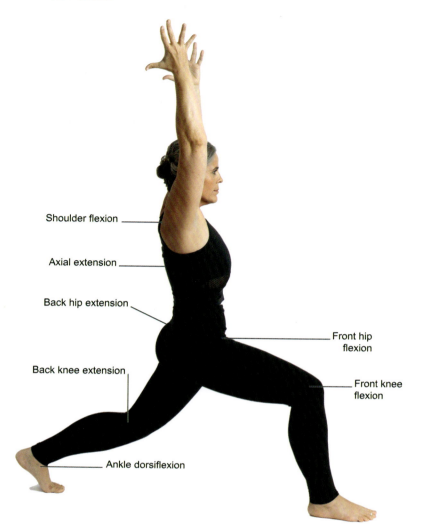

Figure 14.1. High Lunge.

High Lunge

High Lunge
Crescent Lunge
Anjaneyasana

High Lunge is a fiery standing posture which requires a little more balance than others since the back heel is lifted. It is a **closed-hip** posture.

Begin with a long stance front to back. Place your feet near hip-width distance apart left to right so you feel stable and supported. Lunge into your front leg with your front shin near vertical. Aim all ten toes straight forward. Extend your back leg long while keeping a slight bend in your back knee. Keep an active lift in your back heel to maintain strength through the entire back leg. Stay squared forward from your toes all the way up through your crown and hands. Keep your spine neutral, and maintain all the natural curves of your back while drawing your tailbone slightly toward the ground. Reach your arms up energetically, and gaze straight ahead.

STANDING POSTURES | CHAPTER 14

High Lunge. What am I feeling?

HOW DO I GET THERE?	WHAT IS STRENGTHENING?	WHERE COULD I NOTICE TIGHTNESS?	IS COMPRESSION POSSIBLE?
Axial extension	Axial extensors, fig. 5.10	Entire trunk	
Shoulder flexion	**Shoulder flexors, fig. 6.4**	Shoulder extensors, fig. 6.5	✓ Fig. 6.3
Scapular elevation and upward rotation	Elevators and upward rotators of the scapulae, p. 54 *Natural placement with arm positioning*	Depressors and downward rotators of the scapulae, p. 54	
Elbow extension	Elbow extensors, fig. 10.2	Elbow flexors, fig. 10.3	
Back-leg knee extension	**Back-leg knee extensors, fig. 8.2**	Knee flexors, fig. 8.3	
Back-leg hip extension	Back-leg hip extensors, fig. 7.6	**Back-leg hip flexors, fig. 7.5**	
Front-leg knee flexion	**Knee extensors, fig. 8.2** *Even though the knee is bent, extensors stabilize eccentrically and/or isometrically to oppose gravity.*		
Front-leg hip flexion	**Front-leg hip flexors, fig. 7.5** *While lowering into the lunge, hip extensors work eccentrically to oppose gravity. While holding, they work isometrically.*		
Back-leg ankle dorsiflexion	**Back-leg ankle dorsiflexors, fig. 9.3**	**Back-leg ankle plantar flexors, fig. 9.4**	✓ Fig. 9.2

My discoveries:

I have highlighted the most common tendencies I see in my students. It is possible to feel strengthening or to notice tightness in any of the muscle groups listed within their respective columns.

PART THREE | THE POSTURES

Special Considerations

Foot, ankle, hip, spine, or shoulder injury can limit this pose.

A rotator cuff injury makes it challenging to lift the arms beyond parallel to the ground. (See chapter 6, "The Shoulder," fig. 6.16.) Simply keep your hands in Prayer if this is an issue for you.

This pose is a great substitute for Warrior I, offering increased spaciousness in the pelvis and lumbar spine. The unanchored back heel allows for more mobility in the back leg, pelvis, and spine. Consequently, if you suffer from sacroiliac (fig. 5.15) misalignment or low back pain, High Lunge is a good replacement for Warrior I.

Keeping the back knee bent allows for additional mobility of the pelvis while the spine is upright. Locking the back leg straight will also lock the pelvis in place, typically in an anterior tilt. An anterior tilt of the pelvis can't occur without extending or backbending the lumbar spine (fig. 14.6). With a locked back leg and anterior tilt of the pelvis, the range of lumbar backward bend is probably maxed out with the spinous processes compressed. In "The Anatomy of Backbending," chapter 18, I discuss the benefits of keeping some spaciousness in the lumbar spine. Bending the back knee releases the pelvis so the sacrum can be drawn down a bit, bringing the spine out of maximum extension and compression. This relationship changes as the pelvis and spine angle forward for the Twist variation. As the torso tilts forward in preparation for the Twist, firmly straightening the back leg will provide an anchor for the pose and will support a neutral spine and pelvis.

Those with hypermobile lumbar spines, tend to "hang out" in a maxed-out lumbar backbend in High Lunge. It is important to maintain the back-knee bend along with posterior tilt of the pelvis, not eliminating lumbar curve but rather maintaining some spaciousness and staying out of extreme backward bending.

Modifications

Take your arms down.

Lower your back knee to the mat.

Try Cactus arms if you are experiencing shoulder compression or discomfort.

Variations

Use varying arm positions.

Build additional Cylindrical Core (fig. 13.17) strength by leaning and reaching forward.

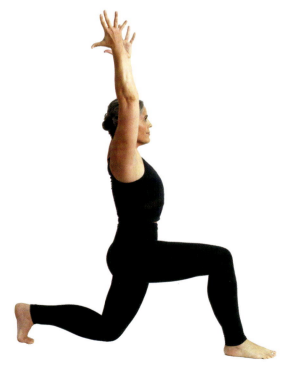

Figure 14.2. High Lunge modification with back knee down.

STANDING POSTURES | CHAPTER 14

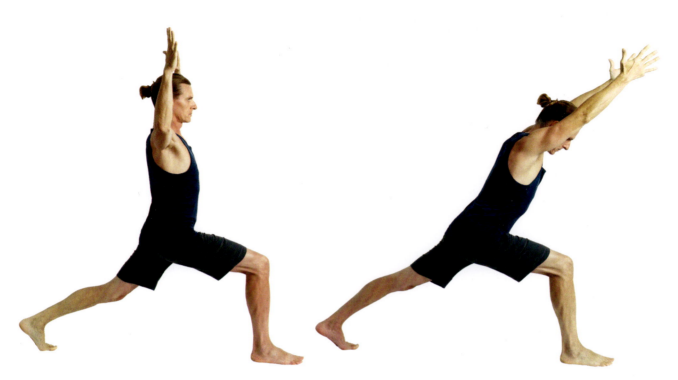

Figure 14.3. High Lunge with Cactus arms.

Figure 14.4. High Lunge variation, reach-and-lean power lunge.

Exploration/Possible Cues

Try the pose with your back leg firm and straight, and notice the lack of pelvic mobility. You can feel this by attempting to draw your tailbone down toward the ground (posterior tilt) and then by trying to send your tailbone back behind you (anterior tilt). It might help to think of Cat/Cow movements in your hips. Now bend the back knee a bit, and feel the increased pelvic mobility this allows. With a bent back knee, lift the pit of your belly up while dropping your sitting bones toward the ground.

Instead of just lifting your arms straight up, try turning your palms face up and then lifting your arms for an external rotation of the humerus. This might give you more shoulder spaciousness.

Take your feet as wide as needed left to right for stability.

Get tall from the pit of your belly to the center of your chest.

Imagine the pit of your belly holding on to the bottom of your spine.

161

PART THREE | THE POSTURES

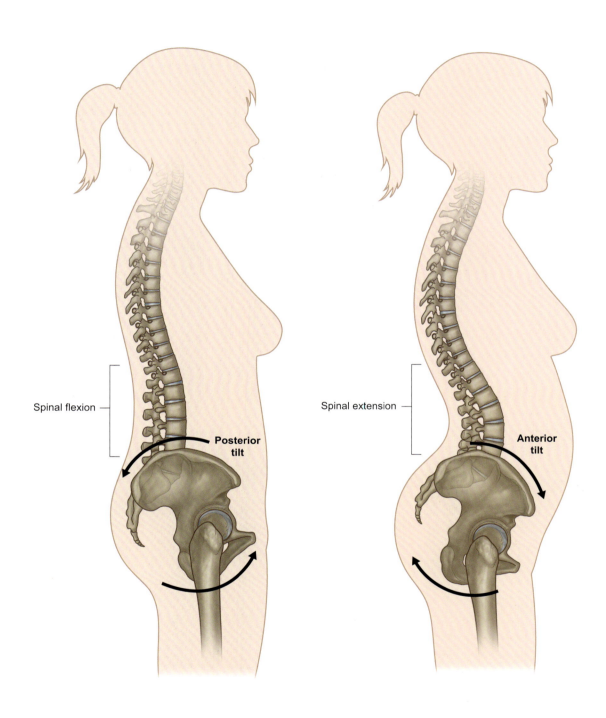

Figure 14.5. Posterior pelvic tilt.

Figure 14.6. Anterior pelvic tilt.

STANDING POSTURES | CHAPTER 14

Consider...

The more we study and understand the body's design, the more we can dial in to the alive, felt experience of moving within our own bodies. Noticing how actions feel in the moment is crucial. For example, attempting to move the fronts of your vertebral bodies apart is not nearly as concrete and perceptible as tilting the pelvis anteriorly or posteriorly. Even this pelvic tilting can be elusive if it's something you've never considered. Here we will look at two similar, yet very different actions that are sometimes confused. This clarification will be helpful when fine tuning your postures.

"Tilt your pelvis" and "lead with your pelvis" are common yoga cues. First, you need to know that the pelvis is the entire bony structure containing the ilium, ischium, pubis, coccyx, and sacrum (fig. 5.15). These cues could refer to two distinct actions: pelvic tilt or torso tilt.

Pelvic tilt describes moving the pelvis independently of the spine, *changing the shapes of the spine and the intervertebral discs.* For example, anterior tilt of the pelvis results in increased spinal extension or backward bend (fig. 14.6). Posterior tilt causes increased spinal flexion or forward rounding (fig. 14.5). It is an active engagement of the lower abdominals. Skillfully using posterior tilt can reduce excessive lumbar spinal extension in backward bends and standing postures. When combined with Cylindrical Core (fig. 13.17), posterior tilt also helps stabilize the spine in postures like Plank and inversions.

Teaching these motions to my students, I use several different descriptions because what resonates with one person doesn't always help another. One way to find it is to lie down with your knees bent and your feet on the floor. From this position, press your sacrum into the floor while straightening your lumbar curve. This is posterior tilt. Here are a few additional ways to cue posterior tilt of the pelvis in a standing posture:

- Draw your tailbone toward the floor.
- Draw your sacrum toward the floor.
- Activate your lower abdominal muscles.
- Anchor your sitting bones toward the floor.
- Lift your pubic bone toward your navel.
- Lift your front hip points upward.

Here are some sample cues for anterior tilt of the pelvis:

- Stick your bum back.
- Aim your sitting bones back behind you.
- Aim your tailbone back behind you.
- Take your front hip points down and forward.

Torso tilt is moving the pelvis and spine dependently, as one unit. As the pelvis tilts, the spine goes with it. You can think of it as moving from the pelvis while keeping the spine in Mountain pose. Sometimes referred to as hinging from the hip, this requires tilting the pelvis on the femoral heads to create hip flexion. We tilt the torso moving into poses such as Triangle, Side Angle, and Forward Fold. These are two possible cues for torso tilt:

- Draw the hip crease(s) back, and hinge the pelvis forward (or laterally for Triangle or Side Angle).
- Tilt from the pelvis, and keep the spine in Mountain.

PART THREE | THE POSTURES

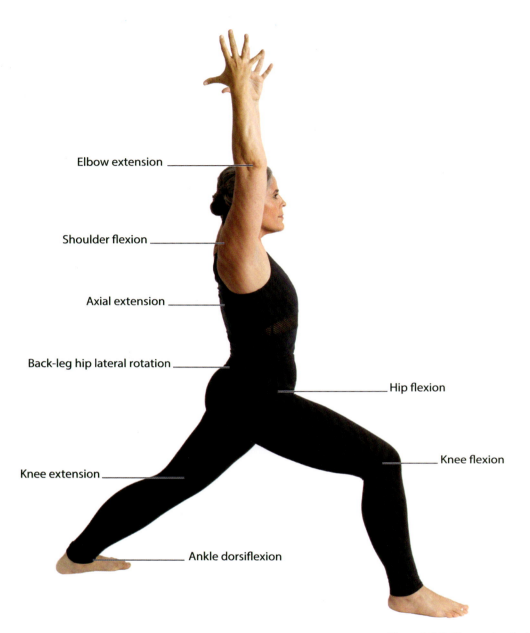

Figure 14.7. The anatomical actions of Warrior I.

Warrior I

Warrior I
Virabhadrasana I

Warrior I is a strong standing posture useful for strengthening, for releasing, and for establishing a sense of sturdiness. It also provides an effective hip flexor stretch for the back leg. I teach this pose as neither a closed- nor open-hip posture, but rather as a blend of the two.

STANDING POSTURES | CHAPTER 14

Warrior 1. What am I feeling?

HOW DO I GET THERE?	WHAT IS STRENGTHENING?	WHERE COULD I NOTICE TIGHTNESS?	IS COMPRESSION POSSIBLE?
Axial extension	Axial extensors, fig. 5.10	Entire trunk	
Front-leg hip flexion	**Front-leg hip extensors, fig. 7.6** *While lowering into the lunge, hip extensors work eccentrically to oppose gravity. While holding, they work isometrically.*		
Front-leg knee flexion	**Knee extensors, fig. 8.2** *Even though the knee is bent, extensors stabilize isometrically to oppose gravity.*		
Back-leg hip extension	**Back-leg hip extensors, fig. 7.6**	**Back-leg hip flexors, fig. 7.5**	
Back-leg hip lateral rotation *Due to back foot placement*	Hip lateral rotators, fig. 7.12	**Hip medial rotators, fig. 7.11**	✓ Fig. 7.10
Back-leg knee extension	**Back-leg knee extensors, fig. 8.2**	Knee flexors, fig. 8.3	
Back-leg ankle dorsiflexion	Back-leg ankle dorsiflexors, fig. 9.3	**Back-leg ankle plantar flexors, fig. 9.4**	✓ Fig. 9.2
Shoulder flexion	**Shoulder flexors, fig. 6.4**	**Shoulder extensors, fig. 6.5**	✓ Fig. 6.3
Scapular elevation and upward rotation	Elevators and upward rotators of the scapulae, p. 54 *Natural placement with arm positioning*	Depressors and downward rotators of the scapulae, p. 54	
Elbow extension	**Elbow extensors, fig. 10.2**	Elbow flexors, fig. 10.3	

My discoveries:

PART THREE | THE POSTURES

Begin with a long stance front to back, lunging strongly into your front leg. You can vary the length of your stance depending on your chosen effort level. A longer front-to-back stance creates a lower lunge, typically requiring more effort. Keep your front shin bone near vertical with your front toes aiming forward. Activate and engage your back leg while placing your back foot near a 45-degree angle. Allow your hips to remain slightly side facing, and align your feet wide enough left to right for stability. The width left to right will depend on your unique structure. Somewhere near hip-width distance apart is typical. Squeeze and lift your back arch to avoid landing pressure in your back-knee joint. Draw your sacrum down toward the floor, and then actively lift through your crown and arms creating axial extension. Gently aim your chest toward forward, and gaze straight ahead. Simply stand, and breathe into your strength, steadfastness, and readiness.

Special Considerations

SI joint injury (p. 38) can limit this pose.

As the arms lift in poses like this, the shoulder flexors work concentrically (shortening). If the arms are held up, the same muscles work isometrically (statically). As the arms are slowly lowered forward and down, the shoulder flexors work eccentrically (lengthening).

This pose may present some biomechanical issues because it can create asymmetry in the pelvis. The forward leg encourages the pelvis to action forward while the back leg creates an anchoring back. This uneven leveraging force can land in the SI joints and/or lumbar spine

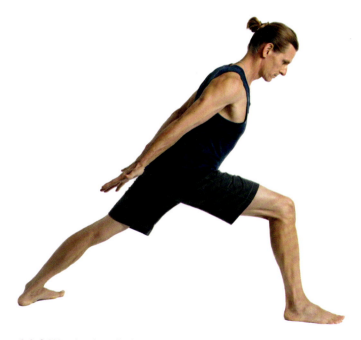

Figure 14.8 Warrior I variation with Airplane reach.

if overdone. It is crucial to allow freedom in foot placement and not to be adamant about squaring the hips forward. Forcing the hips to square forward with an anchored back heel will exaggerate the torque pressure across the pelvic bones and in the back knee. As in most poses, it is best first to align the pelvis in a spacious position and then to adjust the foundation accordingly, rather than building the pose from the foundation up.

If you have an existing sacroiliac injury or tendency toward this, avoid Warrior I altogether. Simply do High Lunge instead.

Occasionally an ankle injury (p. 84) will prevent anchoring the back foot at an angle. The solution here is High Lunge or back knee down.

When this pose is taught with a blend of open- and closed-hip alignment, the pelvis angles to the side. In this case, the hips are slightly abducted.

Modifications

Try varying your arm positions.

Find a wider stance, and/or try varying your foot and leg positions.

Do High Lunge instead.

Variations

Airplane variation brings additional Cylindrical Core strengthening. This position can be challenging if you have back and core weakness or injury.

Exploration/Possible Cues

Start with your feet about hip-width distance apart.

Angle your back foot somewhere around 45 degrees, maybe a little more or less.

Notice how the pose lands in your back knee. Readjust to maintain sound stability.

Instead of working to square your hips forward, allow your pelvis to stay slightly open, and gently square your chest forward.

Anchor your sitting bones down toward the ground.

Stay strong and engaged in your legs, sending stability down through your feet to the ground.

Lift up and away through the entire length of your spine while avoiding backward bending.

Set your **drishti** straight ahead and slightly lifted.

THE POSTURES

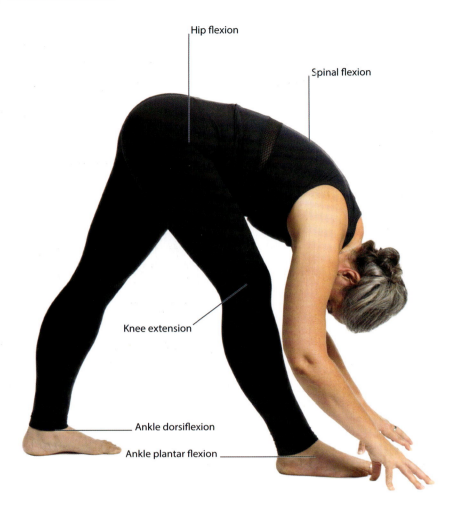

Figure 14.9. The anatomical actions of Pyramid.

Pyramid

Pyramid
Parsvottanasana

Pyramid pose provides an entire back-body stretch along with leg toning and strengthening. It is a **closed-hip** posture.

From Mountain, step your left foot back three to four feet. Your feet should land about hip-width distance apart left to right with your back toes angled forward. Your back foot placement will be similar to Warrior I with toes angled more forward, depending on your body. Actively reach up with your hands while anchoring your sacrum toward the floor. Draw your hips back as you slowly fold forward over your front leg. Take your fingertips or hands to the ground on either side of your front foot. Keep your legs active, and keep your hips toward squared forward. Maintain an even grounding through both feet. Powerfully lift and engage the front of your quadriceps and hip flexors to encourage a release of the back-body musculature. Simply breathe, and access the perfect combination of strength and ease.

STANDING POSTURES | CHAPTER 14

Pyramid. What am I feeling?

HOW DO I GET THERE?	WHAT IS STRENGTHENING?	WHERE COULD I NOTICE TIGHTNESS?	IS COMPRESSION POSSIBLE?
Spinal flexion	*Passive*	**Spine extensors, fig. 5.3** *Entire back body*	
Hip flexion *More on front leg than back leg*	**Hip extensors, fig. 7.6** *Front-leg hip extensors work eccentrically going into the pose to oppose gravity.*		✓ Fig. 7.4
Knee extension	**Knee extensors, fig. 8.2**	**Knee flexors, fig. 8.3** *Front leg predominantly*	
Back-leg ankle dorsiflexion	*Passive with position and gravity*	Ankle plantar flexors, fig. 9.4	
Front-leg ankle plantar flexion	*Passive with position and gravity*	Ankle dorsiflexors, fig. 9.3	✓ Fig. 9.2

My discoveries:

Special Considerations

Avoid working *hard* to even out the hips as this can put too much strain on the sitting bones' tendon attachments and too much strain overall on the pelvis. As with all intense stretches, find subtle movements which land most of the stretch in the middle of the muscles rather than at their attachment points. Always remember that a little goes a long way.

If you have hamstring tendonitis (fig. 7.14), intervertebral disc inflammation (fig. 5.12), or sciatica (p. 33), keep your front knee bent, and place blocks underneath your hands to maintain a Halfway Lift position in your torso. Or skip the pose altogether.

PART THREE | THE POSTURES

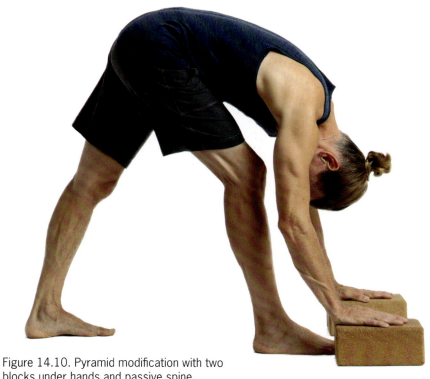

Figure 14.10. Pyramid modification with two blocks under hands and passive spine.

Modifications

Place a block or two under your hands.

Maintain a lengthened, active spine instead of passively folding forward.

Slightly vary your foot placement to accommodate your unique hip range of motion.

Bend either knee, or unanchor your back heel by lifting it slightly.

Variations

Vary your arm positions to change the dynamics of the pose.

Try an arm bind to open the anterior shoulder, wrist flexor, and chest.

STANDING POSTURES | CHAPTER 14

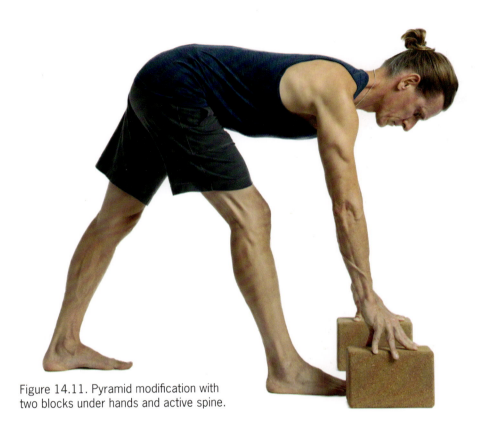

Figure 14.11. Pyramid modification with two blocks under hands and active spine.

Exploration/Possible Cues

Readjust your feet to accommodate your pelvis. Go as wide as needed to square your hips forward.

Before folding, reach up actively, and lift out of your waist. Slowly fold forward while reaching your hips back.

Play with different angles of back foot placement to see which fits your pelvis best.

With your hands on blocks and your back lengthened, gently draw your front hip back and your back hip forward.

Distribute your weight evenly into the three corners of your feet.

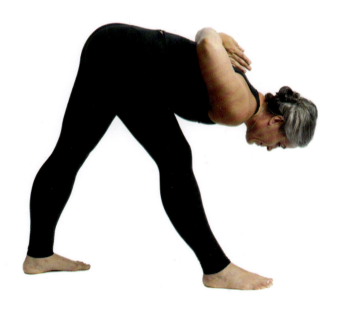

Figure 14.12. Pyramid modification with Reverse Prayer hands.

PART THREE | THE POSTURES

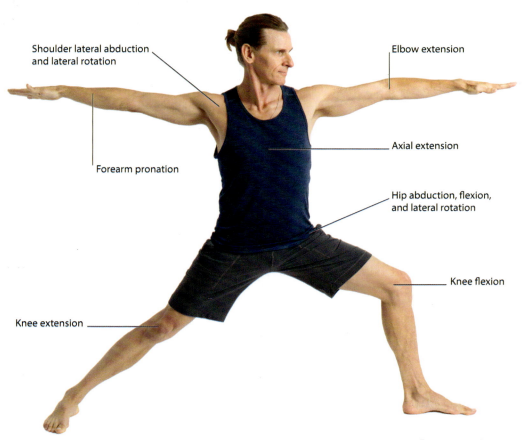

Figure 14.13. The anatomical actions of Warrior II.

Warrior II

Warrior II
Virabhadrasana II

Warrior II is a powerful stance which strengthens the upper and lower body while stretching the hips, groin, and chest. It is an **open-hip** posture.

Begin in a wide, side-facing Five-Pointed Star stance. Turn your front toes forward, and come into a lunge with your front shin near vertical. Action your front knee slightly toward your front pinky toe to keep it from collapsing toward the midline. Place your back foot near parallel to the back edge of your mat while engaging along a strong line through your back ankle, knee, and hip joint. Hold your arms parallel to the ground, reaching actively front to back. Maintain the natural curvatures of your spine while drawing your sacrum slightly downward toward the floor for spaciousness in the lumbar spine. As your hip range of motion allows, keep your hips facing to the side. Gaze at a point beyond your front hand. Experience the sensations of steadiness in your body, breath, and mind.

STANDING POSTURES | CHAPTER 14

Warrior II. What am I feeling?

HOW DO I GET THERE?	WHAT IS STRENGTHENING?	WHERE COULD I NOTICE TIGHTNESS?	IS COMPRESSION POSSIBLE?
Axial extension	**Axial extensors, fig. 5.10**	Entire trunk	
Hip abduction	**Hip abductors, fig. 7.9**	**Hip adductors, fig. 7.8**	✓ Fig. 7.7
Front-leg hip flexion	**Front-leg hip extensors, fig. 7.6** Hip extensors work eccentrically and/or isometrically to oppose gravity.		
Lateral rotation of front-leg hip	Hip lateral rotators, fig. 7.12	**Hip medial rotators, fig. 7.11**	✓ Fig. 7.10
Back-leg knee extension	**Knee extensors, fig. 8.2**	Knee flexors, fig. 8.3	
Front-leg knee flexion	**Knee extensors, fig. 8.2** While lowering into the pose, front-leg knee extensors work eccentrically to oppose gravity. While holding, they work isometrically.		
Shoulder lateral abduction	**Shoulder lateral abductors, fig. 6.7**	Shoulder lateral adductors, p. 45	
Shoulder lateral rotation	Shoulder lateral rotators, fig. 6.14	**Shoulder medial rotators, fig. 6.11**	
Forearm pronation	Forearm pronators, fig. 10.5	Forearm supinators, fig. 10.4	
Elbow extension	**Elbow extensors, fig. 10.2**	Elbow flexors, fig. 10.3	

My discoveries:

Special Considerations

As with all standing postures, dictating the posture's shape by making the foundation the most important alignment piece is difficult. Instead, tune in to how the posture is affecting the hips and spine, and then adjust the feet accordingly. Maintaining some spaciousness in the pelvis and lumbar spine is desirable. At times, allowing the pelvis to remain slightly angled is more effective than forcing it to square to the side. Remember that the overall experience of awareness is more important than achieving an aesthetic ideal.

Modifications

Keep your arms down.

Shorten your stance from front to back.

Slightly vary your foot placement to accommodate your unique hip range of motion.

Variations

Try varying arm positions such as Eagle arms.

Exploration/Possible Cues

Take up lots of space as you reach front to back.

Allow your reach to be felt across your chest.

Create more length from your crown to your tail without going into backward bend.

Drop your lowest front ribs back into your belly.

Activate your legs and core by pressing strongly into both feet and pulling them toward each other. Now try pulling them away from each other. Notice the shift in sensation.

STANDING POSTURES | CHAPTER 14

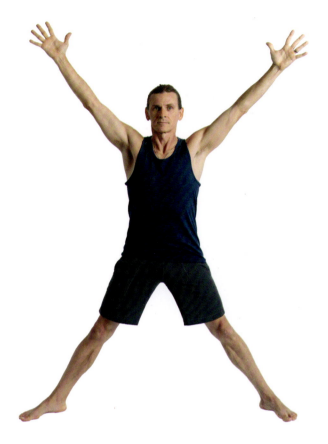

Figure 14.14. Five-Pointed Star.

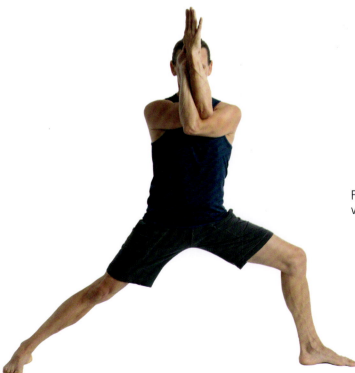

Figure 14.15. Warrior II variation with Eagle arms.

175

PART THREE | THE POSTURES

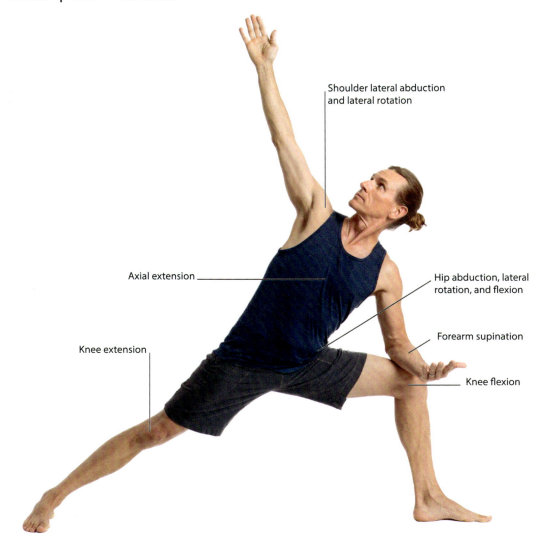

Figure 14.16. The anatomical motions of Side Angle.

Side Angle

Side Angle
Extended Side Angle
Utthita Parsvakonasana

When approached properly, this pose strengthens the entire body. It also effectively stretches the sides of the body. Side Angle is an **open-hip** posture.

Begin in Warrior II with your left leg forward. Tilt your torso forward (p. 163), laterally flexing your pelvis toward your front leg. Place your left forearm lightly on your left thigh. Maintain Mountain alignment throughout your entire torso. Stay evenly grounded through the three corners of each foot. Reach your right arm straight up from your shoulder, toward the ceiling. If you feel like going lower with your left hand, you can hold your inner ankle, or place your hand on the ground near your foot. Rotate your gaze up toward your reaching arm. Remain evenly active through both legs, light in the front arm and hand. Breathe into the lateral side stretch.

STANDING POSTURES | CHAPTER 14

Side Angle. What am I feeling?

HOW DO I GET THERE?	WHAT IS STRENGTHENING?	WHERE COULD I NOTICE TIGHTNESS?	IS COMPRESSION POSSIBLE?
Axial extension	Axial extensors, fig. 5.10	Entire trunk	
Hip abduction	**Hip abductors, fig. 7.9**	**Hip adductors, fig. 7.8**	✓ Fig. 7.7
Lateral rotation of front-leg hip	Hip lateral rotators, fig. 7.12	**Hip medial rotators, fig. 7.11**	✓ Fig. 7.10
Front-leg hip flexion	**Front-leg hip extensors, fig. 7.6** Hip extensors work eccentrically and/or isometrically to oppose gravity.	**This torso tilt stretches the top-side, lateral spinal flexors. fig. 5.6**	
Back-leg medial hip rotation *Or strong neutral*	Hip medial rotators, fig. 7.11	Hip lateral rotators, fig. 7.12	✓ Fig. 7.10
Back-leg knee extension	**Knee extensors, fig. 8.2**	Knee flexors, fig. 8.3	
Front-leg knee flexion	**Knee extensors, fig. 8.2** Even though the knee is bent, the extensors work eccentrically and/or isometrically to stabilize the knee against gravity.		
Shoulder lateral abduction	**Shoulder lateral abductors, fig. 6.7**	Shoulder lateral adductors, p. 45	
Shoulder lateral rotation	Shoulder lateral rotators, fig. 6.14	Shoulder medial rotators, fig. 6.11	
Forearm supination	Forearm supinators, fig. 10.4	Forearm pronators, fig. 10.5	

My discoveries:

PART THREE | THE POSTURES

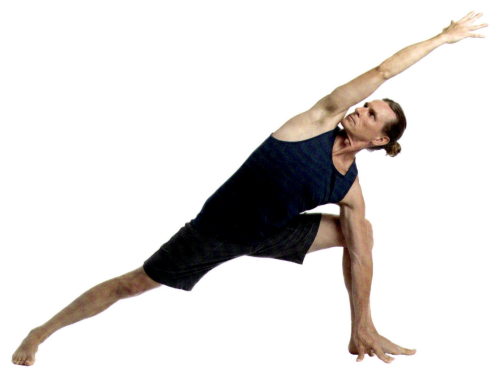

Figure 14.17. Extended Side Angle.

Special Considerations

Foot, knee, hip, back, or shoulder injury can limit this pose.

Some teach this as a lateral bend with a slight twist. I teach this pose with Mountain alignment of the torso. Compare the anatomical actions of this pose and Warrior II (fig. 14.13). The main difference is the addition of front hip lateral flexion as the torso tilts forward (p. 163). To maintain axial extension and Mountain alignment in the trunk, you must tune in and feel what is happening in your front hip crease. Once the range of motion is maxed out with the lateral tilt of the pelvis toward the femur, you can't go any farther without losing Mountain alignment. This will show up in either a laterally rounded spine, a backward bend, or a jutted-back front hip.

Notice the inner sensation of your lateral hip flexion. Once you've reached your stopping point, don't go any farther. Be mindful of your range of motion as you place your front hand. Keep spaciousness in your front hip crease rather than jamming it closed trying to take your hand lower toward the floor.

Where you place your bottom hand will also partly depend on your body proportions. Can you see how someone with longer arms compared to torso length might reach the floor more easily? Combine this with skeletal lateral range of motion, soft-tissue tightness, and length of stance, and you can see that many factors contribute to posture variation.

Variations

Reach your top arm over your head to increase the emphasis on stretching the sides of your body. You may encounter shoulder skeletal compression here. Reaching your arm from a different direction, as in sweeping the arm down and then forward, may help you get around the compression.

Exploration/Possible Cues

Stay spacious in your front hip crease rather than closing it completely.

As you tilt your torso forward, fire up your back leg and foot even more to stay balanced from front to back.

Stay light in your front shoulder and wrist.

Keep length in both lateral sides of your body.

Create an active line of energy from the center of your back heel all the way through your reaching hand.

PART THREE | THE POSTURES

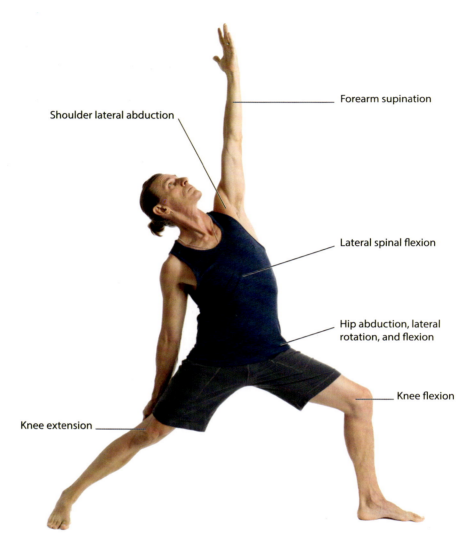

Figure 14.18. The anatomical actions of Reverse Warrior.

Reverse Warrior

Reverse Warrior
Exalted Warrior
Viparita Virabhadrasana

Reverse Warrior is a variation from Warrior II alignment; therefore, it is an **open-hip** posture. We are simply adding a lateral side bend with a reach upward. It offers effective lower-body strengthening with an added side-torso stretch.

From Warrior II position, sweep your front arm straight up while placing your back hand lightly on your back leg. Stay anchored in your front lunge and active in both legs. Keep an expanding, lifting action in both sides of your ribs to avoid over-compressing the back lateral bend. Keep your gaze up toward your lifted hand or down toward your back foot.

STANDING POSTURES | CHAPTER 14

Reverse Warrior. What am I feeling?

HOW DO I GET THERE?	WHAT IS STRENGTHENING?	WHERE COULD I NOTICE TIGHTNESS?	IS COMPRESSION POSSIBLE?
Lateral spinal flexion	Lateral spinal flexors, fig. 5.6 *Back side*	**Lateral spinal flexors, fig. 5.6** *Front side*	
Hip abduction	**Hip abductors, fig. 7.9**	**Hip adductors, fig. 7.8**	✓ Fig. 7.7
Front-leg hip flexion	**Front-leg hip extensors, fig. 7.6** Hip extensors work eccentrically and/or isometrically to oppose gravity.		
Lateral rotation of front-leg hip	Hip lateral rotators, fig. 7.12	Hip medial rotators, fig. 7.11	✓ Fig. 7.10
Back-leg medial hip rotation *Or strong neutral*	Hip medial rotators, fig. 7.11	Hip lateral rotators, fig. 7.12	✓ Fig. 7.10
Back-leg knee extension	**Knee extensors, fig. 8.2** Knee extensors are working concentrically and/or isometrically on the back leg.	Knee flexors, fig. 8.3	
Front-leg knee flexion	**Knee extensors, fig. 8.2** Even though the knee is bent, the extensors stabilize the knee against gravity.		
Front-shoulder lateral abduction	Shoulder lateral abductors, fig. 6.7	Shoulder lateral adductors, p. 45	✓ Fig. 6.3 ✓ Fig. 6.6
Front-forearm supination	Forearm supinators, fig. 10.4	Forearm pronators, fig. 10.5	

My discoveries:

PART THREE | THE POSTURES

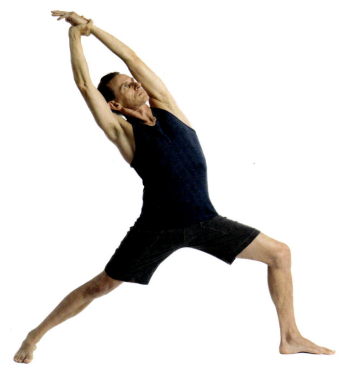

Figure 14.19. Reverse Warrior variation holding front wrist.

Special Considerations

Ankle, foot, knee, hip, spine, or shoulder injury can limit this pose.

Often this pose is practiced with excessive reaching back which lands in collapsed compression on the back side. Focus on the upward component as if someone were holding both sides of your ribs and lifting you up.

Modifications

Take a shorter Warrior stance.

Variations

For a different sensation and increased lateral side stretch, use your back hand to grasp and gently pull your front wrist.

STANDING POSTURES | CHAPTER 14

Exploration/Possible Cues

Drive your front heel into the ground, and let that propel your reach up and back.

Put more energy into reaching up than into reaching back.

Stay spacious in both sides of your ribs.

Keep your belly facing toward the side.

As you reach, create more space between your front-bottom-side ribs and thigh.

Try looking down at your back foot instead of up for a nice side-neck stretch.

PART THREE | THE POSTURES

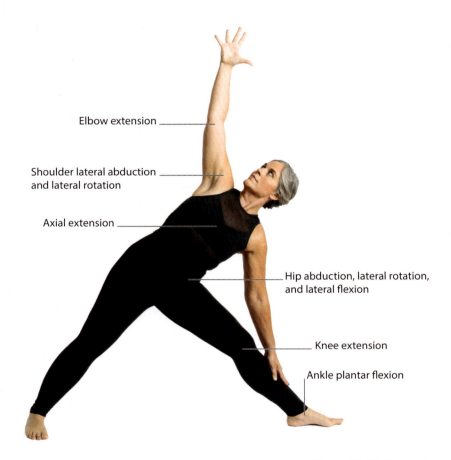

Figure 14.20. The anatomical actions of Triangle.

Triangle

Triangle
Extended Triangle
Utthita Trikonasana

Triangle pose stretches and tones the lower body while creating a sense of openness in the upper body, especially along the sides. It is an **open-hip** posture.

From Warrior II (fig. 14.13) alignment, straighten your front leg, and then tilt your torso (p. 163) toward your front thigh bone while extending and reaching forward with the front hand. Reach and elongate out of your front hip crease. Keep both quadriceps actively engaged. Place your front hand on your leg or on a block outside of your calf to maintain an uphill line in your spine. From here, reach your top hand straight up and away from your bottom arm, extending long from hand to hand. Keep a soft bend in your legs for healthier alignment in your knees and ankles. Actively integrate your shoulder blades into your torso by drawing them down your back and slightly together. This will help maintain an openness across your chest. Lengthen in all directions.

STANDING POSTURES | CHAPTER 14

Triangle. What am I feeling?

HOW DO I GET THERE?	WHAT IS STRENGTHENING?	WHERE COULD I NOTICE TIGHTNESS?	IS COMPRESSION POSSIBLE?
Axial extension	**Axial extensors, fig. 5.10**	Entire trunk	
Hip abduction	**Hip abductors, fig. 7.9**	**Hip adductors, fig. 7.8**	✓ Fig. 7.7
Lateral rotation of front-leg hip	Hip lateral rotators, fig. 7.12	**Hip medial rotators, fig. 7.11**	✓ Fig. 7.10
Front-leg hip flexion	**Front-leg hip extensors, fig. 7.6** *Hip extensors work eccentrically and/or isometrically to oppose gravity.*	*This torso tilt stretches the top-side lateral spinal flexors. fig. 5.6*	
Back-leg medial hip rotation *Or strong neutral*	Hip medial rotators, fig. 7.11	Hip lateral rotators, fig. 7.12	
Knee extension	**Knee extensors, fig. 8.2**	**Knee flexors, fig. 8.3** *Front leg predominantly*	
Front-leg ankle plantar flexion	Front-leg ankle plantar flexors, fig. 9.4	Ankle dorsiflexors, fig. 9.3	✓ Fig. 9.2
Shoulder lateral abduction	**Shoulder lateral abductors, fig. 6.7**	Shoulder lateral adductors, p. 45	
Shoulder lateral rotation	Shoulder lateral rotators, fig. 6.14	**Shoulder medial rotators, fig. 6.11**	
Elbow extension	Elbow extensors, fig. 10.2	Elbow flexors, fig. 10.3	

My discoveries:

PART THREE | THE POSTURES

Special Considerations

This pose is often taught with a "jutting" of the hips back while the front hand slides forward. This action changes the relationship between the front femur and the hip socket. This may or may not be beneficial, depending on your unique hip-socket structure.

Once the forward hip joint flexion is maxed out, your front hand can't go any lower without lateral spinal flexion and/or backbending. This can result in bearing too much weight in the front hand, arm, or foot. The key to healthy alignment is feeling when your front hip flexion is maxed out and not attempting to go deeper. This pose is an example of using Torso Tilt rather than Pelvic Tilt (p. 163). Torso Tilt entails maintaining a stable, neutral Mountain spine.

Some people may experience pain behind the ankle in the front leg. If this is the case, your ankle extension has probably maxed out, and you are feeling compression with plantar flexion (fig. 9.2). A shorter stance or a soft bend in the front knee will help.

If you suffer from hamstring tendonitis, you should take a shorter stance, and keep a slight bend in your front knee to alleviate pulling on the ischial tuberosity tendon attachment (fig. 7.14) as your pelvis tilts away from your front foot. Also stay up higher with your bottom hand.

Modifications

If you are needing to slow your heart rate, rest your top arm along your side instead of reaching up.

Stay higher with your bottom hand.

Place a block or two under your bottom hand.

Slightly vary your foot placement to accommodate your unique hip range of motion.

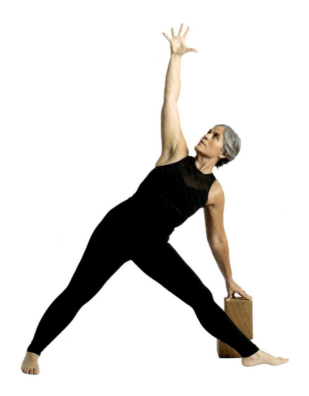

Figure 14.21. Triangle variation with two blocks.

Variations

Try varying arm positions.

Reach your bottom hand forward to activate your Cylindrical Core more. It is very important here to avoid backward bending or forward rounding. Maintain axial extension.

Exploration/Possible Cues

Create more length from your crown to your tail without going into backward bend.

Drop your front, lowest ribs back into your belly.

Distribute your weight evenly into the three corners of your feet.

Go for stacked shoulders rather than folding toward the inside of your front leg.

Experiment with actively hugging feet toward each other to provide lift and support up and away from the ground.

Reach your tailbone back and down toward your back heel for a spine anchor.

Engage your back-leg glutes firmly. Use a strong back-leg, glute, and heel activation when lifting up out of the pose.

Radiate out in all directions!

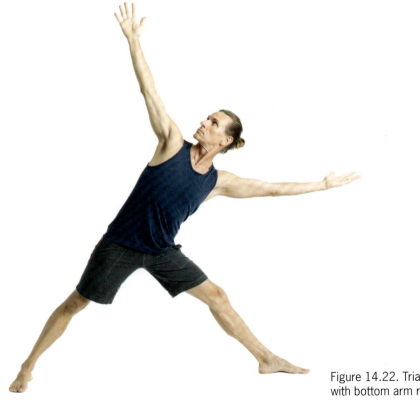

Figure 14.22. Triangle variation with bottom arm reach.

PART THREE | THE POSTURES

Chapter 15

Twists

The Anatomy of Twists

Twisting is an integral part of any great yoga practice, and for good reason. The spine is our architectural center as well as the home of the body's electrical superhighway, the spinal cord. Twists are not only helpful for maintaining structural mobility, but they also provide a gentle wringing massage to all the soft tissues and vital organs of the trunk. Although the spine is at the core center of twists, the entire body is involved.

To examine the action of spinal rotation, we need to look closely at how the vertebrae interact with each other in this motion. The twisting articulation takes place at the facet joints on the sides of the vertebral bodies. Observing the facet joints within the lumbar spine, we see these joints are shaped to prevent or block twisting. In other words, the lumbar spine is not designed to twist (fig. 15.1). Now look at the facet joints of the thoracic spine (fig. 15.2), and see how they are designed to facilitate twisting. The ribs maintain a sturdy structure for the thoracic spine and keep it from rotating too far. So, the spine's range of motion in a twist is gathered from the thoracic area and the neck. Twists are wonderful for maintaining thoracic mobility.

To protect the intervertebral discs, it is important to keep the spine in an uphill line for

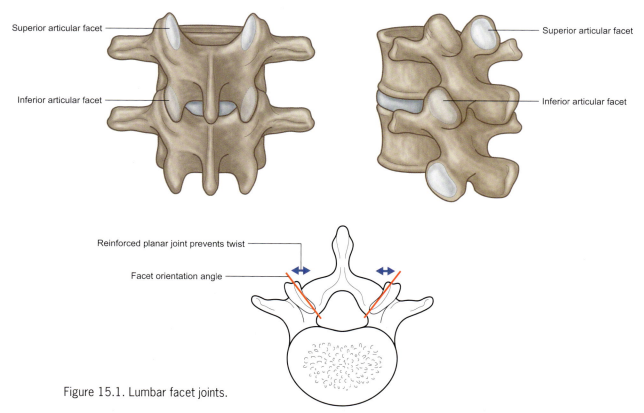

Figure 15.1. Lumbar facet joints.

TWISTS | CHAPTER 15

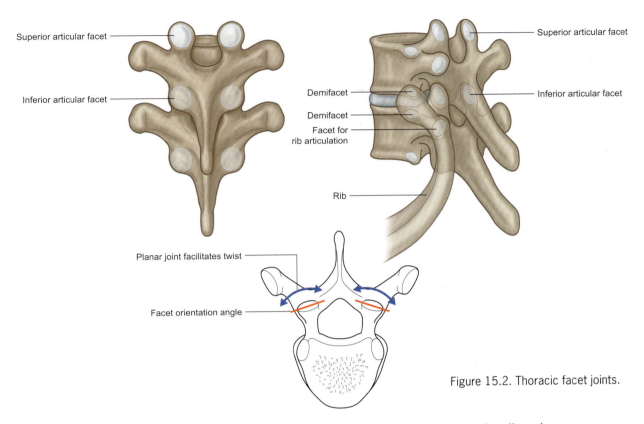

Figure 15.2. Thoracic facet joints.

twisting. A downhill line in the spine will often lead to spinal flexion, putting the discs in a compromised position when twisting. See figure 5.4 to review the spine and intervertebral discs in flexion.

Considering how the twist is anchored within the body is also important. For most yoga poses, the anchoring point of stability is the hips. Keeping the hips stable and square is an attempt to maintain a sound structure across the sacroiliac (SI) joints (fig. 5.15) and the lumbar spine. *This stabilization can be effective as long as too much force is not put into the twisting action.* Excessive force happens with overuse of a lever, such as taking the arm outside the thigh in Chair Twist and "cranking" from the arms to get farther into the twist.

When the hips are being held adamantly square along with a forceful twist, at some point something must give way architecturally. This *giving way* often lands in the SI joints or the facet joints as destabilization or injury. If a forceful, leveraged twist is happening (I don't recommend this), it would be safer to allow the hip to follow the twist rather than remaining square. This would provide a release valve for the force landing in the spine and sacrum. An example would be allowing one knee to gently move forward of the other in Chair Twist.

Bottom line: *It is effective to hold the hips square if the twist is not being forced or leveraged.* I typically teach students to use the exhale and the trunk muscles to guide the twist rather than using force. Refer to the muscles of spinal rotation as a reminder (fig. 5.9).

Remember, how we do anything is how we do everything. If we tend to overdo in our lives, constantly pushing to our max, this will also show up in our practice. Always zoom out and ask, "How is my practice serving me?" and, "What is this for?" Your most effective and relevant practice will arise when you are closely observing yourself with curiosity and honesty.

PART THREE | THE POSTURES

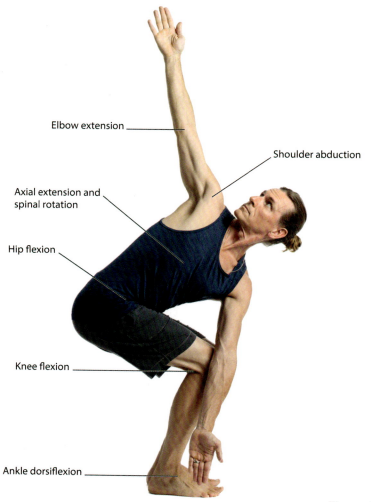

Figure 15.3. The anatomical actions of Chair Twist.

Chair Twist

Chair Twist
Revolved Chair
Parivrtta Utkatasana

Chair Twist is a fiery posture that strengthens the legs and core. It also offers a wringing-out action to the entire torso.

From Chair pose alignment, bring your hands to the center of your heart in Prayer position. Draw your sacrum slightly toward your heels. Then elongate up and away through your crown. From this expanded, lengthened position, turn your chest toward the right for the twist. It is

TWISTS | **CHAPTER 15**

Chair Twist. What am I feeling?

HOW DO I GET THERE?	WHAT IS STRENGTHENING?	WHERE COULD I NOTICE TIGHTNESS?	IS COMPRESSION POSSIBLE?
Axial extension	Axial extensors, fig. 5.10	Entire trunk	
Spinal rotation	**Spinal rotators, fig. 5.9**	**Spinal rotators, fig. 5.9** Opposite side	✓ Fig. 5.7 ✓ Fig. 5.8
Shoulder abduction	Shoulder abductors, fig. 6.7	Shoulder adductors, p. 45	✓ Fig. 6.6
Elbow extension	Elbow extensors, fig.10.2	Elbow flexors, fig. 10.3	
Knee flexion	**Knee extensors, fig. 8.2** While lowering into Chair, knee extensors work eccentrically to oppose gravity. While holding, they work isometrically. Standing out of the pose is concentric contraction of the knee extensors.		
Hip flexion	**Hip extensors, fig. 7.6** While lowering into Chair, hip extensors work eccentrically to oppose gravity. While holding, they work isometrically.	Remember, when you see an eccentric contraction, those muscles are also lengthening.	
Ankle dorsiflexion	Ankle dorsiflexors, fig. 9.3	Ankle plantar flexors, fig. 9.4	✓ Fig. 9.2

My discoveries:

I have highlighted the most common tendencies I see in my students. It is possible to feel strengthening or to notice tightness in any of the muscle groups listed within their respective columns.

PART THREE | THE POSTURES

important to maintain an uphill spine, avoiding any forward rounding. As you settle into the twist, make sure that your knees and hips stay in a neutral, steady alignment. Place your left arm or hand outside your outer right thigh for gentle guidance while reaching your right arm directly out of your shoulder.

As mentioned in the "Anatomy of Twists," let the exhale guide the twist rather than using forceful leverage.

Special Considerations

Students often attempt to get the bottom hand to the floor, but this typically puts the spine in a downhill slope. Healthier alignment is staying angled upright.

If you have shoulder injuries, placement of the top arm can be challenging. Resting your top hand on your low back is an option.

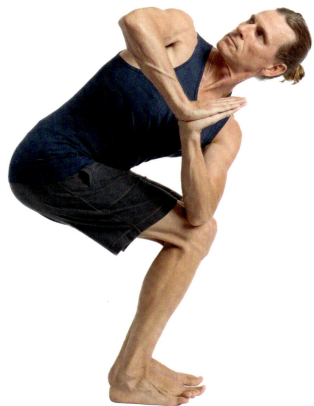

Figure 15.4. Chair Twist modification with Prayer hands.

Modifications

Stay more upright.

Use varying arm positions.

Lay your forearm across your thighs for support.

Variations

A variation I call "Arm Bar" helps establish a greater sense of stability and strength in the lower body while awakening the muscles of hip adduction (fig. 7.8).

Strengthening the hip adductors and abductors is an often overlooked yet very important part of pelvic stability and hip health. Doing the "Arm Bar" Chair, putting a block between the thighs, or working with a strap around the thighs for abduction work can be helpful additions to any practice.

Exploration/Possible Cues

Anchor down through both feet. Then lift through your chest on an inhale before twisting on an exhale.

Put more effort into getting length along your spine, and be gentle with the twist.

Let every exhale invite your bottom lung underneath your top lung.

On your exhales, gently move toward stacked shoulders.

Maintain stability and steadiness from your hips to your toes.

If it feels difficult to take your lifted arm straight out to the side and up, try sweeping down toward the floor, then forward and up.

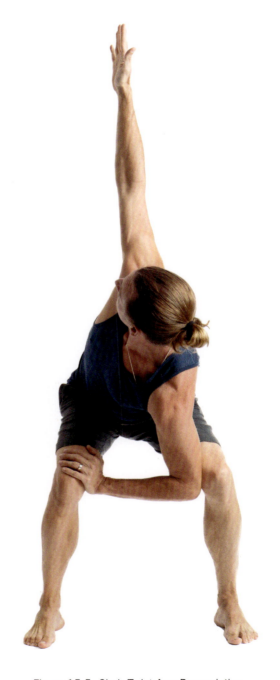

Figure 15.5. Chair Twist Arm Bar variation.

PART THREE | THE POSTURES

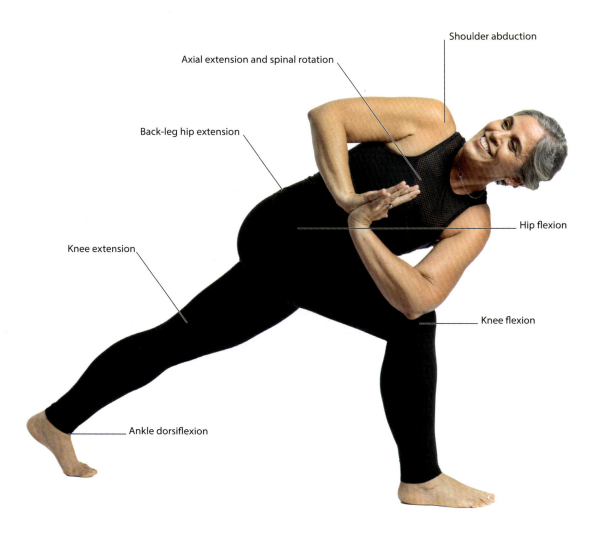

Figure 15.6. The anatomical actions of Crescent Twist.

Crescent Twist

Crescent Twist
Revolved Crescent Lunge
Revolved High Lunge
Parivrtta Anjaneyasana

Crescent Twist is an incredibly strengthening pose. It offers beautiful stimulation and release to the entire inner and outer torso, outer hip muscles, and iliotibial band.

From Crescent Lunge, bring your hands together in Prayer position. Pushing your palms together gently, integrate your shoulder blades by bringing them slightly together and toward your back pockets, feeling expansion across your chest. Draw your sacrum down toward the floor. Inhale, and lift your crown upward and away from your lower belly. From this expanded,

TWISTS | CHAPTER 15

Crescent Twist. What am I feeling?

HOW DO I GET THERE?	WHAT IS STRENGTHENING?	WHERE COULD I NOTICE TIGHTNESS?	IS COMPRESSION POSSIBLE?
Axial extension	Axial extensors, fig. 5.10	**Entire trunk**	
Spinal rotation	**Spinal rotators, fig. 5.9**	**Spinal rotators, fig. 5.9** *Opposite side*	✓ Fig. 5.7 ✓ Fig. 5.8
Shoulder abduction	Shoulder abductors, fig. 6.7	**Shoulder adductors, p. 45**	✓ Fig. 6.6
Elbow extension *If arms are extended*	Elbow extensors, fig. 10.2	Elbow flexors, fig. 10.3	
Front-leg knee flexion	**Front-leg knee extensors, fig. 8.2** Even though the knee is bent, the extensors work eccentrically and/or isometrically to oppose gravity.		
Front-leg hip flexion	**Front-leg hip extensors, fig. 7.6** While lowering into the lunge, hip extensors work eccentrically to oppose gravity. While holding, they work isometrically.		
Back-leg knee extension	**Back-leg knee extensors, fig. 8.2**	Back-leg knee flexors, fig. 8.3	
Back-leg hip extension *Varies depending on torso angle*	**Back-leg hip extensors, fig. 7.6**	**Back-leg hip flexors, fig. 7.5**	
Ankle dorsiflexion	Ankle dorsiflexors, fig. 9.3	Ankle plantar flexors, fig. 9.4 *Back leg predominantly*	✓ Fig. 9.2 Back-leg ankle

My discoveries:

lengthened position, shift your spine forward into a diagonal, reaching action. Then turn your chest toward the right for the twist. Your left elbow or arm can be placed outside of your front thigh for gentle twist support. Reach your right arm directly out of your right shoulder, or keep your hands at Prayer. Keep your back foot and leg firm and active, with your hips steady and even. Let your breath be your guide as you ride the wave of this pose.

Special Considerations

Some instructors may emphasize getting the shoulder over and around the front knee/thigh for twisting leverage. This setup definitely isn't for everyone because it tends to create an "over-cranking" of the twist. As noted in the "Anatomy of Twisting," forced leverage can lead to injury in vulnerable joints if you attempt to go beyond your natural range of motion. We should always zoom out and ask what we are trying to accomplish with our practice.

The asymmetrical leg placement puts tension on the pelvis in two different directions, forward and back. This tension is combined with added forces rotating and pulling the spine (along with the sacrum) away from the pelvis. These combined actions can create unnecessary shear torque on the sacroiliac joints (fig. 5.15), leading to injury. In this sort of posture, you should aim for stability and steadfastness instead of forcing beyond your natural range of motion. This illustrates the importance of truly *embodying* the posture rather than trying to fit some textbook or magazine cover ideal. Listen to what's happening in your body. Challenge yourself, but respect your structure.

Modifications

Instead of taking your arm or elbow over your front thigh, try placing your hand on a block or on the floor under your shoulder.

Drop your back knee down.

Keep your hands at Prayer.

Place your hand or block wider to the left if the twist is too intense.

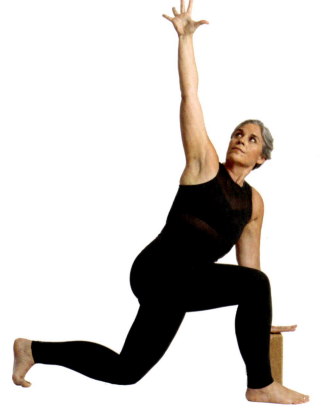

Figure 15.7. Crescent Twist modification with back knee down.

TWISTS | **CHAPTER 15**

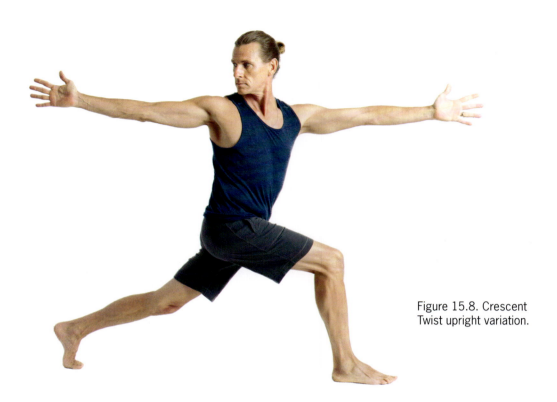

Figure 15.8. Crescent Twist upright variation.

Variations

Keeping your torso upright, reach your arms wide for the twist.

Exploration/Possible Cues

Anchor down through both feet. Then lift through your chest on an inhale before twisting on an exhale.

Maintain length in your spine, and be gentle with the twist.

Let every exhale invite your bottom lung underneath the top lung.

On your exhales, gently move toward stacked shoulders.

Maintain stability and steadiness from your hips to your toes.

If it feels difficult to take your lifted arm straight out to the side and up, try sweeping it down toward the floor, and then forward and up.

Maintain an uphill spine.

Keep your back leg strong with toes aiming straight forward. If your back foot starts turning, you have maxed out your spinal twist, and you are gathering range of motion from your hips.

PART THREE | THE POSTURES

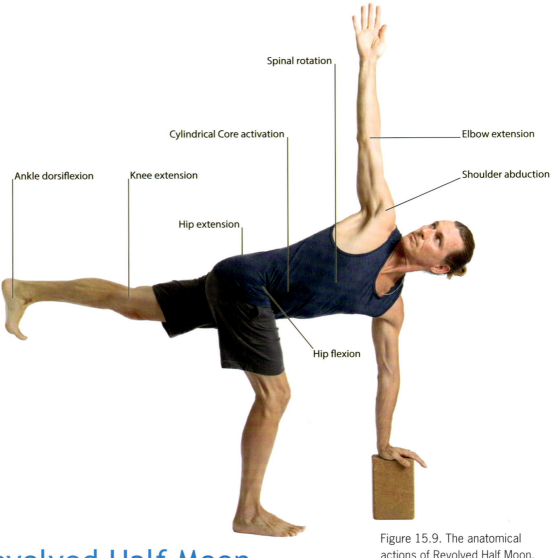

Figure 15.9. The anatomical actions of Revolved Half Moon.

Revolved Half Moon

Revolved Half Moon
Parivrtta Ardha Chandrasana

Revolved Half Moon is a fun, challenging pose. It is like the other twisting postures but also includes the added element of balance.

Begin in Half Moon alignment with your left leg and arm lifted. Square your hips toward the floor, and place your left hand on a block or on claw fingertips directly under your left shoulder. Aim your spine slightly uphill for a healthy twist. Keep your left leg lifted straight back behind you near hip height while reaching your right arm out to the side. Activate both legs strongly. Push through both heels. Twist your left lung under, and move toward stacked ribs and stacked shoulders. As your shoulders move toward stacked, either allow your top arm to continue reaching up and out, or you can place your top hand on your back. Now radiate out into all the spaces around you.

TWISTS | CHAPTER 15

Revolved Half Moon. What am I feeling?

HOW DO I GET THERE?	WHAT IS STRENGTHENING?	WHERE COULD I NOTICE TIGHTNESS?	IS COMPRESSION POSSIBLE?
Cylindrical Core activation	**Cylindrical Core, fig. 13.17**		
Spinal rotation	**Spinal rotators, fig. 5.9**	**Spinal rotators, fig. 5.9** *Opposite side*	✓ Fig. 5.7 ✓ Fig. 5.8
Shoulder abduction	**Shoulder abductors, fig. 6.7**	**Shoulder adductors, p. 45**	✓ Fig. 6.6
Elbow extension	Elbow extensors, fig. 10.2	Elbow flexors, fig. 10.3	
Standing-leg hip flexion	**Standing-leg hip extensors, fig. 7.6** *Hip extensors are working eccentrically and/or isometrically to oppose gravity.*		
Lifted-leg hip extension	**Lifted-leg** hip extensors, fig. 7.6	Lifted-leg hip flexors, fig. 7.5 *Predominantly in bound version, fig. 15.10*	
Knee extension	**Knee extensors, fig. 8.2**	Knee flexors, fig. 8.3	
Ankle dorsiflexion	Ankle dorsiflexors, fig. 9.3	Ankle plantar flexors, fig. 9.4 *Back-leg predominantly*	

My discoveries:

PART THREE | THE POSTURES

Special Considerations

If you lack sufficient leg and core strength, this can be a very challenging pose.

If you have any back injury or weakness, the long lever of the back leg may be too much for your core to support. Try shortening the lever by bending your lifted leg.

In most standing twists, I recommend keeping the spine at least slightly uphill to avoid any spine rounding/flexing and to maintain axial extension. Because your back leg is not anchored in this pose, you may find it easy to maintain axial extension with your spine parallel to the ground. So, either spine slightly uphill or spine parallel to ground can work, depending on your body.

Modifications

Place your bottom hand on a block or two.

Place your hand or block wider to the left if the twist is too intense.

Keep both hands on a block, and simply work on lifting your back leg.

Keep your top hand on your low back.

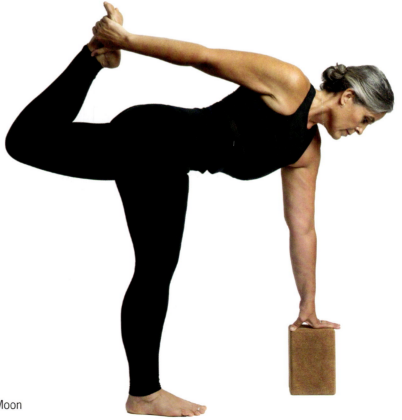

Figure 15.10. Revolved Half Moon variation with bind.

Variations

Adding a bind by catching your lifted leg typically brings in the backward-bend dynamic.

Place your lifted foot on a wall for support.

Exploration/Possible Cues

As you set up the pose, place your lifted hand on the back of your hips to check for evenness.

Use your exhales to roll the bottom lung underneath the top lung, just as in any other twist.

Your back leg will want to drop. This is what makes this pose fun and challenging. Remain activated through your core, and imagine pressing your foot into a wall behind you.

Aim to keep your hips level. Once the spinal rotation has maxed out, the lifted-leg hip might drop, trying to gather more range of motion from the hips. A dropping hip may also indicate hip-stabilizer muscle weakness.

If you can reach the upper-leg bind, it actually makes the pose much easier. The leg bind typically brings in a little backward-bend element.

Smile as you feel your strength expanding.

PART THREE | THE POSTURES

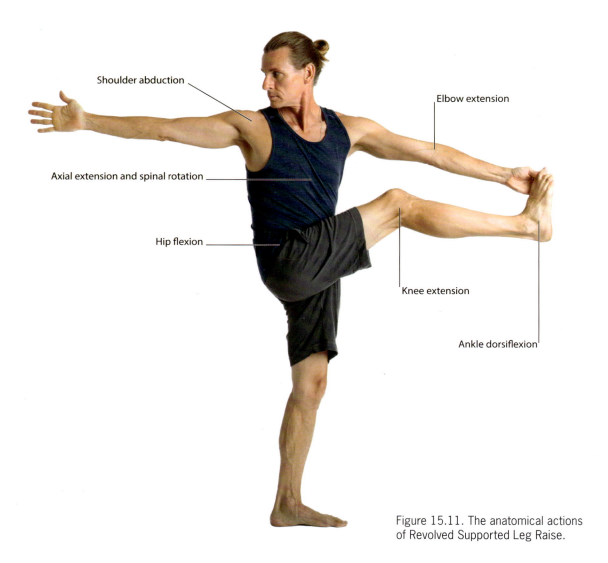

Figure 15.11. The anatomical actions of Revolved Supported Leg Raise.

Revolved Supported Leg Raise

Revolved Supported Leg Raise
Dancing Shiva
Parivrtta Hasta Padangusthasana

Revolved Supported Leg Raise is a balancing act, providing opportunities for cultivating patience and acceptance. This pose offers overall body strengthening along with all the twist benefits.

Start from Supported Side Leg Raise (fig. 16.8) with your right leg lifted. Bring your lifted leg forward, and catch your foot/toes with your left hand. Aim toward keeping your spine in Mountain pose. You might need to bend your lifted leg if your spine and chest are beginning

TWISTS | CHAPTER 15

Revolved Supported Leg Raise. What am I feeling?

HOW DO I GET THERE?	WHAT IS STRENGTHENING?	WHERE COULD I NOTICE TIGHTNESS?	IS COMPRESSION POSSIBLE?
Axial extension	**Axial extensors, fig. 5.10** *Especially the erector spinae in opposition to forward rounding*	**Entire trunk**	
Spinal rotation	**Spinal rotators, fig. 5.9**	**Spinal rotators, fig. 5.9** *Opposite side*	✓ Fig. 5.7 ✓ Fig. 5.8
Shoulder abduction	Shoulder abductors, fig. 6.7	**Shoulder adductors, p. 45**	✓ Fig. 6.6
Elbow extension	Elbow extensors, fig. 10.2	Elbow flexors, fig. 10.3	
Lifted-leg hip flexion	**Lifted-leg hip flexors, fig. 7.5**	**Lifted-leg hip extensors, fig. 7.6**	
Knee extension	**Knee extensors, fig. 8.2**	**Knee flexors, fig. 8.3** *Predominantly on lifted-leg side*	
Ankle dorsiflexion	Ankle dorsiflexors, fig. 9.3	Ankle plantar flexors, fig. 9.4	
Ankle stabilization	**Ankle stabilizers, fig. 9.3, fig. 9.4**		

My discoveries:

to round forward. Action your lifted foot forward as you draw your right lung back toward axial rotation. Nudge your left lung forward while you gently draw your right lung back. Reach your right arm back, following the twist. Gaze past your right hand. Stand tall, and don't hold your breath. Remember that learning to balance is all about compassionately navigating the imbalances.

PART THREE | THE POSTURES

Special Considerations

Bending your lifted leg will allow slack in the hamstring and in the entire back body.

If you have lumbar disc inflammation, you will want either to avoid this pose or to hold your lifted knee rather than your foot.

Remember, aim for doing this pose as a variation of Mountain.

Modifications

If your hip range of motion or hamstring flexibility is limited, keep your lifted leg bent, and hold your knee.

Variations

Placing a strap loop around your lifted foot is helpful if you can't quite reach it. This also shifts the physics of the pose even if you can reach your toes.

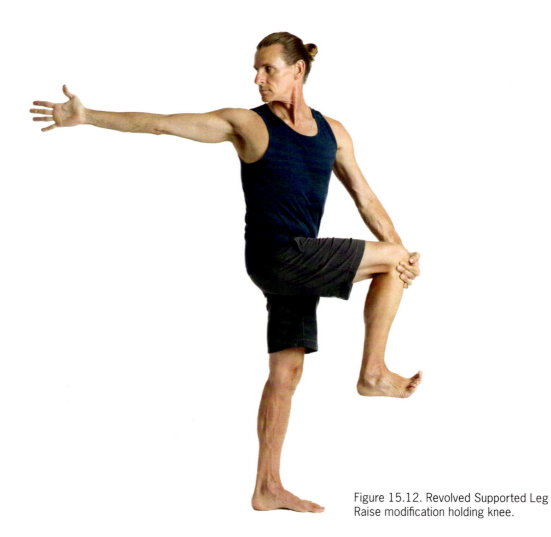

Figure 15.12. Revolved Supported Leg Raise modification holding knee.

TWISTS | CHAPTER 15

Exploration/Possible Cues

See if you can find Mountain pose in your shoulders and hips. Feel the subtle shifts to return there.

Stand tall, and take up the space around you.

Reach actively left to right, beyond where your body lands.

Increase the space between your standing heel and your crown.

Imagine a strong vertical pole from your standing foot through the crown of your head; now gently revolve around it for the twist.

Compassionately navigate the imbalance. If you fall out, smile and begin again.

PART THREE | THE POSTURES

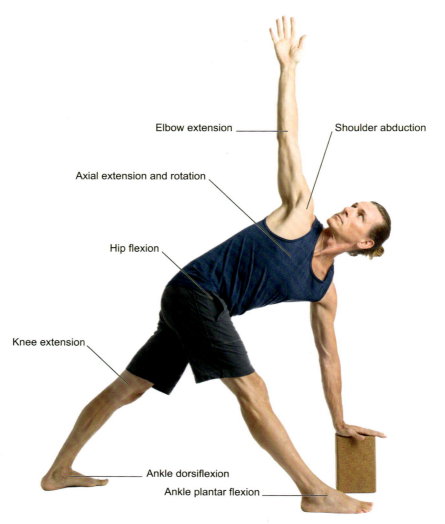

Figure 15.13. The anatomical actions of Revolved Triangle.

Revolved Triangle

Revolved Triangle
Parivrtta Trikonasana

Some might say that Revolved Triangle is one of the most advanced yoga postures. Requiring patience and coordination, this pose cultivates full-body strength while providing the same wringing release as the other twists. While all twists offer some iliotibial band stretch, this pose especially stretches the front leg's iliotibial band and outer hip muscles.

With your right leg forward in Warrior I alignment, straighten your front leg. Then arrange your feet as needed to square your hips evenly forward. Your feet will be somewhere near hip-width distance apart left to right, and your back toes will angle forward anywhere from 25 to

TWISTS | CHAPTER 15

Revolved Triangle. What am I feeling?

HOW DO I GET THERE?	WHAT IS STRENGTHENING?	WHERE COULD I NOTICE TIGHTNESS?	IS COMPRESSION POSSIBLE?
Axial extension	Axial extensors, fig. 5.10	Entire trunk	
Spinal rotation	**Spinal rotators, fig. 5.9**	**Spinal rotators, fig. 5.9** *Opposite side*	✓ Fig. 5.7 ✓ Fig. 5.8
Shoulder abduction	Shoulder abductors, fig. 6.7	**Shoulder adductors, p. 45**	✓ Fig. 6.6
Elbow extension	Elbow extensors, fig. 10.2	Elbow flexors, fig. 10.3	
Hip flexion *More on front leg than back leg*	**Hip extensors, fig. 7.6** Hip extensors engage eccentrically and/or isometrically to oppose gravity toward further hip flexion.	*Remember, when you see an eccentric contraction, those muscles are also lengthening.*	
Knee extension	**Knee extensors, fig. 8.2**	**Knee flexors, fig. 8.3** *Front-leg side predominantly*	
Back-leg Ankle dorsiflexion	Back-leg ankle dorsiflexors, fig. 9.3	**Back-leg ankle plantar flexors, fig. 9.4**	
Front-leg ankle plantar flexion	Front-leg ankle plantar flexors, fig. 9.4	Ankle dorsiflexors, fig. 9.3	✓ Fig. 9.2

My discoveries:

45 degrees. Once you are in this stance, reach both arms up while breathing in, and elongate up and out of your legs. Draw your sacrum down toward the floor. Actively reach both arms forward and long as you draw your hips back. Maintaining an uphill spine, place your left hand on claw fingertips or on a block beneath your left shoulder, close to your right foot. Your individual body proportions and length of stance front to back will determine what you need to do to keep your spine uphill. Now turn your chest toward the right for spinal rotation, and allow your right arm to follow the twist, extending straight out of your right shoulder. Stay and breathe. Fill the spaces of your body with your breath and awareness.

Special Considerations

This pose is sometimes called Revolved Pyramid, depending on the length and width of stance along with the angle of the back foot. I believe the practitioner's unique anatomy dictates these variable elements, so I teach Revolved Pyramid and Revolved Triangle as variations of the same pose.

Spine, hamstring, shoulder, foot, or ankle injury can limit this pose.

This pose may cause excess tension in the sacroiliac joints and/or lumbar spine. *For full details, see the "The Anatomy of Twists" section (p. 188) along with the explanation under Special Considerations in Crescent Twist (p. 196).*

If you have sacroiliac dysfunction or lumbar spine injury, lifting your back heel can release tension in your pelvis and lumbar spine. Or you might need to avoid the pose.

If you have hamstring tendonitis in the front leg, lessen the degree of hip flexion by putting two stacked blocks under your hand, or do the twist upright. If this doesn't relieve the tension, avoid the pose for now.

The twisting poses present unique interaction with the shoulder as the arm is abducted out to the side and up. For some people, skeletal structure makes this uncomfortable. It can be helpful to take a different entry pathway. Instead of taking your arm straight out and up, try sweeping it down and forward, and then up. Rotating the direction of your palm may help you navigate around this compressive point.

Rotator cuff injuries will also make this movement challenging. In this case, it is better not to lift your arm. Place the lifted hand on your low back instead.

Modifications

Placing your bottom hand on two stacked blocks may help you access this pose, specifically if you are having trouble maintaining axial extension (fig. 5.10) while reaching your hand to a single block.

Place your hand or the block wider to the left if the twist is too intense.

Lift your back heel.

Bend your front knee.

Resting your top hand on your back is a great option if you have any shoulder injury.

Variations

For a different approach to the twist, try practicing it upright with a vertical spine. Let your arms reach long, directly out of your shoulders.

Rolling the front foot onto its outer edge can increase the stretch of the front leg's iliotibial band and outer hip compartment. If you choose this variation, decrease the intensity of the twist, and focus on steadiness and stability.

Exploration/Possible Cues

The variable pieces in Revolved Triangle are
- how long your stance is front to back,
- how wide your feet are left to right, and
- how much your back foot is angled forward.

Play with all these variables, and feel the perfect shape for your body.

Instead of setting your feet first, find a neutral, squared-forward pelvis, and then set your feet accordingly.

Individual body proportions highly affect all yoga postures. Whether or not you need a block will often be determined by your arm length or arm-torso-leg-length ratios. Decide what you need to maintain an uphill spine in this pose.

Draw your hips back as you elongate your crown forward.

Place your hand on your front-leg outer hip. Gently draw it back. Notice the stretch that lands in the outer hip and iliotibial band.

PART THREE | **THE POSTURES**

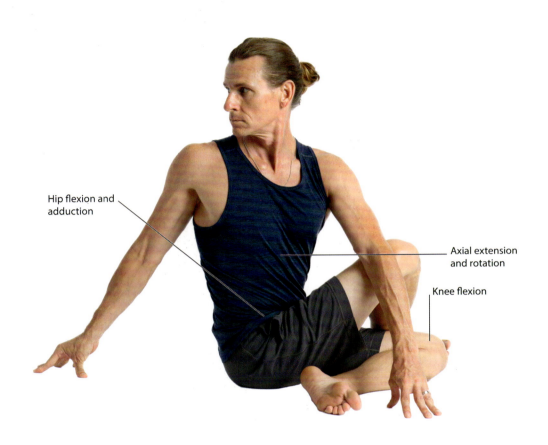

Figure 15.14. The anatomical actions of Seated Twist.

Seated Twist

Seated Twist
Half Lord of the Fishes Pose
Ardha Matsyendrasana

Seated Twist provides a gentle wringing out without expending lots of effort or having to balance on one leg as with the standing twists. This variation creates a nice stretch for the top-leg outer thigh, iliotibial band, and glutes.

Begin seated upright with your hips even on the floor. Bending your right knee, place your right leg over your left, and stand your right foot on the ground outside your left thigh. Draw your left foot toward your right hip, allowing your left thigh to rest on the floor. Your right knee will point straight up. Now shift around to get your hips even on the floor again. If your lumbar

TWISTS | CHAPTER 15

Seated Twist. What am I feeling?

HOW DO I GET THERE?	WHAT IS STRENGTHENING?	WHERE COULD I NOTICE TIGHTNESS?	IS COMPRESSION POSSIBLE?
Axial extension	**Axial extensors, fig. 5.10**	**Entire trunk**	
Spinal rotation	**Spinal rotators, fig. 5.9**	**Spinal rotators, fig. 5.9** *Opposite side*	✓ Fig. 5.7 ✓ Fig. 5.8
Knee flexion	Knee extensors, fig. 8.2	Knee flexors, fig. 8.3	
Hip adduction	Hip adductors, fig. 7.8	Hip abductors, fig. 7.9	✓ Fig. 7.7
Hip flexion	Hip flexors, fig. 7.5	**Hip extensors, fig. 7.6** *Top-leg side*	✓ Fig. 7.4

My discoveries:

spine is rounding too much, or if you are uncomfortable, try folding your mat a few times and placing it underneath your buttocks. Wrap your left arm around your right leg, and place your right hand as a kickstand on the floor behind your spine. Lengthen and lift through your crown as you breathe in, and twist from your ribs as you breathe out. Allow your gaze to follow the twist. Don't force your neck range of motion.

Special Considerations

If this pose is difficult for you because your hip or knee range of motion makes you uncomfortable, you have other options for Seated Twist. See Modifications below.

This pose is often taught with the front arm leveraged outside the thigh. Do not overtorque the leverage if you take this variation. (See "Anatomy of Twists," p. 188.)

Modifications

Sit in Easy Pose with legs crossed for the twist instead of planting your top foot on the ground.

Sit on a small cushion, block, or folded blanket.

Exploration/Possible Cues

Allow your weight to evenly distribute through both hips into the ground.

As you inhale, imagine your spine telescoping up and out of your hips.

As you exhale, invite a soft twist around your thoracic spine.

Gently take the twist all the way up to the top of your neck.

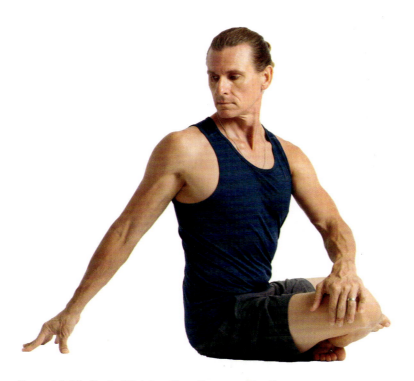

Figure 15.15. Seated Twist as Easy Pose modification.

TWISTS | CHAPTER 15

I have been a seeker, and I still am, but I stopped asking the books and the stars. I started listening to the teaching of my Soul.

—Rumi

PART THREE | **THE POSTURES**

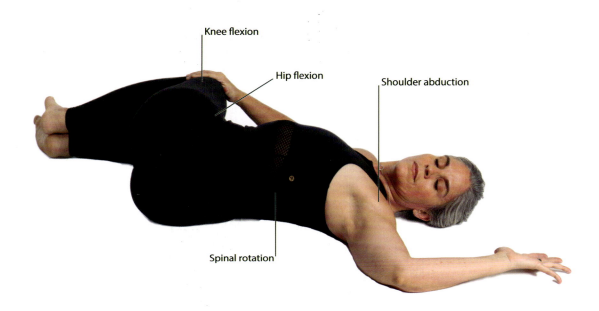

Figure 15.16. The anatomical actions of Supine Twist.

Supine Twist

Supine Twist
Reclined Spinal Twist
Supta Matsyendrasana

Supine Twist typically arrives in class after all the work is done. It is practiced with the quality of letting go.

Begin lying on your back in a comfortable position with your knees bent and feet on the floor. Shift your hips several inches to the left. Hug both knees into your chest. Take your knees over to the right side of your body while turning your hips until stacked. Move your left shoulder blade back toward the floor, and reach your right arm out to the side, or place it on your top leg. Look toward the left, but don't force your neck range of motion. Let yourself simply be.

TWISTS | CHAPTER 15

Supine Twist. What am I feeling?

HOW DO I GET THERE?	WHAT IS STRENGTHENING?	WHERE COULD I NOTICE TIGHTNESS?	IS COMPRESSION POSSIBLE?
Spinal rotation	Passive	Spinal rotators, fig. 5.9 Opposite side	✓ Fig. 5.7 ✓ Fig. 5.8
Knee flexion	Passive	Knee extensors, fig. 8.2	
Hip flexion	Passive	Top-leg hip extensors, fig. 7.6	
Shoulder abduction	Passive	Shoulder adductors, p. 45	

My discoveries:

Special Considerations

Instructors sometimes cue to keep both shoulders anchored to the ground. This may be fine for some students, but if your twist range of motion is not there, it's best not to force it.

Keeping the pelvis stacked will help maintain more stability and encourage thoracic mobility.

Modifications

If you have sacroiliac joint instability, knees together with a block placed between them is typically more comfortable and effective. This assures stability and equanimity in the pelvis.

Variations

Varying your leg and hand positions will change the overall dynamic of this pose by increasing or decreasing the amount of spinal twist and by adding in different stretch elements.

Exploration/Possible Cues

Encourage your muscles to let go so that your body can get heavy on the floor.

Let the weight of your body go.

Notice the change in your breath capacity in this shape.

Feel your breath. Allow it to gently invite the twist.

Allow the back of your ribs to release toward the floor.

Chapter 16
Standing Balance Postures

Standing Balance Posture Overview

These postures are very similar to the standing postures with one major difference—you are balancing on one foot. Bearing weight on one leg not only strengthens your body, but it also sharpens the balancing centers in your brain. Additionally, standing on one leg is a great way to strengthen the often-forgotten outer-hip stabilizers, the gluteus medius, the gluteus minimus, and the tensor fascia latae (fig. 7.9). These muscles are very important for the health of the entire kinetic chain downward through the iliotibial band, the knee, and the ankle.[36] An evidence of hip stabilizer weakness is "dumping" into one hip in a balancing pose. Here are four tips for practicing the balance postures: 1) focus on evenness in the pelvis, 2) keep a soft bend in your standing-leg knee, 3) use your gaze or drishti, and 4) don't forget to breathe. Like the standing postures, I categorize these as open-hip and closed-hip postures.

Open-Hip Standing Balance Postures

These poses require hip **abduction** (fig. 7.9), or an open relationship between the femurs and the pelvis. These poses are practiced with hips facing to the side. Either the pelvis opens away from the femur, as in moving the hips toward stacked in Half Moon Balance (fig. 16.11), or the femur opens away from the pelvis, as in drawing the thigh out to the side in Tree (fig. 16.9).

- Half Moon
- Tree
- Supported Side Leg Raise

Closed-Hip Standing Balance Postures

Closed-hip postures are those in which we keep the thigh bones somewhat neutral with the pelvis, so there is a closed relationship between the thighs and pelvis. We can think of these as the poses in which the hips are facing forward.

- Eagle
- Supported Front Leg Raise
- Warrior III

PART THREE | THE POSTURES

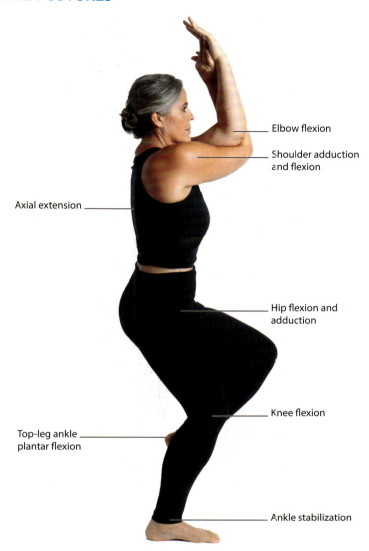

Figure 16.1. The anatomical actions of Eagle.

Eagle

Eagle
Garudasana

Eagle is a unique balance pose producing a strong sense of hugging into our own bodies for stability. No other yoga posture utilizes the wrapping and drawing in of limbs in quite the same way. This is a **closed-hip** posture.

Begin in Mountain pose. Sweep both arms up, and then wrap your right elbow under your left elbow, bringing your hands together, fingertips to palm. Hold your elbows near shoulder level. Press your hands forward until your forearms are near vertical. Wrap your right leg over your left leg, and bend your standing leg as in Chair pose. If your foot can wrap around your calf, do that; if not, squeeze it in as close to your leg as possible. Gaze straight ahead while riding the waves of balance and imbalance.

STANDING BALANCE POSTURES | CHAPTER 16

Eagle. What am I feeling?

HOW DO I GET THERE?	WHAT IS STRENGTHENING?	WHERE COULD I NOTICE TIGHTNESS?	IS COMPRESSION POSSIBLE?
Axial extension	**Axial extensors, fig. 5.10**	Entire trunk	
Shoulder flexion	Shoulder flexors, fig. 6.4	**Shoulder extensors, fig. 6.5**	✓ Fig. 6.3
Shoulder adduction	**Shoulder adductors, fig. 6.9**	**Shoulder horizontal abductors, p. 46**	✓ Fig. 6.8
Possible lateral rotation shoulders	Shoulder lateral rotators, fig. 6.14	Shoulder medial rotators, fig. 6.11	
Elbow flexion	Elbow flexors, fig. 10.3	Elbow extensors, fig. 10.2	
Hip flexion	**Standing-leg hip extensors, fig. 7.6** Although the hip is flexed, the standing-leg hip extensors are working isometrically during a hold to oppose gravity. This will vary depending on the amount of hip flexion.		
Hip adduction	**Hip adductors, fig. 7.8**	**Hip abductors, fig. 7.9**	
Knee flexion	**Knee extensors, fig. 8.2** While lowering, knee extensors work eccentrically to oppose gravity. While holding, they work isometrically.		
Standing-leg ankle stabilization	**Standing-leg ankle stabilizers, fig. 9.3, fig. 9.4**		
Top-leg ankle plantar flexion	Top-leg ankle plantar flexors, fig. 9.4	top-leg ankle dorsiflexors, fig. 9.3	

My discoveries:

I have highlighted the most common tendencies I see in my students. It is possible to feel strengthening or to notice tightness in any of the muscle groups listed within their respective columns.

219

Special Considerations

The following elements can limit this pose:
- Leg size limiting the wrap and/or ankle-to-leg connection
- Arm size limiting the wrap and/or hand connection
- Leg, ankle, foot, knee, spine, and shoulder injuries
- Physiological factors affecting balance

The arm position in this pose provides an opportunity for release within all the soft tissues attached to the scapulae. You can increase this by allowing the scapulae to protract (fig. 6.17).

You can work the muscles of adduction in the shoulders and hips by squeezing toward the midline. Or you can work the muscles of abduction by using the binds to activate a pulling away from the body midline.

Modifications

Simply do half of the pose—just the arms or just the legs.

If the arm wrap is too difficult, try a simple top-arm shoulder stretch instead, or grab your opposite shoulders.

Place a block under your top-leg toes for more stability.

Exploration/Possible Cues

Do this pose as a variation of Mountain, maintaining all the natural curves of your spine.

Use the arm and leg bind to spark an internal squeeze into the core of your body.

Experiment with holding your elbows lower and higher, noticing the change in your upper-back sensation.

Soften your grip on the balance, allowing yourself to ebb and flow with the imbalance.

STANDING BALANCE POSTURES | CHAPTER 16

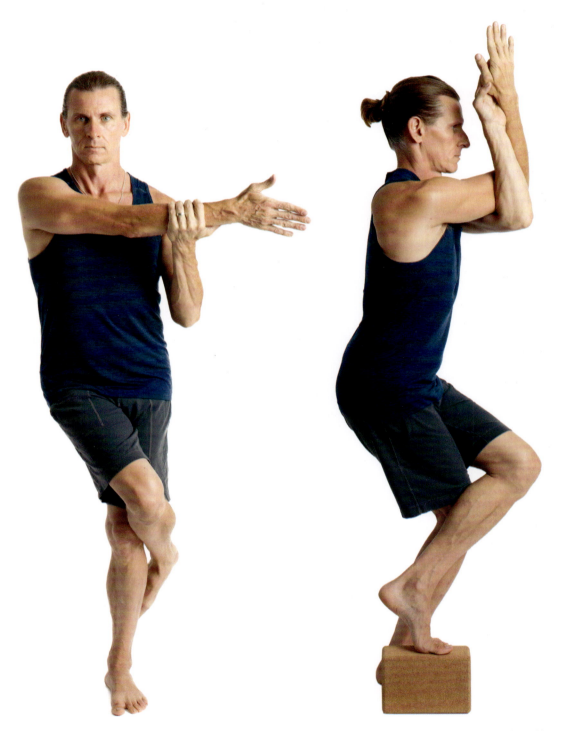

Figure 16.2. Eagle modification with top-arm shoulder stretch.

Figure 16.3. Eagle modification with block under toes.

221

PART THREE | THE POSTURES

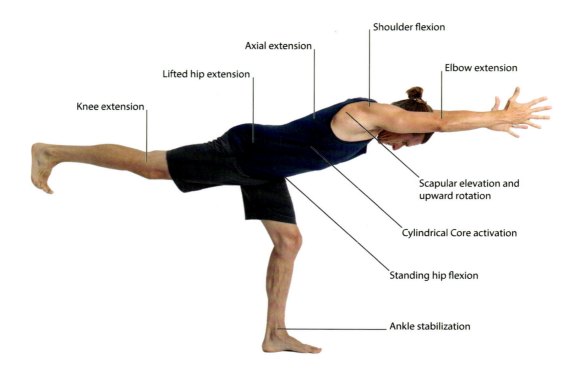

Figure 16.4. The anatomical actions of Warrior III.

Warrior III

Warrior III
Virabhadrasana III

Warrior III is one of the best functional strengthening poses available. Be sure to review and incorporate Cylindrical Core (fig. 13.17) with this **closed-hip** posture.

Begin in High Lunge (fig. 14.1) with your left leg forward. With a neutral spine, draw your front lower ribs into your belly. Lean forward and balance on your left foot. Then actively reach your right toes straight back. Activate your legs and the lifted-leg glutes to lift weight out of your standing hip, knee, and ankle. Keep your hips as squared as possible. Reach strongly, and aim to have your biceps beside your ears. Hold your body as close to parallel to the floor as you can. Gaze at the floor, keeping your neck long and neutral.

STANDING BALANCE POSTURES | CHAPTER 16

Warrior III. What am I feeling?

HOW DO I GET THERE?	WHAT IS STRENGTHENING?	WHERE COULD I NOTICE TIGHTNESS?	IS COMPRESSION POSSIBLE?
Cylindrical Core activation *This increases as the torso moves more toward parallel to the floor.*	**Cylindrical Core, fig. 13.17**		
Shoulder flexion	**Shoulder flexors, fig. 6.4**	**Shoulder extensors, fig. 6.5**	✓ Fig. 6.3
Scapular elevation and upward rotation	**Elevators, upward rotators of the scapulae, p. 54**	Depressors, downward rotators of the scapulae, p. 54	
Elbow extension	**Elbow extensors, fig. 10.2** *Elbow extensors are working concentrically and/or isometrically to keep arms straight.*	Elbow flexors, fig. 10.3	
Standing-leg hip flexion	**Standing-leg hip extensors, fig. 7.6** *The extensors work eccentrically and/or isometrically to oppose gravity. This varies depending on the degree of hip flexion.*		
Lifted-leg hip extension	**Lifted-leg hip extensors, fig. 7.6** *The hip extensors work isometrically to stabilize the lifted leg and hip.*	Lifted-leg hip flexors, fig. 7.5	
Knee extension	**Knee extensors, fig. 8.2**	**Knee flexors, fig. 8.3**	
Ankle stabilization	**Ankle stabilizers, fig. 9.3, fig. 9.4**		

My discoveries:

Special Considerations

This pose demands Cylindrical Core strength. If you are weak here, it is better to modify the pose so that your spine can be more supported until you build additional strength.

Sliding the shoulder blades toward the ears while reaching the arms forward will provide a much more stable support at the glenohumeral joint (fig. 6.1). Many yogis are improperly trained to "take the shoulders away from the ears" in all actions. As discussed in chapter 6, "The Shoulder," in "Shoulder Stability and Scapular Movements," this isn't always the most stable shoulder position.

Bending the standing leg more lowers the center of gravity and makes the pose easier.

Modifications

This is what I call a "long lever" pose. Reaching the arms and/or legs this far away from the centerline of the body can be challenging if you have back/core injury or weakness. The solution is to shorten the levers as needed to reduce the workload on the spine. Levers can be shortened in two ways:
- Draw your hands to Prayer, or reach your hands back beside the body.
- Or bend your back leg to shorten the lever.

Place tall blocks under your hands, or place two stacked blocks under each hand.

Keep your torso higher, not taking your body parallel to the floor.

Variations

Hold a strap between your reaching hands to add support to your body overall.

Press your lifted foot into a wall to feel what strong foot and leg activation bring to the pose.

STANDING BALANCE POSTURES | CHAPTER 16

Exploration/Possible Cues

Use your full body strength. Connect legs to belly to back to arms.

Anchor through the three corners of your foot. Think of your foot as a tripod. Anchor through the big-toe ball mound, pinky-toe ball mound, and the heel.

Wake up your fingers and toes.

Expand into the space around you.

Let your breath provide structural support.

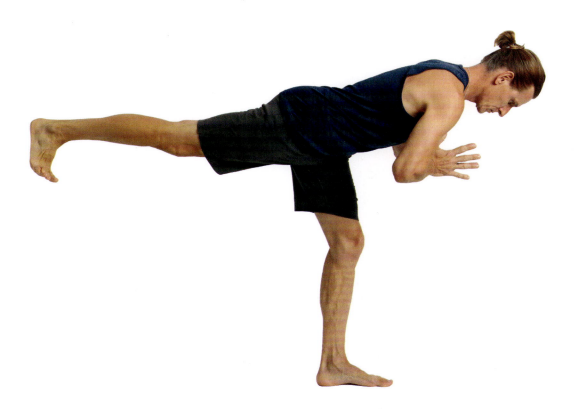

Figure 16.5. Warrior III modification with hands at Prayer.

PART THREE | **THE POSTURES**

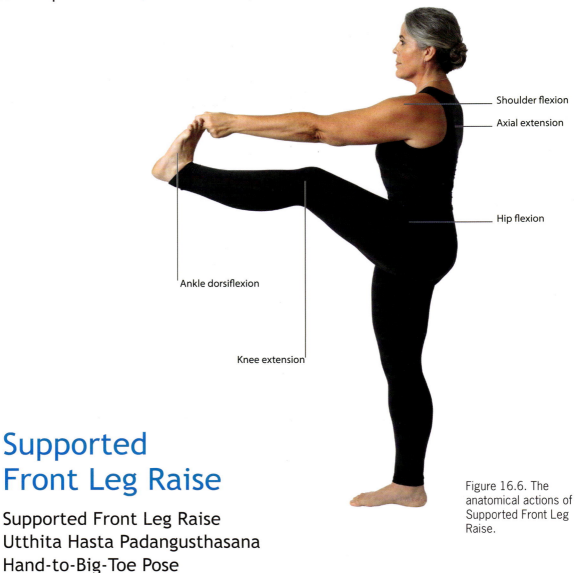

Figure 16.6. The anatomical actions of Supported Front Leg Raise.

Supported Front Leg Raise

Supported Front Leg Raise
Utthita Hasta Padangusthasana
Hand-to-Big-Toe Pose

This effective, strengthening balance posture will test the range of motion and flexibility in your lower body. Supported Front Leg Raise is a **closed-hip** posture.

Begin standing in Mountain. Lift your left leg up, and loop the first two fingers of your left hand around your big toe. Place your right hand on your right hip for stability. Extend your leg as straight as you can out in front of you. If straightening your leg causes you to round your spine, back out by bending your knee as much as needed to keep your back lengthened. Draw your lifted sitting bone down to level your hips. Aim to maintain Mountain pose quality.

Special Considerations

In this posture's full variation, extending the lifted leg and grabbing the toe puts quite a demand on the body's back-side soft tissues. Any excessive tightness will cause the spine to round forward. If you can't maintain a Mountain spine here, it is best to bend your knee a bit, to grab your knee, or to use a strap.

STANDING BALANCE POSTURES | CHAPTER 16

Supported Front Leg Raise. What am I feeling?

HOW DO I GET THERE?	WHAT IS STRENGTHENING?	WHERE COULD I NOTICE TIGHTNESS?	IS COMPRESSION POSSIBLE?
Axial extension	**Axial extensors, fig. 5.10** *Especially erector spinae, to counter any forward flexing in the trunk*	Entire trunk	
Shoulder flexion in arm holding foot or knee	Shoulder flexors, fig. 6.4	Shoulder extensors, fig. 6.5	
Lifted-leg hip flexion	Lifted-leg hip flexors, fig. 7.5	**Lifted-leg hip extensors, fig. 7.6** *Entire back body*	
Knee extension	**Knee extensors, fig. 8.2**	**Knee flexors, fig. 8.3** *Predominantly lifted leg*	
Ankle stabilization	**Ankle stabilizers, fig. 9.3, fig. 9.4**		
Lifted-leg ankle dorsiflexion	Ankle dorsiflexors, fig 9.3	**Ankle plantar flexors, fig. 9.4**	
My discoveries:			

Modifications

Hold your knee instead of your toe.

Use a looped strap to hold your foot.

Exploration/Possible Cues

Aim both your chest and your gaze straight forward.

Only straighten your leg as much as you can while maintaining Mountain in your spine.

Expand from your standing heel to your crown.

Draw your right shoulder back in line with your left.

Place your left hand on your hip bone to feel support.

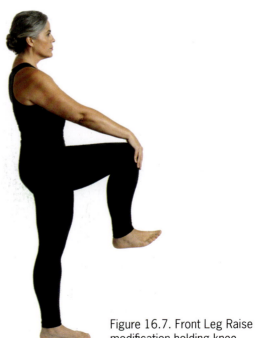

Figure 16.7. Front Leg Raise modification holding knee.

PART THREE | THE POSTURES

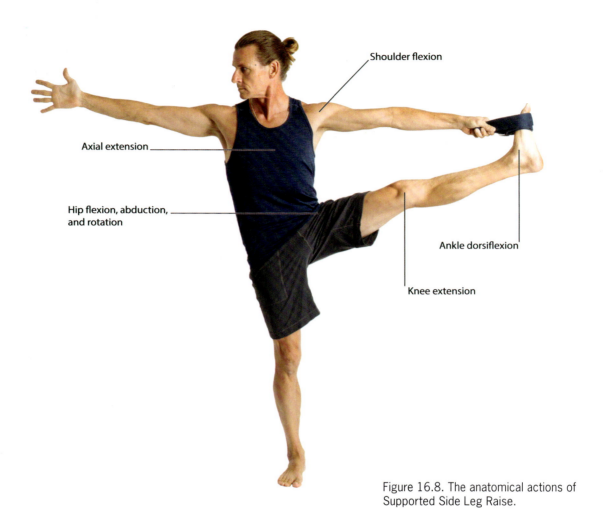

Figure 16.8. The anatomical actions of Supported Side Leg Raise.

Supported Side Leg Raise

Supported Side Leg Raise
Utthita Hasta Padangusthasana
Extended Hand-to-Big-Toe Pose

This pose is typically done in conjunction with its partner, Supported Front Leg Raise (fig. 16.6). Supported Side Leg Raise is an **open-hip** posture. It will test your balance as well as the flexibility of the body's back side.

Begin in Supported Front Leg Raise. Using your left hand, hold your left big toe with your first two fingers, or hold a strap looped around your outstretched foot. Maintaining a tall, stable stance, take your leg out to the left. Stay firmly rooted in your standing foot and leg while drawing your left sitting bone *toward* even with the right. Place your right hand on your right hip for support or reach out to the side. Gaze to the right, away from the lifted foot.

STANDING BALANCE POSTURES | CHAPTER 16

Supported Side Leg Raise. What am I feeling?

HOW DO I GET THERE?	WHAT IS STRENGTHENING?	WHERE COULD I NOTICE TIGHTNESS?	IS COMPRESSION POSSIBLE?
Axial extension	**Axial extensors, fig. 5.10** *Especially erector spinae, to counter any forward rounding*	Entire trunk	
Shoulder flexion	Shoulder flexors, fig. 6.4	Shoulder extensors, fig. 6.5	
Lifted-leg hip flexion	Lifted-leg hip flexors, fig. 7.5	**Lifted-leg hip extensors, fig. 7.6**	✓ Fig. 7.4
Knee extension	**Knee extensors, fig. 8.2** *Knee extensors are working concentrically and/or isometrically to hold the leg straight.*	**Knee flexors, fig. 8.3** *Predominantly lifted leg*	
Lifted-leg hip abduction	**Lifted-leg hip abductors fig. 7.9**	**Lifted-leg hip adductors, fig. 7.8**	✓ Fig. 7.7
Lifted-leg hip lateral rotation	Lifted-leg hip lateral rotators fig. 7.12	**Lifted-leg hip medial, fig. 7.11**	✓ Fig. 7.10
Ankle stabilization	**Ankle stabilizers, fig. 9.3, fig. 9.4**		
Lifted-leg ankle dorsiflexion	Ankle dorsiflexors, fig 9.3	**Ankle plantar flexors, fig. 9.4**	

My discoveries:

PART THREE | THE POSTURES

Special Considerations

Just a reminder: With any pose having movement within the hip socket, in addition to soft tissue tightness, the unique skeletal complex will determine end ranges of motion, such as where the femur can be comfortably moved without shifting the pelvis. Because of this, you may or may not be able to keep your hips level in this pose.

Your unique skeletal hip complex will determine your experience with flexing, rotating, and abducting the lifted leg. Some will max out this range sooner than others, and either the leg won't go as far, or the pelvis will shift with the leg placement.

If you are holding your toe in this pose, back-body tightness can be navigated by changing the bend in the lifted knee. You know you have met your limit when you can't maintain a Mountain spine. *In all poses, back-body tightness can be minimized by bending the knees.*

Modifications

Hold your knee instead of your toe.

Use a looped strap around your lifted foot.

Reach your opposite arm out to the side for counterbalance.

Exploration/Possible Cues

Press down firmly through your standing foot while reaching up through your crown.

Take up space from left to right, reaching beyond where your body lands.

Energetically pull apart left to right from your gaze point to your outstretched foot or knee.

STANDING BALANCE POSTURES | CHAPTER 16

The Breeze at Dawn

The breeze at dawn has secrets to tell you.
Don't go back to sleep.
You must ask for what you really want.
Don't go back to sleep.
People are going back and forth across
the doorsill
Where the two worlds touch.
The door is round and open.
Don't go back to sleep.

—Rumi

PART THREE | THE POSTURES

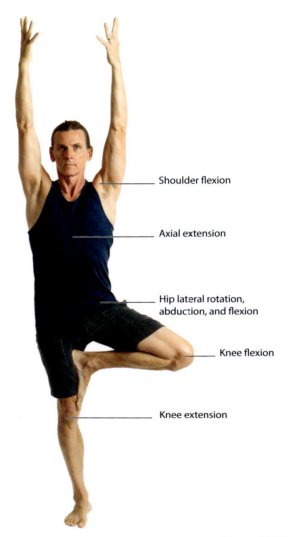

Figure 16.9. The anatomical actions of Tree.

Tree

Tree
Vrikshasana
Vrksasana

Standing in Tree has the quality of standing in True North, ready and willing for whatever comes your way. Tree provides foot, hip, and core strengthening like all standing balance postures. It is an **open-hip** posture.

Begin in Mountain. Lift your left leg, and place the sole of your foot in a stable position on the inside of your right leg. Keep your weight balanced in the three corners of your standing foot while squeezing your lifted foot and standing leg together. Reach your arms up and away,

STANDING BALANCE POSTURES | CHAPTER 16

Tree. What am I feeling?

HOW DO I GET THERE?	WHAT IS STRENGTHENING?	WHERE COULD I NOTICE TIGHTNESS?	IS COMPRESSION POSSIBLE?
Axial extension	**Axial extensors, fig. 5.10**	Entire trunk	
Shoulder flexion	**Shoulder flexors, fig. 6.4**	Shoulder extensors, fig. 6.5	✓ Fig. 6.3
Lifted-leg hip flexion	Lifted-leg hip flexors, fig. 7.5	Lifted-leg hip extensors, fig. 7.6	✓ Fig. 7.4
Lifted-leg hip abduction	**Lifted-leg hip abductors fig. 7.9**	**Lifted-leg hip adductors, fig. 7.8**	✓ Fig. 7.7
Lifted-leg hip lateral rotation	Lifted-leg hip lateral rotators fig. 7.12	Lifted-leg hip medial, rotators, fig. 7.11	✓ Fig. 7.10
Standing-leg knee extension	Standing-leg knee extensors, fig. 8.2	Standing-leg knee flexors, fig. 8.3	
Lifted-leg knee flexion	Lifted-leg knee flexors, fig. 8.3	Lifted-leg knee extensors, fig. 8.2	
Ankle stabilization	**Ankle stabilizers, fig. 9.3, fig. 9.4**		

My discoveries:

PART THREE | THE POSTURES

creating an energetic line of action from hands to feet. Stand tall, and gaze forward.

Special Considerations

If you have any knee tenderness, avoid pressing your heel into it. Although the cue "Place your foot above or below but never on the knee" is very commonly used, I have found many students like the stability of placing the arch of their foot on their knee with the heel pressing above and the ball mound pressing below. Like everything else, it depends on the individual.

Depending on the range of motion in your lifted hip, you may or may not be able to abduct your knee straight out to the side. Once you have met the end of your range of motion, your pelvis will turn with your knee as you move it out. Aim to keep your pelvis aligned in neutral and straight forward, even if your knee isn't straight out to the side.

Modifications

Try varying arm positions as needed, such as Cactus or arms wide in a V.

Keep your hands in Prayer.

Place your lifted-leg toes on the ground like a kickstand if balance is difficult, or place your toes on a block.

Exploration/Possible Cues

Drive down through your standing foot while reaching up and away.

Find more stabilization by adding more energy into your reach.

Play with different arm variations. Feel the sensations of your body returning to balance.

Instead of focusing on pressing your lifted foot into your thigh, engage your standing leg adductors (inner thigh) to press into your foot.

Strongly squeeze your glutes for stabilization, and then stretch your spine straight up toward the ceiling.

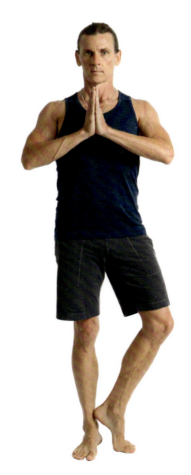

Figure 16.10. Tree modification with toes on ground.

STANDING BALANCE POSTURES | CHAPTER 16

To be nobody but yourself in a world which is doing its best night and day to make you everybody else means to fight the hardest battle which any human being can fight and never stop fighting.

—e. e. cummings

PART THREE | THE POSTURES

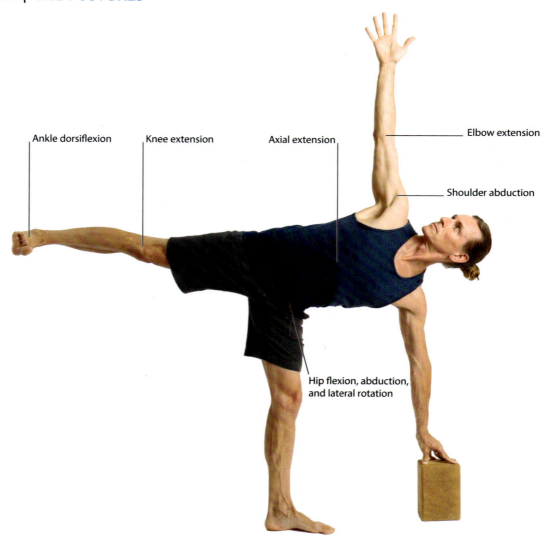

Figure 16.11. The anatomical actions of Half Moon.

Half Moon

Half Moon
Ardha Chandrasana
Ardha Chandrasana Chapasana/Sugarcane/Bound Half Moon

This powerful pose cultivates mental and physical stamina while providing incredible strengthening of your feet, ankles, and legs. Half Moon is an **open-hip** posture.

Begin in left side Warrior II (fig. 14.13). Keeping your hips open toward the right, look down at your left toes. Place a block about a foot forward and a little to the left of your left toes. With your left hand on the block, lift your spine and back leg up parallel to the ground in one active line. Move your top hip toward stacked over the bottom hip. Stand strong in your supporting leg. Reach actively through both feet, firmly tightening the leg muscles and glutes. Maintain your Cylindrical Core engagement (fig. 13.17), and extend out through both hands. Gaze upward toward your lifted hand.

STANDING BALANCE POSTURES | CHAPTER 16

Half Moon. What am I feeling?

HOW DO I GET THERE?	WHAT IS STRENGTHENING?	WHERE COULD I NOTICE TIGHTNESS?	IS COMPRESSION POSSIBLE?
Cylindrical Core activation *More so if the bottom hand is floating rather than resting on the floor or on a block*	Cylindrical Core, fig. 13.17		
Axial extension	Axial extensors, fig. 5.10	Entire trunk	
Shoulder abduction	Shoulder lateral abductors, fig. 6.7	Shoulder lateral adductors, p. 45	
Elbow extension	Elbow extensors, fig. 10.2	Elbow flexors, fig. 10.3	
Standing-leg hip flexion	Standing-leg hip extensors, fig. 7.6 *Hip extensors work eccentrically and/or isometrically to oppose gravity.*		✓ Fig. 7.4
Standing-leg hip lateral rotation	Standing-leg hip lateral rotators, fig. 7.12	Standing-leg hip medial rotators, fig. 7.11	✓ Fig. 7.10
Standing-leg hip abduction	Standing-leg hip abductors, fig. 7.9	Standing-leg hip adductors, fig. 7.8	✓ Fig. 7.7
Lifted-leg hip extension	Lifted-leg hip extensors, fig. 7.6 *Hip extensors work isometrically to stabilize the lifted hip and leg.*	Lifted-leg hip flexors, fig. 7.5	
Knee extension	Knee extensors, fig. 8.2	Knee flexors, fig. 8.3 *Predominantly standing leg*	
Standing ankle stabilization	Standing-leg ankle stabilizers, fig. 9.3, fig. 9.4		
Lifted-leg ankle dorsiflexion	Lifted-leg ankle dorsiflexors, fig. 9.3	Ankle plantar flexors, fig. 9.4	

My discoveries:

Special Considerations

Tilting the body in space can make the anatomical motions a bit confusing at times. Remember that hip joint movements can result from either the femur head rotating within the hip socket or the pelvis rotating about the femur head.

With fatigue or weakness, you may lose Cylindrical Core engagement, resulting in backward-bending collapse.

Your unique hip complex will determine whether or not you can keep your standing toes straight forward while stacking your hips. Skeletal compression in the hip socket may cause your standing toes to turn in while stacking.

You can either flex or point your lifted foot. Flexing engages the muscles on the front of the lower leg, while pointing engages the muscles on the back of the lower leg. The important thing is giving the feet an assignment, so they stay active. Review the muscles of plantar flexion (fig. 9.4) and dorsiflexion (fig. 9.3). This principle applies to many poses.

Here, as in every other posture, we should consider what is happening in the load-bearing joints. The ankle, knee, and hip of the standing leg are holding the body's weight through a vertical line of force. The more active the Cylindrical Core and the reaching foot and hand remain, the less force will be transferred downward. Engaging the outer hip muscles is also key. So, it is important to remain active. If you have any weakness or injury in these weight-bearing joints, it is better to avoid long, one-leg standing postures or sequences of strung-together, one-leg standing postures on the same leg. Only you will know when enough is enough, by paying close attention. Sometimes it is hard to discern, but if you feel yourself fatiguing so weight is collapsing downward, it is time to back out. Or come out for a moment, and then go back in when able.

If you have hip weakness or injury, it is also important not to combine long, one-leg holds with shifting between open-hip and closed-hip positions. An example would be going from a long Half Moon hold to a Standing Split or possibly even to a fold. The combination of fatigue, weight bearing in the hip, and rotating the pelvis down can lead to further degradation of structure in a hip that is already weak or compromised.

Modifications

Keep your top arm resting on your side.

Practice the pose against a wall.

Press your lifted foot into a wall.

Use two blocks instead of one for limited range of motion.

Variations

Try Bound Half Moon, bending your lifted leg to reach back and catch for a bind. If it is difficult to reach, try bringing your lifted knee toward your chest slightly to catch your ankle, foot, or shin. This variation invites in an element of backward bend or spinal extension. Tightness in your front body line, specifically in your hip flexors and quadricep, may limit you.

Exploration/Possible Cues

Explore your skeletal structure. Begin with your standing toes aimed forward. Place your top hand on your hip as you guide this hip to stack over the bottom. Can you achieve stacked hips without your toes moving inward toward the center line? Do you feel a point where you can't go any farther without your supporting foot moving? What does this feel like? Can you tell what is happening within? Is your sturdiest balance point with your foot turned in?

Once sturdy, expand out in all directions. Take up lots of space.

Activate your outer hips, and hover your bottom hand to stay lifted out of your standing hip socket.

Draw your tailbone toward your lifted heel to elongate the lumbar spine.

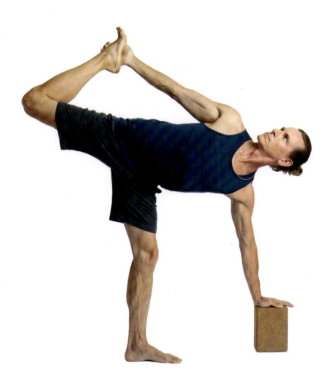

Figure 16.12. Bound Half Moon variation.

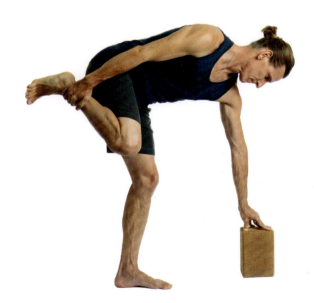

Figure 16.13. Bound Half Moon variation optional setup.

PART THREE | THE POSTURES

Chapter 17
Forward Folds

The Anatomy of Forward Folding

Forward folding entails closing the front of the body, gathering most of the movement from the hip joint. Many postures with forward-folding elements are not discussed in this section, for instance Halfway Lift. Here I've only included those postures having the deepest forward-folding qualities: Standing Forward Fold, Standing Wide-Leg Forward Fold, and Seated Forward Fold. In these poses the legs are straight or slightly bent with maximum front hip flexion. I've also included Boat, a pose not typically considered a forward fold, to broaden your perspective of the relationships between yoga poses.

Forward folding is repeated over and over in most vinyasa classes, so noticing how it is happening in your body is important. As with any other movement, it helps to recognize your unique range of motion. When you stand in Mountain pose and fold forward to touch your toes, two main anatomical actions are occurring, hip flexion and spinal flexion.

Hip Flexion

Hip flexion in forward folding is achieved with torso tilting. (See p. 163 for detailed information on pelvic tilt vs. torso tilt.) Torso tilt involves moving the pelvis and spine together as one unit, maintaining Mountain pose quality in the spine (fig. 13.13). These factors influence the degree of torso tilt:

- The unique shape of the skeletal hip complex will determine how much hip flexion can occur before reaching compression between the hip and the femur (fig. 7.2, fig. 7.3, fig. 7.4).
- Soft-tissue tightness in the back of the hip (hip extensor muscles, fig. 7.6) and along the entire back side of the body will also determine the amount of fold.

Spinal Flexion

Once forward tilt of the torso is maxed out due to skeletal compression in the hip or due to soft-tissue tightness, rounding the spine forward into flexion is the only pathway to folding farther without making adjustments. We will discuss these adjustments below.

We don't want to avoid rounding the spine altogether because spinal flexion can provide

FORWARD FOLDS | CHAPTER 17

a nice stretch to the soft tissues of the back. However, it is best not to bear weight with excessive rounding in the spine. The key is always increasing awareness of your movement patterns. Are you rounding purposefully, or are you unaware that rounding is happening? If you have excessive **kyphosis**, or a rounded spinal posture, it might be best to focus on maintaining a long spine in your folds to train your body into a new pattern.

If lumbar intervertebral disc injury is present, you should primarily avoid lumbar flexion (rounding), especially with any sort of weight bearing, momentum, or force. (See "Intervertebral Disc Herniation," p. 32).

What is your target?

Aim for getting as much torso tilt as possible, and then allow a small amount of spinal flexion as needed, or stay higher in the fold maintaining a long spine. Review the actions of hip flexion (p. 58) and spinal flexion (p. 24).

When initiating any fold, begin with your knees softly bent. This immediately gives you a little slack along your back side. (We could say that there are two main anatomical actions for folding, hip flexion and spinal flexion, along with one supplemental action, knee flexion.) Lead with the anterior tilt of your torso, hinging at your hips. If and when you reach a point of limitation, notice where it is in your body. Chapter 12, "Navigating the Posture," will help you distinguish between tension and compression.

If you determine that compression in the front of the hip joint is stopping you, play with the angles by placing your feet and legs differently. This could mean taking your feet a little wider apart, moving them closer together, or angling them differently. If you realize that soft-tissue tightness is limiting you, try bending your knees even more to find just the right amount of stretch.

Remember, it's fine if you can't feel where the limitation is happening within your body right away. The main thing is to begin feeling and experimenting. Just the act of tuning in to your own sensory experience will increase your ability to be aware on your mat and in all aspects of your life.

PART THREE | THE POSTURES

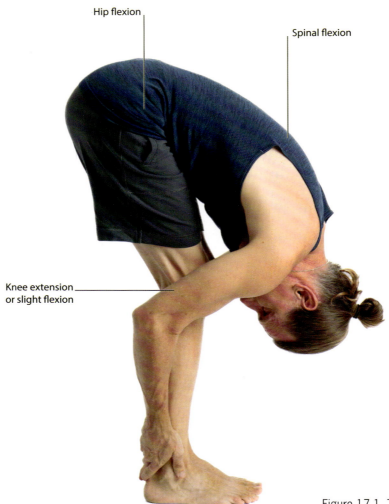

Figure 17.1. The anatomical actions of Standing Forward Fold.

Standing Forward Fold

Standing Forward Fold
Uttanasana

Standing Forward Fold embodies the perfect combination of steadfastness and easiness from the very beginning of a practice. A common linking pose within a yoga flow, it offers leg strengthening along with a total back-body release, spinal traction, internal-organ stimulation, and all the benefits of an inversion.

Begin in Mountain (fig. 13.13). Fold forward by reaching your hips up and back while drawing your spine long and forward. Keep your knees softly bent. Energetically engage the front of your legs to encourage the back of your legs to release. Continue folding until the crown of your head is aiming down. Activate from the soles of your feet up through your hips, and strongly elongate your torso.

FORWARD FOLDS | CHAPTER 17

Standing Forward Fold. What am I feeling?

HOW DO I GET THERE?	WHAT IS STRENGTHENING?	WHERE COULD I NOTICE TIGHTNESS?	IS COMPRESSION POSSIBLE?
Spinal flexion	Spinal flexors, fig. 5.5 Active or passive	**Spinal extensors, fig. 5.3** Entire back body	
Hip flexion	**Hip extensors, fig. 7.6** Hip extensors work eccentrically on the way into the pose to oppose gravity.		✓ Fig. 7.4
Knee extension or slight flexion	**Knee extensors, fig. 8.2** Knee extensors work isometrically in a hold. The more the knees are bent, the more they must work to oppose gravity.	**Knee flexors, fig. 8.3**	

My discoveries:

Special Considerations

The smaller the hip flexion range of motion is, the greater the spinal flexion will be.

If you have hamstring tendonitis (p. 68), it's best to modify this pose by decreasing the angle of hip flexion, avoiding a full fold.

If you have spinal disc injury (p. 32), proceed with caution. You should avoid rounding your spine in the fold. Using blocks under your hands and not going down all the way can help.

Modifications

Place blocks under your hands for the reasons mentioned above.

If you have lots of space between your belly and chest, try bending your knees more, and/or change the angles of your feet. Excess space between your belly and chest is a sure indication that you have maxed out your hip flexion (see "Anatomy of Forward Folding," p. 240).

If you have excess tightness along the back side of your body, bend your knees even more.

PART THREE | **THE POSTURES**

Variations

Rag Doll is a variation of Standing Forward Fold. It is typically a more passive posture, held longer. Keep your legs active with your knees bent while the torso "Rag Dolls" down.

Exploration/Possible Cues

For Standing Forward Fold:

At the bottom of the fold, allow the rounding quality of Cat pose.

Use the active fold to support your exhale.

Exhale dynamically to encourage the fold.

Lift up through your hip creases as you draw your crown down.

Try different hand placements: fingertips to the floor, hands to the outer shins, or hands holding the calves.

Consider...

If you've been to many yoga classes, you may have heard that folding and twisting "massage" the digestive organs. This may not be true for every person, depending on their mobility and unique body shape. But for many people, deep folds and twists may provide a sort of internal squeezing or poking and prodding. Although probably not as intense, these actions are similar to an actual abdominal massage. Research shows that abdominal massage can increase peristalsis, or gut motility, decreasing the discomfort felt with constipation[37].

One frequent claim is that twisting and folding can "wring out toxins." I don't teach this because I haven't seen any science to support it. The fact is, the body has an incredible detoxification system that, in part, involves the liver, kidneys, lungs, skin, and lymphatic system. Yoga can be a wonderful addition to a healthy lifestyle of maintaining the vitality of these organs and supporting the detoxification pathways.

FORWARD FOLDS | CHAPTER 17

For Rag Doll:

Nod your entire torso toward the ground.

Sway a little from side to side to loosen your torso.

Grab your opposite elbows creating a frame around your head.

Find ways to close the space between your belly and chest. This will bring you into more spinal traction.

Clasp your hands behind your back, or use a strap or towel. Let your hands move forward and away from your back, squeezing into your shoulders just a bit.

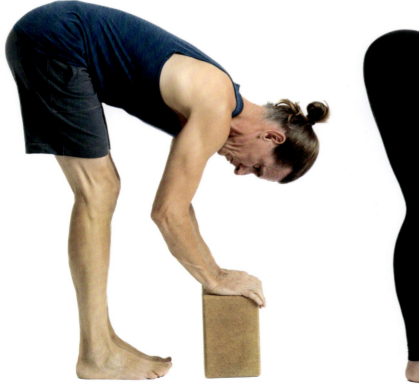

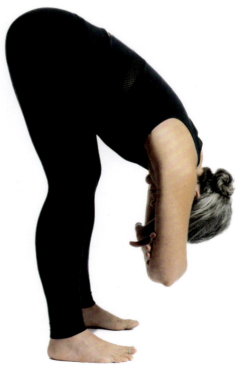

Figure 17.2. Standing Forward Fold modification with blocks under hands and spine actively lifted.

Figure 17.3. Rag Doll.

PART THREE | **THE POSTURES**

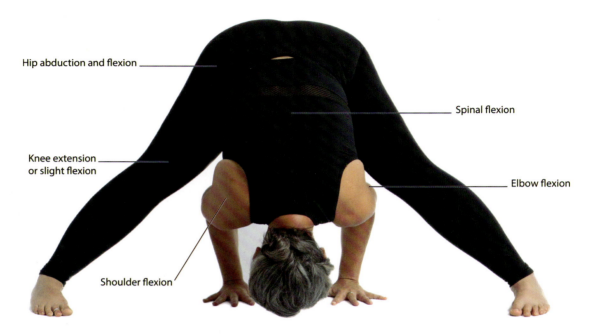

Figure 17.4. The anatomical actions of Standing Wide-Leg Forward Fold.

Standing Wide-Leg Forward Fold

Standing Wide-Leg Forward Fold
Prasarita Padottanasana
Wide-Leg Straddle Fold

This pose provides powerful awakening to the legs and feet. Like other forward bends, Standing Wide-Leg Forward Fold stretches the entire back body while gently massaging the internal organs. It is often offered just at the right time in a strong standing sequence to provide some much-needed inversion and release.

Stand in Five-Pointed Star position facing sideways on your mat. Take your hands to your hips, and turn your feet parallel to the short edges of your mat. As you inhale, elongate up through the crown, and begin actively drawing your hips back. Slowly begin folding forward. Once you are halfway down, pause to energetically elongate your torso. Draw your hips back, and beam your crown forward. This is an example of torso tilting as described on p. 163.

FORWARD FOLDS | CHAPTER 17

Standing Wide-Leg Forward Fold. What am I feeling?

HOW DO I GET THERE?	WHAT IS STRENGTHENING?	WHERE COULD I NOTICE TIGHTNESS?	IS COMPRESSION POSSIBLE?
Axial extension or spinal flexion	Axial extensors, fig. 5.10	Entire trunk	
Spinal flexion	Spinal flexors, fig. 5.5 Active or passive	**Spinal extensors, fig. 5.3** *Entire back body*	
Shoulder flexion	Passive	Shoulder extensors, fig. 6.5	
Hip flexion	**Hip extensors, fig. 7.6** *Hip extensors work eccentrically on the way into the pose to oppose gravity.*		✓ Fig. 7.4
Hip abduction	Hip abductors, fig. 7.9	Hip adductors, fig. 7.8	✓ Fig. 7.7
Knee extension or slight flexion	**Knee extensors, fig. 8.2**	**Knee flexors, fig. 8.3**	
Elbow flexion	Elbow flexors, fig. 10.3 Active or passive	Elbow extensors, fig. 10.2	

My discoveries:

I have highlighted the most common tendencies I see in my students. It is possible to feel strengthening or to notice tightness in any of the muscle groups listed within their respective columns.

Focusing on hinging at your front hip creases, fold the rest of the way down. Aim your crown toward the floor, and place your palms firmly on the ground moving toward 90-degree bends in your arms. Let your elbows point straight back. Use your palms for traction to elongate your spine downward, away from your lifting hips. Stay very active in your feet, lifting your inner arches as your press into your big toes and outer feet edges. Stay engaged in your quadriceps by keeping a lifting action in your knee caps. Steady your gaze on one point, and feel the sensations of your body and breath.

PART THREE | THE POSTURES

Special Considerations

This pose will feel different than regular Standing Forward Fold due to thigh abduction. Some may experience hip-flexion compression in Standing Forward Fold but not in Wide-Leg Forward Fold. This is simply because the angles between the femurs and hips are changed.

Above, I say to begin with your feet parallel to the edges of the mat. If hip skeletal compression is an issue, you may need to angle your toes in or out. I recently had a woman in my teacher training program who had to approach this pose with her toes turned out. She could only flex her hips when she also externally rotated at the hip. We discovered the same pattern in the rest of her poses.

Remember, if you are ever feeling skeletal compression, the solution is to play with the angles of the joint.

Modifications

One way to play with the angles in this pose is varying your foot position, changing the articulation of your femur in the hip socket. Try angling your toes out wider or turning them inward.

Bending your knees can help if the hamstring stretch is too intense or localized. Remember, bending your knees will release the entire back side of your body.

Place blocks under your hands if you want to avoid going deeply into the fold.

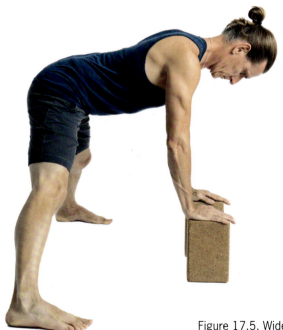

Figure 17.5. Wide-Leg Forward Fold modification with blocks under hands and active spine.

FORWARD FOLDS | CHAPTER 17

Variations

Clasping your hands behind your back can offer a beneficial anterior-shoulder and chest opening.

You can move into Side Lunges from this pose.

Combine this pose with Goddess pose for a nice variation.

Exploration/Possible Cues

Play with the placement of your feet to get the most traction down and forward through your spine. Your feet can be closer together or farther apart, and your toes can angle more or less in either direction.

As you inhale, light up the strength of your legs; as you exhale, release down through your crown.

Let the weight of your head go.

Can you feel the weight of your head providing traction to your upper spine? Middle spine? Lower spine?

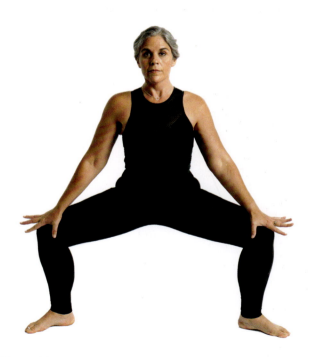

Figure 17.6. Goddess pose.

PART THREE | THE POSTURES

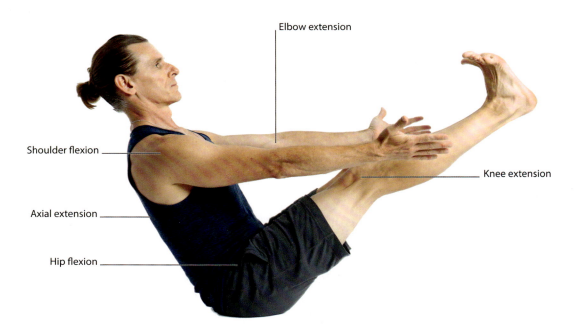

Figure 17.7. The anatomical actions of Boat pose.

Boat

Boat
Navasana
Paripurna Navasana

Although we don't often think of this balance pose as a forward fold, it is. Because it entails a very different gravitational relationship between the trunk, the legs, and the floor, the Cylindrical Core (fig. 13.17) must fire up to support the body in space. This builds significant core strength.

Begin seated with your knees bent and your feet flat on the floor. Hold on to the backs of both thighs. Lengthen from your tailbone to crown as in Mountain. Remain actively lifted through your chest. While slowly leaning back, lift your feet off the ground until your lower legs are parallel to the floor. Energetically reach through your feet and toes. Release your hands, reaching forward while you straighten your legs as much as possible. As you do this, you may need to lean back a little more to stay balanced. Your torso and legs should form a near-45-degree angle with the ground. Your body will look like a V from the side. Remain actively engaged in your legs and trunk while extending longer through your crown and your feet. Keep your chest lifted to avoid collapse. Set your gaze ahead, and breathe into the strength of your body.

FORWARD FOLDS | CHAPTER 17

Boat. What am I feeling?

HOW DO I GET THERE?	WHAT IS STRENGTHENING?	WHERE COULD I NOTICE TIGHTNESS?	IS COMPRESSION POSSIBLE?
Axial extension	Axial extensors, fig. 5.10	Entire trunk	
Hip flexion	Hip flexors, fig. 7.5	Hip extensors, fig. 7.6	
Knee extension	Knee extensors, fig. 8.2 *Even if knees are bent, the activation is toward extension in opposition to gravity.*	Knee flexors, fig. 8.3	
Elbow extension	Elbow extensors, fig. 10.2	Elbow flexors, fig. 10.3	
Shoulder flexion	Shoulder flexors, fig. 6.4	Shoulder extensors, fig. 6.5	
Cylindrical Core activation	Cylindrical Core, fig. 13.17		

My discoveries:

Special Considerations

Whether it is genetic or due to some sort of trauma, occasionally the shape and orientation of the coccyx (tailbone) can make it very difficult to balance in Boat. In this case, you may be able to lean farther back to bear weight differently, or you may need to avoid the pose altogether.

Refer to the Cylindrical Core section (fig. 13.17). Remember, any time the spine is not stacked vertically over the hips or over the hips and legs, more demand is placed on the trunk muscles to support the spine. Activate your Cylindrical Core in Boat to avoid possible forward rounding and collapse of the spine.

Modifications

You can reduce the muscular demand of Boat by keeping your knees bent and/or by holding the backs of your thighs.

Variations

Different arm positions slightly shift the demand in the core. Try lifting your arms, taking them out to the sides, or even clasping your hands in front of you while reaching toward your feet.

Exploration/Possible Cues

Lift the center of your chest like raising a sail.

Keep the periphery of the pose bright, fingertips and toe tips electric.

Your unique structure might require leaning back a little more or less to find balance. Experiment.

Keep your head directly in line with your spine. Don't let it drop forward.

Maintain strong Mountain alignment in your spine.

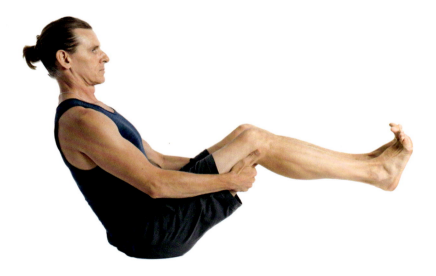

Figure 17.8. Boat modification with hands holding thighs and knees bent.

FORWARD FOLDS | CHAPTER 17

What I am looking for is not out there, it is in me.
—Helen Keller

PART THREE | THE POSTURES

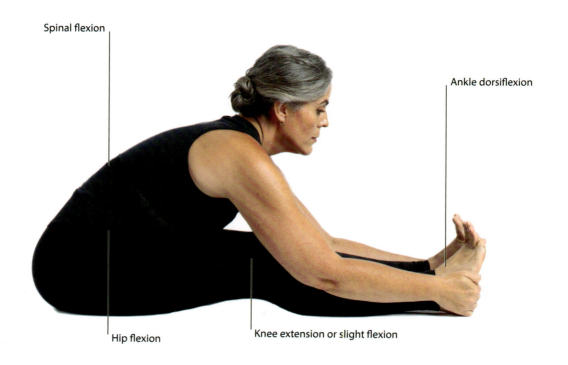

Figure 17.9. The anatomical actions of Seated Forward Fold.

Seated Forward Fold

Seated Forward Fold
Paschimottanasana

The ground supports us in Seated Forward Fold. This can invoke a sense of nurturing and inward focus. Like the standing forward folds, seated folds offer release of the back body and increased awareness of the inner body as you press your abdomen toward or into your legs.

Begin seated with your legs outstretched in front of you, feet about hip-width distance apart. Activate and flex your feet as you extend your legs nice and long. Sit up tall, and reach your arms up overhead. Tilt the front of your hip points forward, and draw your sit bones back. Use torso tilt to begin the fold. Once you can't tilt any farther, you have the option to stay there with an elongated spine. Grab your feet if you can reach them, or loop a strap or towel around them. Continue lifting your chest up and out of your hips, and activate your shoulders back and down. Another option is to allow some passive rounding in your spine as you relax your arms and head. Get still, and enjoy the sensation. Remember, as long as you are feeling it, you are doing enough. A little stretch goes a long way.

FORWARD FOLDS | CHAPTER 17

Seated Forward Fold. What am I feeling?

HOW DO I GET THERE?	WHAT IS STRENGTHENING?	WHERE COULD I NOTICE TIGHTNESS?	IS COMPRESSION POSSIBLE?
Axial extension or spinal flexion	**Axial extensors, fig. 5.10** *In active variation*	Entire trunk	
Spinal flexion	*Passive*	**Spinal extensors, fig. 5.3**	
Hip flexion	Hip flexors, fig. 7.5 *Passive*	**Hip extensors, fig. 7.6**	✓ Fig. 7.4
Knee extension or slight flexion	Knee extensors, fig. 8.2 *Active or passive*	**Knee flexors, fig. 8.3**	
Ankle dorsiflexion	Ankle dorsiflexors, fig. 9.3 *Active or passive*	**Ankle plantar flexors, fig. 9.4**	

My discoveries:

Special Considerations

It is best to avoid lumbar flexion/rounding if you have intervertebral disc injury.

If you have hamstring tendonitis, avoid this pose.

Modifications

Bend your knees.

Place a block or rolled towel behind the backs of your knees.

Loop a strap or towel around your feet.

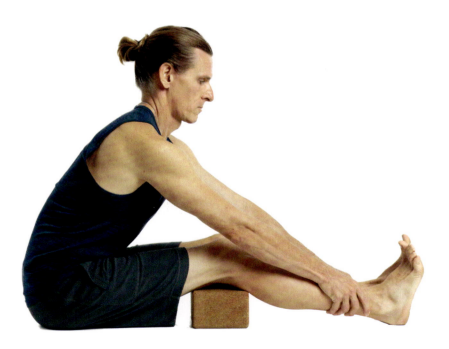

Figure 17.10. Seated Forward Fold modification with blocks under knees.

FORWARD FOLDS | CHAPTER 17

Variations

Wide-Leg Seated Forward Fold is the same pose with legs spread wide in a V shape. Most people will experience quite a difference when they change the relationship between their femurs and hips. If you have limited hip flexion due to skeletal compression in regular Seated Forward Fold, this position may provide some relief.

Exploration/Possible Cues

Before folding, reach your legs so strongly forward that your heels lift off the ground.

As you fold, draw both front hip creases back evenly as if you are reaching your sitting bones back behind you.

Lead with your pelvis.

Try pointing and then flexing your feet; notice the different sensations.

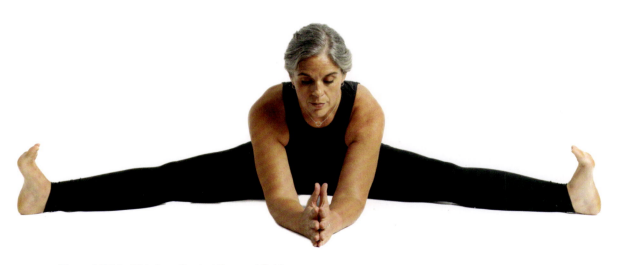

Figure 17.11. Wide-Leg Seated Forward Fold.

PART THREE | THE POSTURES

The success of Yoga does not lie in the ability to perform postures but in how it positively changes the way we live our life and our relationships.
—T. K. V. Desikachar

Chapter 18

Backward Bends

The Anatomy of Backbending

Backward bending, or spinal extension, is one of the unique musculoskeletal actions that makes yoga extremely beneficial. Texting, driving, working on the computer—most of our daily actions—require forward reaching or rounding. We can think of backbends as the much-needed counter stretch to life.

Let's look at a few elements helpful to understanding how to backbend safely and effectively.

How do we access backbends?

As with all postures, our body gathers range of motion from several places, but two predominant anatomical actions are required for backbends: hip extension and spinal extension.

Hip Extension (p. 60)

All backbend postures require hip extension, or opening the front of the hip joint. Your unique hip structure will determine how much range of motion you have with hip extension. Both skeletal and soft-tissue components will contribute. (See figures 7.4 and 7.6 for the anatomical action of hip extension.)

Spinal Extension (p. 22)

As the spine extends, the spinous processes will eventually compress against each other allowing no deeper movement. The backbend is predominantly gathered from the lumbar spine with the most range of motion typically between the eleventh thoracic vertebra and the first lumbar vertebra, or the **thoracolumbar junction**. The lumbar spine is much more mobile with extension than the thoracic spine. Even so, aim to extend your entire spine in the backbend, encouraging whatever thoracic spinal mobility you have because we tend to lose this range of motion if we don't use it. When the thoracic spine is excessively immobile, too much pressure can land in the lumbar spine with extension. The uniqueness of your skeleton,

PART THREE | THE POSTURES

specifically how much space exists between the spinous processes, will primarily determine what your spine looks like in extension. Any tightness on the body's front side will also limit spinal extension. (See figures 5.2 and 5.3 for the anatomical action of spinal extension.)

The Components of a Healthy Backbend

Conservative Lumbar Spinal Extension

Sometimes it is difficult to feel what is happening within the details of your body, but cultivating this ability is at the heart of Embodied Posture alignment. When we learn how to intimately listen to what our body is telling us, we tune in to another level of wisdom from within. Feeling the spine's positioning is a sense that takes time to develop. Because the pelvis is skeletally linked to the spine through the sacrum (fig. 5.15), we can gauge the positioning of the spine—especially the lumbar spine—by focusing on the pelvis; you can't move your pelvis without also moving your spine. Moving the lumbar spine toward extension or backward bending equals anterior tilt of the pelvis (fig. 14.6). In this position, the lumbar spinous processes move closer together.

To avoid injury, do not push to maximum ranges of motion in every pose, especially when force and/or weight bearing are involved. In backward bends, maxing out spinal range of motion involves compressing the spinous processes together while using the legs and/or arms to add forced pressure. Since the lumbar spine has more ability to extend than the thoracic spine, students tend to push to extremes there with full anterior pelvic tilt.

One way to minimize lumbar extension is to tilt the pelvis posteriorly before moving into the backbend. Posterior tilt of the pelvis (fig 14.5) equals moving the lumbar spine toward flexion or rounding while actively engaging the lower abdominals. In this position, the spinous processes move farther apart. It is structurally impossible to remain in a strong posterior tilt while backward bending, but this initial action will keep you from forcibly pushing directly into maximum lumbar compression.

The second way to maintain lumbar spine spaciousness is to focus on making the pose longer (fig. 18.1) from front to back by increasing the distance between your chest and legs.

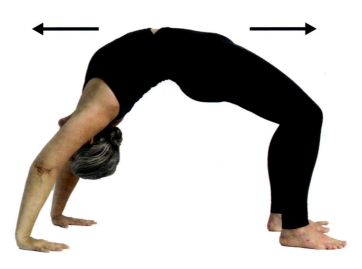

Figure 18.1. Wheel pose with arrows showing directions of activation.

This will keep you from pressing farther and farther into the lumbar spine which happens when you aim to take the pose higher, as in Bridge or Wheel.

When extension of the lumbar spine is minimized in these two ways, the thoracic spine is encouraged toward more extension and greater mobility. Due to lifestyles and biomechanics, many people lose thoracic spine mobility over time.[38] Being conservative with lumbar extension encourages thoracic extension and sustained spinal mobility. Train your body to do this.

Stable Leg Positioning

To honor your unique pelvic structure in any pose, place your feet and/or legs so that they support the shape of your hip joints. This relates to foot placement in poses like Bridge and Wheel, but to leg or knee placement in poses like Camel, Bow, or Up Dog. Hip-width distance apart is a good starting place. You may find that feet or legs slightly wider is better for you. Optimal foot placement depends on your soft tissues and on your unique bone shapes and orientations. In Bridge or Wheel, toes straight forward may work best for some, but toes slightly angled out may be better for others. (Refer to chapter 12, "Navigating the Posture.") Toes angled out slightly doesn't mean that your knees and legs are splayed out widely; that can put excessive pressure on the sacroiliac joints (fig. 5.15). Whatever foot and leg placement you choose, actively pressing toward your inner arches will keep your legs from externally rotating or splaying. Finding your ideal leg placement is where pose *embodiment* comes into play. You will know you are there when you *feel* stable and strong. As with all poses, keeping a curious, investigative approach to your alignment is key.

Balanced Strength

Most backbends contain an element of leveraged force, such as pressing with the hands and feet in Wheel. Relying solely on leveraged force, or just pushing into the backbend, causes an unsupported spine that is probably maxed out in its range of motion. Moderately engaging the muscles of spinal and hip extension will produce a much more stable, functional pose. (Review the muscles of spinal extension [fig. 5.3] and hip extension [fig. 7.6].) Activating both the glutes and the back muscles to encourage the backward bend is more structurally supportive than just forcefully pushing into the posture with the hands and feet. To further protect the lumbar spine from overextension, also engage the lower abdominals or lower spinal flexors. You will need to feel your way into this coordination of front- and back-body strength. Remember, some hip extensor muscles are also external rotators. Pressing your big toes and inner arches down will counter any possible external rotation of your legs. Stability is your goal.

In postures like Bridge (fig. 18.14), and Wheel (fig. 18.21), the legs are moving toward knee extension due to the body's position in space and the required actions, so the quadriceps will be firing. Hip extension also stretches the quadriceps muscles. This can get tricky. The aim is not to over-engage the quadriceps, but to balance them with the hip extensors. The only way to know how much to engage or release is to listen to your body and experiment. Develop a strong sense of interoceptive awareness, feeling from within.

PART THREE | THE POSTURES

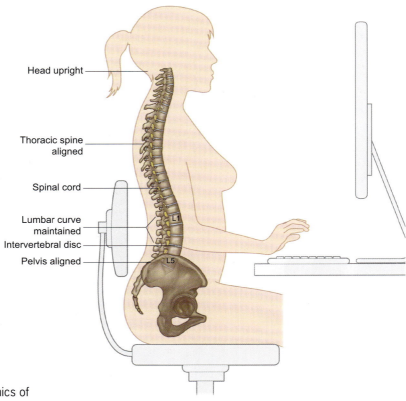

Figure 18.2. Biomechanics of healthy seated posture.

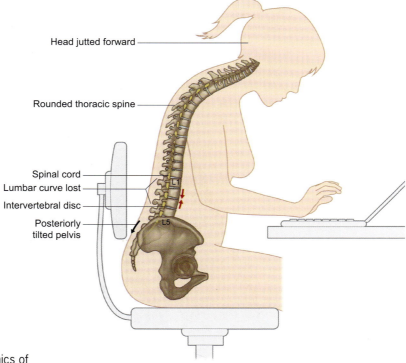

Figure 18.3. Biomechanics of unhealthy seated posture.

BACKWARD BENDS | CHAPTER 18

Consider...

Overall musculoskeletal balance should be a primary objective of yoga class sequencing. If long-term functional wellness is the goal, common lifestyle tendencies and resulting postural patterns must be considered. Most of us would agree that prolonged sitting is almost unavoidable in our culture. Even if you are lucky enough to have a job that doesn't require sitting most of the day, you probably use some sort of technological device that affects your posture.

Many say that sitting is the new smoking, causing back pain and detrimentally affecting health. Others say that even the hunter-gatherers sat for extended periods, but in that era people also engaged in more high-intensity physical activity. Is it possible that it's not sitting itself that causes back pain, but rather it's the way we sit? The hunter-gatherers presumably sat on the ground or on rocks. Now we have all sorts of cushy, comfy chairs. However, we can't simply focus on one lifestyle aspect to determine what provokes back issues or other physical maladies. Whether or not we sit, how often we sit, and how we sit are just pieces of this puzzle.

Regardless of the history of sitting, the human body works through the principle of tensional integrity (p. 32). Imbalanced structure leads to imbalanced load bearing, which then leads to eventual degradation if not corrected. Sitting can shorten and tighten the body's front side while the back side loosens and becomes increasingly lax. This muscular imbalance profoundly affects our skeletal structural balance.

Consider the effects of the head being held in a chronically jutted-forward position.[39] The human head weighs ten to eleven pounds, a heavy load to bear—especially if it is off balance. Notice the postures of those sitting around you. Chances are, they are in rounded-forward postures with their shoulders turned forward, heads forward, and spines rounded (fig. 18.4). This spinal flexion (fig. 5.4) puts pressure on the posterior, or back side, of the intervertebral discs (fig. 5.11).[40] Years and years of this pressure will weaken the back side of the discs, putting them at risk for herniation (fig. 5.12). Consequently, my first suggestions to anyone with back pain are to sit less and to change the way they are sitting. The best yoga program in the world can't compete with excessive time spent in a slouched seated posture.

Start revamping your sitting style by focusing on the pelvis. Most people sit with their pelvis in a posterior tilt (fig. 14.5), or tailbone tucked under. Shift your tailbone back toward an anterior tilt (fig. 14.6) without overdoing it. This will bring natural curvature into your low spine, so the rest of the spine will stack beautifully. It is difficult to sit in a slouched-forward position when the pelvis is aligned properly (fig. 18.2). Along with changing the way you sit, pay more attention to the nuances of how you are holding your body while using your smartphone (fig. 18.4). Little imbalances can add up over time, causing upper-back, shoulder, neck, and head pain.[41] Refrain from jutting your head forward. Hold your phone higher, sit up taller, and balance your head on top of your spine. Awareness is key.

In addition to your new and improved sitting and tech habits, here are some ideas to help balance your body with yoga:

> 1. Practice postures that require engaging the back muscles, including Locust variations, Halfway Lift, Airplane variations, and Warrior III.

> 2. Experiment with more hip extensor engagement (fig. 7.6) in backward bends and in asymmetrical standing postures, for example with the back extended leg in High Lunge (fig. 14.1).

PART THREE | THE POSTURES

> 3. Do more shoulder extension (fig. 6.5) poses to stretch the anterior deltoids, pectoralis major, and biceps brachii, while firing the posterior deltoids, latissimus dorsi, and triceps.
>
> 4. Incorporate more lunge-type postures to stretch the iliopsoas (fig. 18.5) and other muscles of hip flexion (fig. 7.5).
>
> 5. Practice neck strengthening and stretcheimg, targeting the muscles shown in figure 18.4.
>
> 6. Pay more attention to scapular activations (p. 54-55) to stay mobile and strong in the upper back.
>
> I certainly don't think yoga can fix everything. The best solution might be to include more variety of movement on and off the mat. If you do lots of yoga, try adding in various physical activities with different approaches to strengthening. Take your yoga into the weight room, out on the bike, or into a Pilates class. Yoga is truly a state of mind; it can be practiced with any activity, and varied movement might be exactly what your unique body needs to restore and maintain balance.

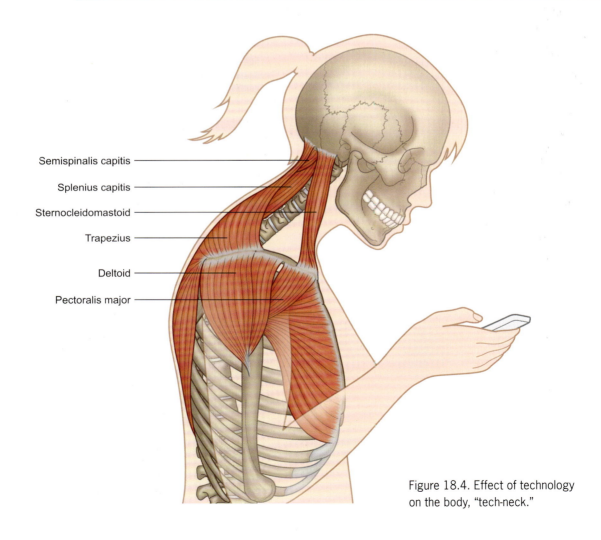

Figure 18.4. Effect of technology on the body, "tech-neck."

BACKWARD BENDS | CHAPTER 18

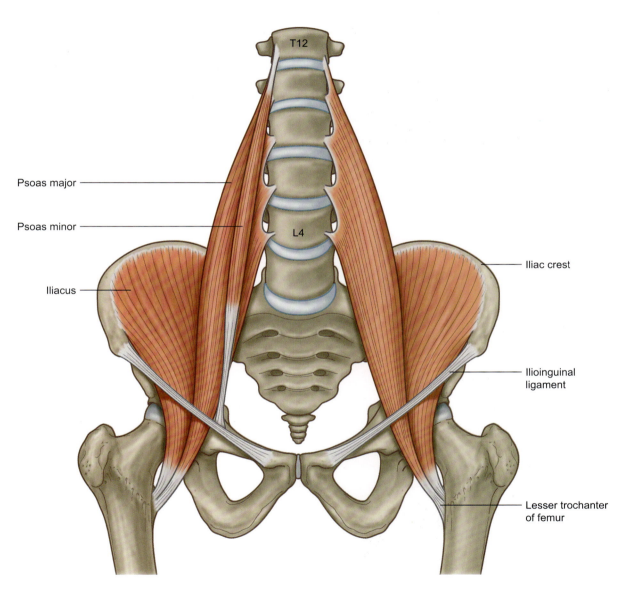

Figure 18.5. Anterior view of the iliopsoas.

PART THREE | THE POSTURES

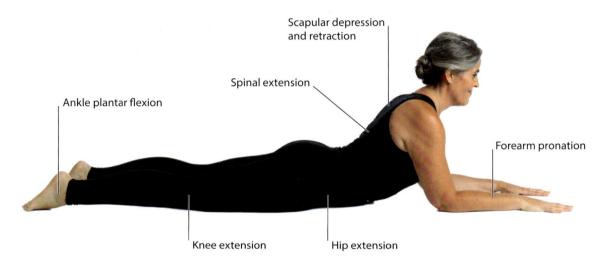

Figure 18.6. The anatomical actions of Sphinx.

Sphinx

Sphinx
Salamba Bhujangasana

Sphinx is a passive pose. Consequently, it has quite a different energy than many other backbends, providing the therapeutic benefits of extension in a restorative way.

Begin lying face down. Lift yourself onto your forearms with your elbows underneath your shoulders. Allow your legs to rest naturally at hip width with your feet face down. Engage your shoulders slightly, keeping them back and down, but remain passive everywhere else in your body. Breathe deeply while allowing your spine to relax into the backbend.

BACKWARD BENDS | CHAPTER 18

Sphinx. What am I feeling?

HOW DO I GET THERE?	WHAT IS STRENGTHENING?	WHERE COULD I NOTICE TIGHTNESS?	IS COMPRESSION POSSIBLE?
Spinal extension	Passive	Spinal flexors, fig. 5.5	
Hip extension	Passive	Hip flexors, fig. 7.5	
Knee extension	Passive	Knee flexors, fig. 8.3	
Scapular depression and retraction	Depressors and retractors of the scapulae, p. 54	Elevators and protractors of the scapulae, p. 54	
Elbow flexion	Passive		
Forearm pronation	Forearm pronators, fig. 10.5	Forearm supinators, fig. 10.4	
Ankle plantar flexion	Passive	Ankle dorsiflexors, fig. 9.3	

My discoveries:

Special Considerations

Back or shoulder injury can limit this pose.

This pose offers effortless backward bending, accessible by most practitioners when other backbends are not.

If you have low-back pain with this pose, engaging your gluteal muscles might help you stabilize and find relief. If not, avoid Sphinx altogether.

While you must strongly engage your legs in other backbends, this is unnecessary in Sphinx due to the minimal spinal extension.

Modifications

Slide your elbows farther forward to lessen the backward bend.

Place blocks under your arms for different levels of backbend.

Variations

Seal (fig. 18.8) is the same pose with increased spinal extension. From Sphinx, walk your hands forward, and straighten your arms.

Exploration/Possible Cues

Think of your arms as pillars, and let the rest of your body drape softly.

Do this pose with as little effort as possible.

Place your gaze wherever needed to keep tension out of your neck and face.

Visualize the shape of your spine in backward bend.

Visualize the shape of the lumbar discs in this position.

Send breath into the back side of your body.

Relax.

BACKWARD BENDS | CHAPTER 18

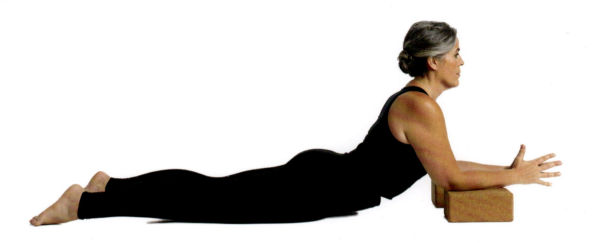

Figure 18.7. Sphinx modification with block under elbows.

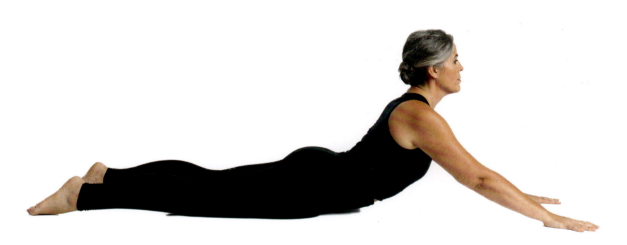

Figure 18.8. Seal.

PART THREE | THE POSTURES

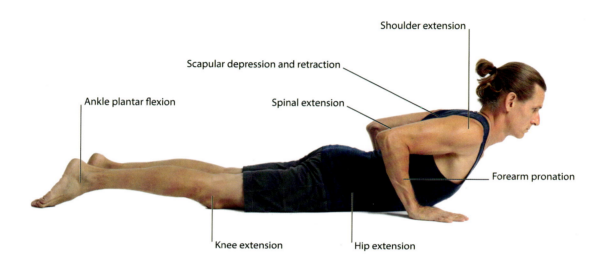

Figure 18.9. The anatomical actions of Cobra.

Cobra

Cobra
Bhujangasana

Cobra is often offered as an Upward-Facing Dog (fig. 18.13) modification, but don't let its "passive" reputation fool you. Because your elbows typically remain more bent, holding it requires greater strength in the back. Only spinal and hip extension are reduced.

Begin lying face down. Place your hands underneath your shoulders with your fingers spread wide and stable. Wrap your arms and shoulders back to activate your back muscles. Pull your chest forward and through. With the tops of your feet down and near hip-width distance apart, activate them by pressing downward. Strongly press your legs and pubis into the floor, and lift your chest higher. Maintain a moderate bend in your elbows. Aim your eyes and chest straight forward.

BACKWARD BENDS | CHAPTER 18

Cobra. What am I feeling?

HOW DO I GET THERE?	WHAT IS STRENGTHENING?	WHERE COULD I NOTICE TIGHTNESS?	IS COMPRESSION POSSIBLE?
Spinal extension	**Spinal extensors, fig. 5.3**	Spinal flexors, fig. 5.5	Since the arms are bent, the likelihood of meeting skeletal compression here is low.
Hip extension	Hip extensors, fig. 7.6	Hip flexors, fig. 7.5	
Shoulder extension	**Shoulder extensors, fig. 6.5**	**Shoulder flexors, fig. 6.4**	
Scapular depression and retraction	**Depressors and retractors of the scapulae, p. 54**	Elevators and protractors of the scapulae, p. 54	
Forearm pronation	Forearm pronators, fig. 10.5	Forearm supinators, fig. 10.4	
Knee extension	**Knee extensors, fig. 8.2**	Knee flexors, fig. 8.3	
Ankle plantar flexion	Ankle plantar flexors, fig. 9.4	Ankle dorsiflexors, fig. 9.3	

My discoveries:

Special Considerations

Back or shoulder injury can limit this pose.

As with most backbends, keep your legs active. In poses like this, students tend to leave their legs inactively resting on the floor. This can lead to lumbar spine instability.

In all backbends, try to keep the lower abdomen slightly engaged. This engagement, combined with anchoring the pubis down, will maintain healthy space within your lumbar spine.

Modifications

Keep your chest lower.

Bend your elbows less.

Try Sphinx (fig. 18.6) instead.

Variations

You can vary how much you bend your elbows, changing the amount of spinal extension or backward bend.

Simply lifting to claw fingertips will also change the overall dynamic of the pose.

Exploration/Possible Cues

Use your connectivity to the ground to focus on your leg strength.

Feel the direct correlation between how much you straighten your arms and how your spine feels moving into extension. Play with tiny lifts and lowers to change this sensation.

Use this opportunity to build strength and balance in your posterior muscles.

Activate your hands like you are drawing your mat back.

Beam your chest forward like a spotlight.

BACKWARD BENDS | CHAPTER 18

PART THREE | THE POSTURES

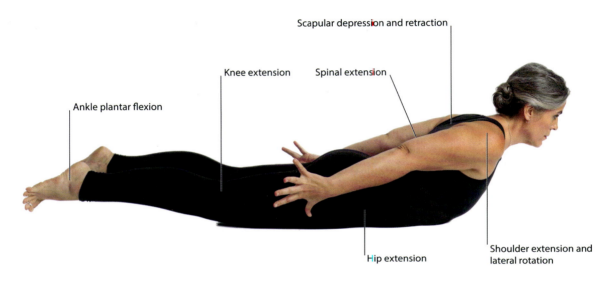

Figure 18.10. The anatomical actions of Locust.

Locust

Locust
Salabhasana

Locust offers essential back-body strengthening to counter all the front-body strengthening in most yoga classes. We work hard building our pushing muscles, often neglecting our pulling muscles. Because many of us also spend a great deal of time sitting, we need to balance our functional strength by incorporating exercises that spark and tone the posterior body.

Begin lying face down with your arms back like Airplane Wings, palms facing the floor. Lift your arms and upper body off the floor. Further engage your back muscles by drawing your shoulder blades back, down, and slightly together. Draw your sacrum and tailbone toward your feet. Lift your legs off the floor while engaging your glutes, hamstrings, and calves. Keep your big toes pointing straight back, countering any external action from the glute activation. Keep your neck nice and long while gazing forward to the floor ahead of your mat.

BACKWARD BENDS | CHAPTER 18

Locust. What am I feeling?

HOW DO I GET THERE?	WHAT IS STRENGTHENING?	WHERE COULD I NOTICE TIGHTNESS?	IS COMPRESSION POSSIBLE?
Spinal extension	**Spinal extensors, fig. 5.3**	Spinal flexors, fig. 5.5	*It is unlikely that you would push into skeletal compression with spinal extension since there is no leveraged force in this backbend.*
Hip extension	**Hip extensors, fig. 7.6**	Hip flexors, fig. 7.5	
Knee extension	**Knee extensors, fig. 8.2**	Knee flexors, fig. 8.3	
Shoulder extension	**Shoulder extensors, fig. 6.5**	Shoulder flexors, fig. 6.4	
Scapular depression and retraction	**Depressors and retractors of the scapulae, p. 54**	Elevators and protractors of the scapulae, p. 54	
Shoulder lateral rotation	**Shoulder lateral rotators, fig. 6.14**	**Shoulder medial rotators, fig. 6.11**	
Forearm supination	Forearm supinators, fig. 10.4	Forearm pronators, fig. 10.5	
Ankle plantar flexion	Ankle plantar flexors, fig. 9.4	Ankle dorsiflexors, fig. 9.3	

My discoveries:

Special Considerations

Locust is unique because it doesn't rely on leveraged force like most other backward bends. It relies solely on back-body engagement.

I always try to include this pose in my daily practice. It not only increases my strength in the moment, but it also reminds me to keep my upper back active while I am going through my day, sitting at the computer, driving, etc.

Tightness in the anterior deltoids and pectoralis major (fronts of shoulders and chest) will make facing the palms down in this pose somewhat challenging. Keeping palms face-down and stretching the thumbs back and away from the chest is a great release for front-body tightness that commonly results from sitting and working with the shoulders rounded forward.

Modifications

If you have discomfort in your hip bones or pubis, fold your mat, or use alternative padding.

Keep your hands on the floor, and/or don't lift as high if your strength is limited.

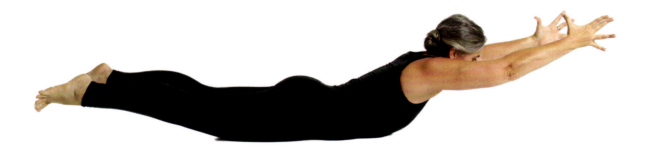

Figure 18.11. Locust variation with Superman arms.

Variations

Vary your arm position. These long levers can change the physics and effort required with any pose when you move them.

Add a dynamic flutter kick with your legs and feet to challenge your back-body strength.

Exploration/Possible Cues

Use all the muscles on the back side of your body to open and lift the front side.

Find greater distance between your fingertips and the center of your chest.

Play with allowing your legs to externally rotate from strong glute activation. Then combine a slight internal rotation by pushing back evenly through your big toes.

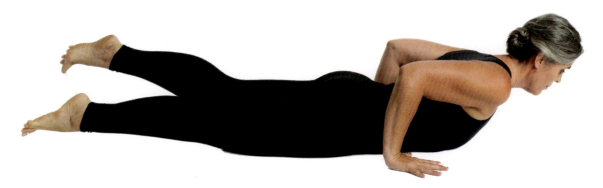

Figure 18.12. Locust variation with flutter kick legs.

PART THREE | THE POSTURES

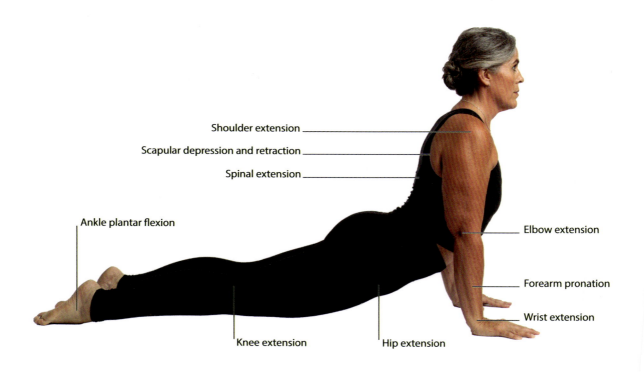

Figure 18.13. The anatomical actions of Upward-Facing Dog.

Upward-Facing Dog

Upward-Facing Dog
Urdhva Mukha Svanasana

Upward-Facing Dog strengthens the back, upper body, and legs, while opening the chest, abdomen, and hip flexors.

Begin lying face down. Place your palms on the floor outside of your ribs (see Special Considerations below). Aim your elbows straight back. Press your palms into the floor, and draw your chest forward. Keep your elbows slightly bent. Press the ground away, and activate your shoulders back and down, taking them away from your ears. Draw your tailbone toward your heels while engaging your lower abdominals. Activate your legs, pushing the tops of your feet into the floor and lifting your knees up off the ground. Gaze straight ahead, and keep the back of your neck nice and long. Shine your heart straight forward.

BACKWARD BENDS | CHAPTER 18

Upward-Facing Dog. What am I feeling?

HOW DO I GET THERE?	WHAT IS STRENGTHENING?	WHERE COULD I NOTICE TIGHTNESS?	IS COMPRESSION POSSIBLE?
Spinal extension	Spinal extensors, fig. 5.3	Spinal flexors, fig. 5.5	✓ Fig. 5.2
Hip extension	Hip extensors, fig. 7.6	Hip flexors, fig. 7.5	
Shoulder extension	Shoulder extensors, fig. 6.5	Shoulder flexors, fig. 6.4	
Scapular depression and retraction	Depressors and retractors of the scapulae, p. 54	Elevators and protractors of the scapulae, p. 54	
Elbow extension	Elbow extensors, fig. 10.2	Elbow flexors, fig. 10.3	
Wrist extension	Wrist extensors, fig. 11.2	Wrist flexors, fig. 11.3	
Forearm pronation	Forearm pronators, fig. 10.5	Forearm supinators, fig. 10.4	
Knee extension	Knee extensors, fig. 8.2	Knee flexors, fig. 8.3	
Ankle plantar flexion	Ankle plantar flexors, fig. 9.4	Ankle dorsiflexors, fig. 9.3	✓ Fig. 9.2

My discoveries:

PART THREE | THE POSTURES

Special Considerations

Back, wrist, shoulder, ankle, or foot injury can limit this pose.

To protect your low back, always engage your legs, even if you are not lifting your knees off the floor.

A slight lower-abdominal engagement will keep your tailbone lengthened toward your heels, maintaining spaciousness in the lumbar spine.

Always keep a soft bend in your elbows. When you lock out your elbows, you diminish the range of motion in your shoulders and put excess strain on your joints.

If your knees are staying on the floor, allow more bend in your elbows to lessen the degree of backbend.

In part, your degree of spinal extension will determine where you place your hands for this pose. The farther back you place them, the greater the demand on your spine. Aim for a placement that does not overextend your wrists, that keeps a nice vertical line from wrists to shoulders, and that feels appropriate for your spine.

Modifications

Sphinx is an option (fig. 18.6).

Come into Cobra instead (fig. 18.9).

Vary the degree you bend your arms.

Keep your knees on the ground while building strength.

Variation

Loop a strap around your thighs above your knees. Make sure it is snug. Strongly abduct your thighs by pressing outward into the strap. Elongate your spine up and away from the strength in your legs. You can keep the strap on for Downward Dog, Plank, Low Push-up, Upward Dog, and back. This is a great way to fire up the often-forgotten hip abductors.

BACKWARD BENDS | CHAPTER 18

Exploration/Possible Cues

Whichever variation you are doing, keep your legs very active.

Engage all your leg muscles, including your glutes.

Telescope your spine forward and away from your legs.

Don't lock out your elbows; keep them soft.

Take your shoulder blades toward your back pockets.

Draw the floor back with your hands while pulling your chest forward and through.

Gather space from the entire length of your spine.

PART THREE | THE POSTURES

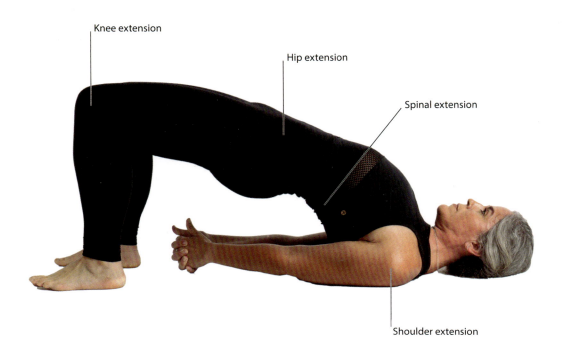

Figure 18.14. The anatomical actions of Bridge.

Bridge

Bridge
Setu Bandha Sarvangasana

Like all backward bends, Bridge opens the entire front side of the body and strengthens the back side. It is quite variable since it can be an active, working pose or a more passive, restorative posture.

From your back, bend your knees until your heels are close to your seat. Have your feet near hip-width distance apart. Draw your sacrum and tailbone toward your knees as you activate your feet and quadriceps to lift your hips up off the ground. Maintain fiery leg engagement, including glute activation. Anchor down through your big toes to counter any external rotation. Leave your arms by your sides, or interlace your hands underneath your body for anterior-shoulder and chest opening.

BACKWARD BENDS | CHAPTER 18

Bridge. What am I feeling?

HOW DO I GET THERE?	WHAT IS STRENGTHENING?	WHERE COULD I NOTICE TIGHTNESS?	IS COMPRESSION POSSIBLE?
Spinal extension	**Spinal extensors, fig. 5.3**	**Spinal flexors, fig. 5.5**	✓ Fig. 5.2
Hip extension	**Hip extensors, fig. 7.6**	**Hip flexors, fig. 7.5**	
Shoulder extension	Shoulder extensors, fig. 6.5	**Shoulder flexors, fig. 6.4**	
Elbow extension	Elbow extensors, fig. 10.2	Elbow flexors, fig. 10.3	
Knee extension	**Knee extensors, fig. 8.2** Although the knees are typically bent, extension is the action that lifts the pose off the ground and into action. During the hold, the extensors engage isometrically.		

My discoveries:

PART THREE | THE POSTURES

Special Considerations

To understand how the intervertebral disks respond to spinal extension/backward bending, review chapter 5, "The Spine" (fig. 5.2).

Resist the urge to push higher and higher. You will lift to a natural height, but then it is better to work toward lengthening the pose. Going higher will only unduly compress the lumbar spine.

Maintain a slight lower-abdominal engagement. This will help you avoid overextending the lumbar spine.

The muscles on the back side of your body are the prime workers to open the front side of your body. Experiment to find the perfect engagement to strengthen and awaken these muscles, combining that with quadriceps engagement. As always, it is a balancing act. Your unique body will determine where you engage more and where you release more.

Outer-knee pain in this pose may possibly be caused by hip-abductor imbalance and/or tight Iliotibial bands (fig. 7.9).

Although the knees are typically flexed in this pose, to activate toward lengthening, the muscles responsible for straightening the knee (knee extensors) will activate. Also, consider the position you begin in on the floor with knees very flexed. To lift off the ground, the knees must move toward extension. The muscles of extension must stay activated to hold the body in space. If they released, the knees would bend completely, and you would return to your starting position on the floor.

Modifications

Place a block underneath your sacrum for Supported Bridge, or place a bolster underneath your hips for a restorative version that can help relieve low-back and hip tightness.

Variations

Try lifting a leg. This requires more strength from the grounded leg while challenging the hip flexor muscles on the lifted side.

BACKWARD BENDS | **CHAPTER 18**

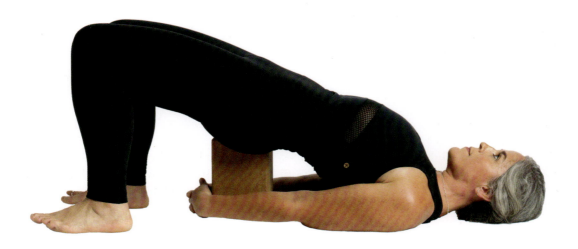

Figure 18.15. Bridge modification supported with block.

Exploration/Possible Cues

Get more spacious from your chest to your legs; pull apart.

Use back-body engagement to open up the front of your body.

Allow your breath to provide a stretch from the inside out.

Watch the rise and fall of your upper abdomen.

PART THREE | THE POSTURES

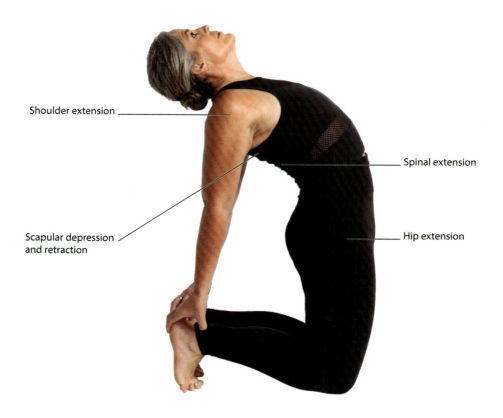

Figure 18.16. The anatomical actions of Camel.

Camel

Camel
Ustrasana

Camel pose has a reputation for sparking intense body sensations. For many people it can be quite a demanding front-body opener.

Begin standing on your knees at near hip-width distance apart. With your legs engaged and your glute muscles firm, place your hands on the backs of your hips. Draw your tailbone down, creating a slight posterior tilt of the pelvis (fig. 14.5). Lift up tall through your chest, and elongate your spine. Look back at your left heel, and place your left hand on it. Now, place your right hand on the center of your chest, guiding your chest toward squared forward again. Look back at your right foot, and place your right hand on it. Stay engaged in your back body to encourage the front body to release. Square your chest and belly forward again, and begin gazing up toward the ceiling. Keep your neck long, and avoid dropping your head back. Aim your hips forward, toward over your knees. Lift up and out of your low spine. Keep your breath full and steady.

BACKWARD BENDS | CHAPTER 18

Camel. What am I feeling?

HOW DO I GET THERE?	WHAT IS STRENGTHENING?	WHERE COULD I NOTICE TIGHTNESS?	IS COMPRESSION POSSIBLE?
Spinal extension	**Spinal extensors, fig. 5.3**	**Spinal flexors, fig. 5.5** Entire front body	✓ Fig. 5.2
Hip extension	**Hip extensors, fig. 7.6**	**Hip flexors, fig. 7.5**	
Shoulder extension	**Shoulder extensors, fig. 6.5**	**Shoulder flexors, fig. 6.4**	
Scapular depression and retraction	**Depressors and retractors of the scapulae, p. 54**	Elevators and protractors of the scapulae, p. 54	
Elbow extension	Elbow extensors, fig. 10.2	**Elbow flexors, fig. 10.3**	
Knee extension Beginning in a kneeling position, the knees extend to come up into Camel.	**Knee extensors, fig. 8.2**	Knee flexors, fig. 8.3	
Ankle plantar flexion or dorsiflexion	Ankle plantar flexors, fig. 9.4 Ankle dorsiflexors, fig. 9.3	Ankle dorsiflexors, fig. 9.3 Ankle plantar flexors, fig. 9.4	

My discoveries:

Special Considerations

The knees are anchored to the ground. This tends to shorten and tighten the front of the body making Camel more demanding than poses in which the feet and legs have more freedom.

As always, *every body* is different, so certain principles will fit some people and not others. I teach and practice not letting the head collapse back in this pose out of concern for
- keeping open air passageways,
- maintaining healthy cervical spine position, and
- avoiding excess tension/pressure on the arteries and nerves of the neck.

Excess pressure on the thoracic cavity, which holds the lungs and heart, could also make achieving full breaths more difficult.

Occasionally practitioners do not like this pose because it makes them feel light-headed or nauseous. Many possible reasons are given for this. When researching, you will find explanations ranging from "excess heart-opening energy," to the carotid arteries flattening when the head is tilted back. I look more to science and physiology when a sudden sensation like nausea or dizziness occurs. If one moment everything is fine, and the next moment dizziness or nausea arises, especially with a specific physical movement, this tells me that the body is responding to the new position. Something caused an imbalance in the cardiovascular or nervous system. The body is simply reacting.

Vasovagal response could be involved. This response immediately slows the heart and drops blood pressure, which would lead to feelings of light-headedness, tunnel vision, clamminess, and nausea. Vasovagal response occurs when the vagus nerve is stimulated by some sudden, traumatic (or perceived-as-traumatic) event. The trigger could be anything from standing up quickly, to becoming extremely angry, to straining from a bowel movement. Whatever causes these uncomfortable feelings, they are sure signs from your body that you should try things differently, or skip this pose altogether.

Modifications

Modifications in Camel aim to lessen the tension/pressure on the front of the body as well as to reduce the degree of spinal extension or backbend.

Keeping your hands at your low back will lessen the spinal extension and will bring release to the front of the body.

If pressing your hips forward to stack over your knees causes too much pressure in the lumbar spine, ease up a bit, and allow your hips to stay back some.

Variations

Placing a block between your thighs will awaken hip adduction as you squeeze into the block for stabilization.

Placing a strap around your thighs will awaken hip abduction as you press outward into the strap for stabilization.

Try this one-arm Camel as a modification or variation. I find that it increases freedom in every aspect of the pose.

BACKWARD BENDS | CHAPTER 18

Exploration/Possible Cues

Don't rush in. Take your time, and feel your way into the backbend.

Your glute muscles are strong stabilizers of the pelvis. Keep them engaged all the way through this pose.

Lift your entire barrel of ribs up and out of the pit of your belly prior to going back at all. Keep lifting up the entire time, rather than collapsing back.

You should be able to maintain your breath here. If you ever lose your breath, back out.

Engage your quadriceps strongly as if you were trying to straighten your legs.

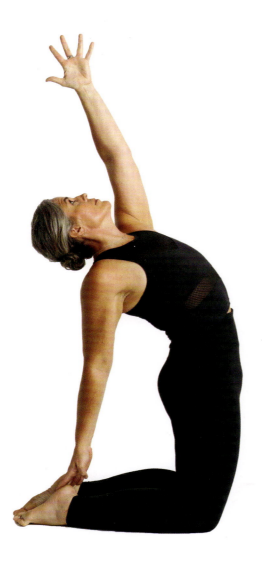

Figure 18.17. Camel variation with one-arm reach.

PART THREE | THE POSTURES

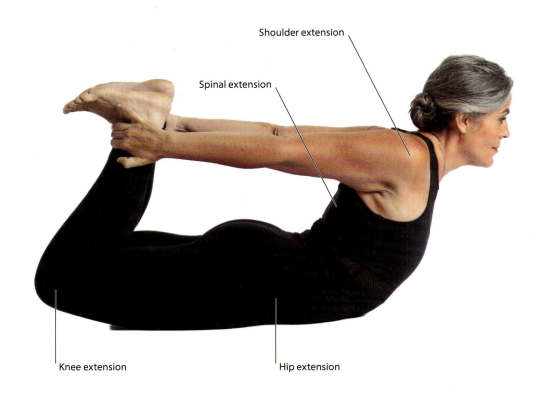

Figure 18.18. The anatomical actions of Floor Bow.

Floor Bow

Floor Bow
Bow
Dhanurasana

Bow pose provides the benefits of all the other backbends plus abdominal massage.

Begin lying face down. Bend both legs, and reach back to catch your outer shins. Your knees should be near hip-width distance apart. Draw your sacrum back and down toward your knees while anchoring your pubis toward the floor. Kick your legs back into your hands, taking your chest forward. Engage your quadriceps, glutes, and back-body muscles to extend and open the entire front body. Allow your neck to remain neutral.

BACKWARD BENDS | CHAPTER 18

Floor Bow. What am I feeling?

HOW DO I GET THERE?	WHAT IS STRENGTHENING?	WHERE COULD I NOTICE TIGHTNESS?	IS COMPRESSION POSSIBLE?
Spinal extension	Spinal extensors, fig. 5.3	Spinal flexors, fig. 5.5	✓ Fig. 5.2
Hip extension	Hip extensors, fig. 7.6	Hip flexors, fig. 7.5	
Knee extension	Knee extensors, fig. 8.2 Although the knees are typically bent, extension is the action that lifts the pose off the ground and into action.	Knee flexors, fig. 8.3	
Shoulder extension	Shoulder extensors, fig. 6.5	Shoulder flexors, fig. 6.4	
Elbow extension	Elbow extensors, fig. 10.2	Elbow flexors, fig. 10.3	

My discoveries:

Special Considerations

Injury or pain in the front of the body or abdomen can limit this pose.

Protruding hip bones or pubis may be uncomfortable. Placing padding under your hips usually helps.

You might notice that you grip your outer shins for Floor Bow rather than the inner shins as in Dancer (fig. 18.24). Although external rotation of the shoulder (inside grip) is better for shoulder extension, this pose offers a different dynamic. First of all, holding on to the outsides of the shins helps keep the legs in a strong neutral position. Secondly, this pose involves both legs, which typically results in less range in the backbend and less extension in the anterior shoulder, thus allowing the outside grip. The outside grip is not a hard-and-fast rule in Bow—nothing I present is—because I have seen some practitioners successfully hold the insides of their shins. As always, everything depends on your unique body.

Feel the pose from within. Let all the information from your teachers, books, and online sources filter through you. Then embody the pose, and find your own way.

Modifications

Do one leg at a time with your opposite-side arm/hand extended forward for support.

Variations

Use a strap in Floor Bow to change the physics and overall feel.

Exploration/Possible Cues

Soften the front of your body while activating your legs.

Create more space between your legs and chest. Pull apart.

Vary your hand placement. Try catching lower down on your shins for a different leverage point. Try holding on to your feet for an extended ankle stretch.

Keep your neck passive rather than engaged.

BACKWARD BENDS | CHAPTER 18

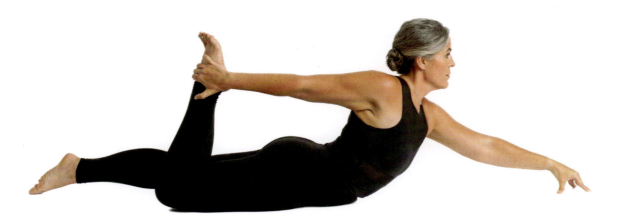

Figure 18.19. Floor Bow modification holding one leg.

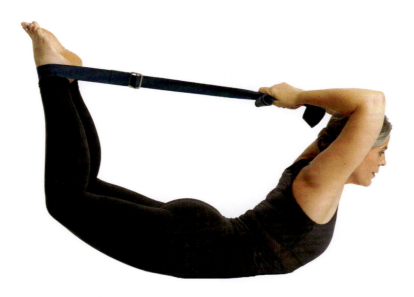

Figure 18.20. Floor Bow variation with strap.

293

PART THREE | THE POSTURES

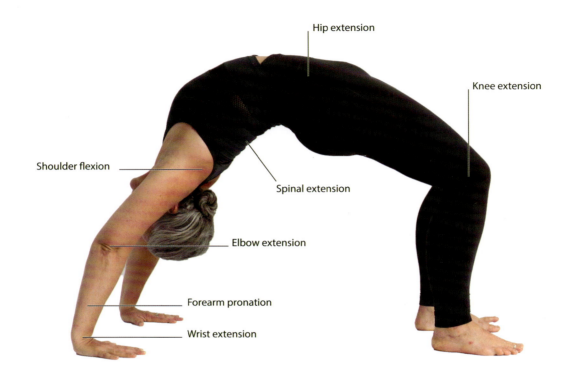

Figure 18.21. The anatomical actions of Wheel.

Wheel

Wheel
Upward Bow
Urdhva Dhanurasana
Chakrasana

Wheel pose, for many, is the ultimate backbend posture. It is an invigorating and awakening body opener.

Start on your back with your heels drawn in close to your body. Place your feet near hip-width distance apart. Reach above your head, and place your hands outside your ears near shoulder-width distance apart. Place your palms flat on the floor with fingertips aimed toward shoulders. Aim your tailbone forward toward your knees, and lift up using your quadriceps, glutes, and upper-body strength. Maintain a slight lower-abdominal engagement. Once up, make minor adjustments to your hands and feet until you feel comfortable and sturdy. Continue drawing your sacrum toward your knees. Pull your chest away from active legs. Continue engaging your glutes, and press down through your big toes. Allow your head to hang free, and cultivate your ability to take big, slow breaths.

BACKWARD BENDS | CHAPTER 18

Wheel. What am I feeling?

HOW DO I GET THERE?	WHAT IS STRENGTHENING?	WHERE COULD I NOTICE TIGHTNESS?	IS COMPRESSION POSSIBLE?
Spinal extension	**Spinal extensors, fig. 5.3**	**Spinal flexors, fig. 5.5**	✓ Fig. 5.2
Hip extension	**Hip extensors, fig. 7.6**	**Hip flexors, fig. 7.5**	
Shoulder flexion	**Shoulder flexors, fig. 6.4**	**Shoulder extensors, fig. 6.5**	✓ Fig. 6.3
Elbow extension	Elbow extensors, fig. 10.2	**Elbow flexors, fig. 10.3**	
Wrist extension	Wrist extensors, fig. 11.2	**Wrist flexors, fig. 11.3**	
Forearm pronation	**Forearm pronators, fig. 10.5**	**Forearm supinators, fig. 10.4**	
Knee extension	**Knee extensors, fig. 8.2** *Although the knees are typically bent, extension is the action that lifts the pose off the ground and into action. During the hold, the extensors engage isometrically.*	Knee flexors, fig. 8.3	

My discoveries:

Special Considerations

As some of the prime movers in this pose, the glutes are external rotators as well as hip extensors. They also work to stabilize the sacroiliac joints and the pelvis overall. The key is combining glute engagement with anchoring down through your big toes to counter any external rotation you feel. Focusing on this sensation will also help you determine how much glute engagement is perfect for you.

Anatomical differences quickly become obvious in Wheel because it demands range of motion from several places in the body. I am always fascinated looking out across my class to see huge deviations in shape from mat to mat during this pose. Apart from strength and stamina, the six areas that contribute most to these differences are:

1. The shape and spaciousness of the spinous processes (see "Anatomy of Backbending" p. 259),

2. The shape and constitution of the shoulder complex (skeletal and soft tissue),

3. The amount of wrist mobility,

4. The amount of thoracic mobility (skeletal and soft tissue),

5. The shape and constitution of the hip complex (skeletal and soft tissue), and

6. The overall anterior-body soft-tissue constitution—the level of tightness or openness.

These are all issues of navigating your uniqueness. You will find that classic textbook Wheel alignment may work fine for you, or you may feel from within and learn that you need to subtly shift placement for your individual structure. A few ways to experiment are listed below.

Modifications

Try angling your hands out and/or placing them wider if you meet skeletal compression in the shoulder when your hands are placed at shoulder-width distance apart. Remember that compression will feel like a stuck or pinching sensation. Review shoulder skeletal variation (fig. 6.2, fig. 6.3).

Angle your toes out slightly, and/or place your feet wider apart. This modification helps accommodate varying hip skeletal structures (fig. 7.2, fig. 7.3). Remember, this is not the same as "splaying" your knees out. While your foot placement may be different, your legs should remain strongly neutral. Pushing down through the big toes can help.

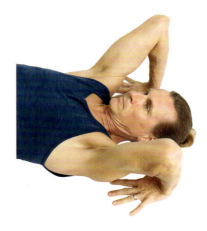

Figure 18.22. Wheel modification with varied hand placement.

BACKWARD BENDS | CHAPTER 18

Bridge (fig. 18.14) is a good option when Wheel is not accessible.

Variations

Once you establish a strong foundation, lift one leg. As always, doing different things with your arms and legs will change the physics and overall experience of the pose. The key is proceeding slowly with awareness so that you maintain foundational stability. I find that adding a leg lift (fig. 18.23) frees up my pelvis, allowing more access to posterior tilt.

Exploration/Possible Cues

Draw your knees forward and your chest back to create length in the posture.

Let your head hang loose and free.

As you lift, feel your posterior muscles working to open the front of your body. Play with varying degrees of firing these muscles. Feel what works most effectively for you.

Keep your breaths long and full.

Engage your quadriceps strongly as if you were trying to straighten your legs.

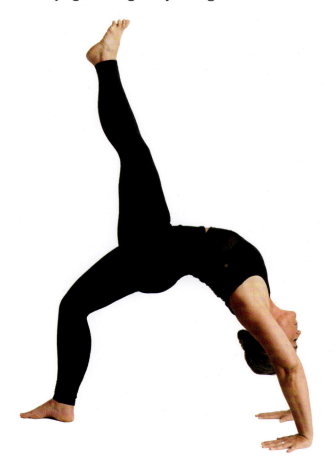

Figure 18.23. Wheel variation with leg lift.

PART THREE | THE POSTURES

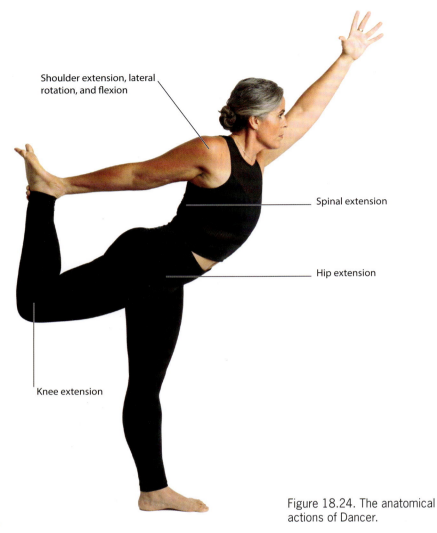

Figure 18.24. The anatomical actions of Dancer.

Dancer

Dancer
Natarajasana
Standing Bow

Dancer pose is a strong standing posture combining backward bending with balance. It offers leg and core strengthening along with front-body release. Additionally, it contains all the amazing spinal extension benefits.

Begin in Mountain pose. Hold your right palm out as if holding a tray. This motion externally rotates the shoulder into a healthy position for extension. Catch the inside of your right shin/ankle. Reach up with your left hand. Stay upright. Maintain a forward-facing neutral position from chest, belly, hips, and thighs. Aim the right knee cap straight down. Draw your tailbone down to slightly expand your lumbar spine. This is posterior pelvic tilt. While keeping your chest forward, kick your lifted leg into your hand. Slowly come into a backward bend as your knee reaches back and away. Remain evenly engaged in both legs while keeping a soft bend in your standing leg.

BACKWARD BENDS | CHAPTER 18

Dancer. What am I feeling?

HOW DO I GET THERE?	WHAT IS STRENGTHENING?	WHERE COULD I NOTICE TIGHTNESS?	IS COMPRESSION POSSIBLE?
Spinal extension	**Spinal extensors, fig. 5.3**	Spinal flexors, fig. 5.5	✓ Fig. 5.2
Lifted-leg hip extension	**Lifted-leg hip extensors, fig. 7.6**	**Lifted-leg hip flexors, fig. 7.5**	
Knee extension	**Knee extensors, fig. 8.2** *Even though the lifted leg is typically bent, the extensors work to kick the leg back toward further extension.*	Knee flexors, fig. 8.3	
Back-arm shoulder extension	Back-arm shoulder extensors, fig. 6.5	**Back-arm shoulder flexors, fig. 6.4**	
Back-arm shoulder lateral rotation	Back-arm shoulder lateral rotators, fig. 6.14	**Back-arm shoulder medial rotators, fig. 6.11**	
Reaching-arm shoulder flexion	Reaching-arm shoulder flexors, fig. 6.4	Reaching-arm shoulder extensors, fig. 6.5	
Elbow extension	Elbow extensors, fig. 10.2	**Elbow flexors, fig. 10.3**	

My discoveries:

PART THREE | THE POSTURES

Special Considerations

Overextending the lumbar spine is common when practitioners don't understand leading with a slight posterior tilt.

Limited ability to catch the shin inside is typically caused by soft-tissue tightness when laterally rotating the arm. This can be from muscles, tendons, ligaments, or joint capsule restriction. In this situation, practitioners tend to internally rotate the arm and catch the inside of the foot; however, this puts the soft tissues of the anterior shoulder at risk with extension. Avoid doing this (See fig. 18.25 for incorrect grip). A better option would be to hold the outside of the shin.

As your leg kicks farther back, you reach a point where the soft tissues in front of the hip flexor are stretched as far as they can go, and/or the extension is maxed out in the lumbar spine. No more backbend is accessible. Then the pelvis goes with the kicking leg, and a side opening or uneven hips result. If you feel your hips opening to the side, stay instead of kicking farther.

Modifications

Catch the outside of the foot or shin if you can't grip the inside.

Place your reaching hand on a wall or on someone else's supportive hand.

Minimize the lift of your back leg.

Variations

Using a strap looped around the foot (fig. 18.26) offers a unique challenge and changes Dancer's physics while making the squared-forward position more easily accessible for some. I like using this variation to teach posterior tilt. In the setup of the pose, before kicking into the backbend, I guide students to draw the sacrum or tailbone down toward the floor. This action will put pressure into the strap and will send the strapped-leg knee slightly forward. From here I guide students to maintain some of that pressure while kicking back into the fullness of the backbend. This ensures that there isn't a collapse into the lumbar spine. It also wires in the sensory experience of posterior tilt for use in other postures.

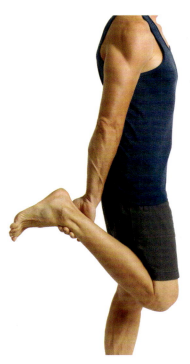

Figure 18.25. Incorrect grip in Dancer.

BACKWARD BENDS | CHAPTER 18

Try catching your foot with both hands for a playful variation testing your balance and hip flexor flexibility. This is a great stretch for the shoulder fronts and chest.

Exploration/Possible Cues

As you begin the pose, find hip extension first. Feel your natural end of range there, and then allow some backward bend.

Feel which portion of the posture is arising from hip extension and which part is from spinal extension.

If you feel your lifted knee wanting to angle out to the side, you are going beyond your natural range of motion. Back out a little bit until your hip and thigh can square forward again.

Try to avoid locking out your standing leg.

Remember, you aren't simply tilting your spine in space as you kick. This is a backward bend. Keep your chest aiming forward.

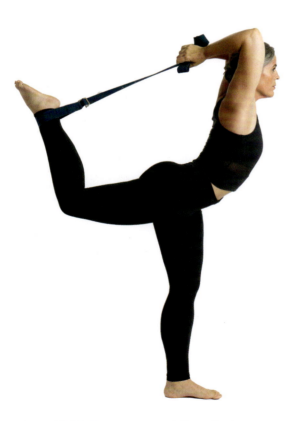

Figure 18.26. Dancer pose variation with strap.

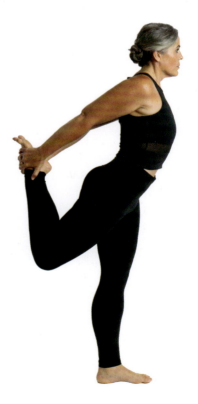

Figure 18.27. Dancer pose variation with both hands holding foot.

PART THREE | THE POSTURES

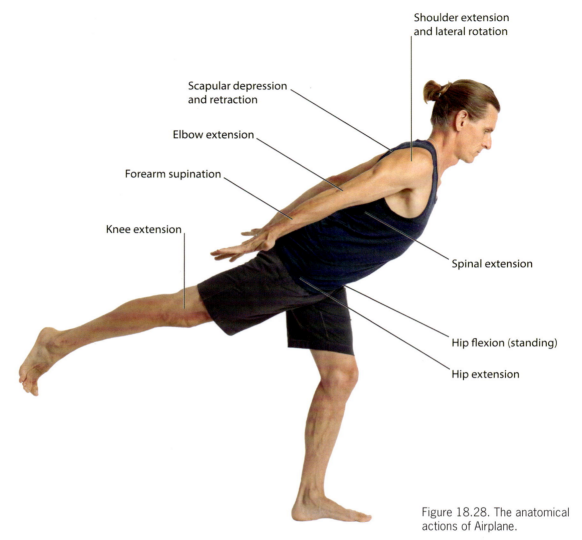

Figure 18.28. The anatomical actions of Airplane.

Airplane

Airplane
Dekasana
Balancing Locust

Some teach this pose as a version of Warrior III with different arms. I prefer to distinguish Airplane from Warrior III by emphasizing spinal extension, much like in Locust. This offers leg and core strengthening while igniting the posterior shoulder and back muscles.

Begin standing in Mountain pose with your arms by your sides and your palms facing forward. Shift your weight into your left foot, and hover your right toes back and off the ground. Keep your right leg straight. Ignite your shoulder blades back, down, and slightly together, while aiming your chest forward. Lean forward with your torso, and lift your right leg higher. Aim your hips toward square. Keep both legs equally engaged all the way up through your glutes. Your chest should stay higher than your hips while aiming forward.

BACKWARD BENDS | CHAPTER 18

Airplane. What am I feeling?

HOW DO I GET THERE?	WHAT IS STRENGTHENING?	WHERE COULD I NOTICE TIGHTNESS?	IS COMPRESSION POSSIBLE?
Spinal extension	**Spinal extensors, fig. 5.3**	Spinal flexors, fig. 5.5	✓ Fig. 5.2
Scapular depression and retraction	**Depressors and retractors of the scapulae, p. 54**	Elevators and protractors of the scapulae, p. 54	
Shoulder extension	**Shoulder extensors, fig. 6.5**	**Shoulder flexors, fig. 6.4**	
Shoulder lateral rotation	**Shoulder lateral rotators, fig. 6.14**	**Shoulder medial rotators, fig. 6.11**	
Forearm supination	Forearm supinators, fig. 10.4	Forearm pronators, fig. 10.5	
Elbow extension	Elbow extensors, fig. 10.2	Elbow flexors, fig. 10.3	
Standing-leg hip flexion	Standing-leg hip extensors, fig. 7.6 *Hip extensors work eccentrically and/or isometrically to stabilize against gravity.*		
Lifted-leg hip extension	**Lifted-leg hip extensors, fig. 7.6**	Lifted-leg hip flexors, fig. 7.5	
Knee extension	**Knee extensors, fig. 8.2**	Knee flexors, fig. 8.3	

My discoveries:

I have highlighted the most common tendencies I see in my students. It is possible to feel strengthening or to notice tightness in any of the muscle groups listed within their respective columns.

Special Considerations

Physiological factors affecting balance can limit this pose.

Leg, ankle, foot, knee, spine, or shoulder injury can limit this pose.

Moving hips toward square is often emphasized in this pose. The natural tendency is to open the lifted hip because it makes weight bearing easier. This is not necessarily wrong; it just changes the physics of the pose and the effort required. As the lifted hip moves toward square, increasing demand is placed on the lifted-leg hip extensors and knee extensors, and on the Cylindrical Core. As always, how you do the pose depends on what you want out of it.

Modifications

Stay more upright in your torso.

Don't lift your back leg as high.

Keep your hands at Prayer.

Allow the lifted hip to roll open slightly.

Variations

Bending your lifted leg brings in more hamstring (knee flexor) focus and shifts the overall physics and sensation.

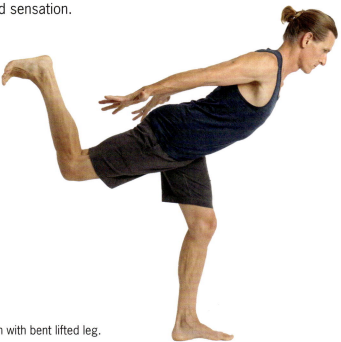

Figure 18.29. Airplane variation with bent lifted leg.

Exploration/Possible Cues

Shine the center of your chest forward to maintain backward bend.

Keeping your hips squared will fire up your Cylindrical Core.

Activate your lifted foot as if you were pressing into a wall to draw your chest forward and up.

Try activating your glutes more, and allow an external rotation of your top leg (instead of squared hips) to experience a different stability. Review the lateral hip rotators (fig. 7.12).

PART THREE | THE POSTURES

Chapter 19
Hip Openers

The Anatomy of Hip Opening

The hip joint has 360 degrees of possible movement. We should practice hip opening in a way that balances the entire joint. To explain how different yoga postures affect various aspects of hip opening, I have separated the hip into three separate compartments: Inner, Outer, and Front. All three compartments contain muscles and/or tendons that cross the hip (or femoroacetabular) joint (fig. 7.1).

The overall tone and balance of all these muscle groups together influence the stability and health not only of the hip joint, but also of the entire pelvis and spine.[42] To maintain balance between the three hip compartments, vary the strengthening and opening postures you are doing from day to day, and vary how you are doing them as well.

HIP OPENERS | CHAPTER 19

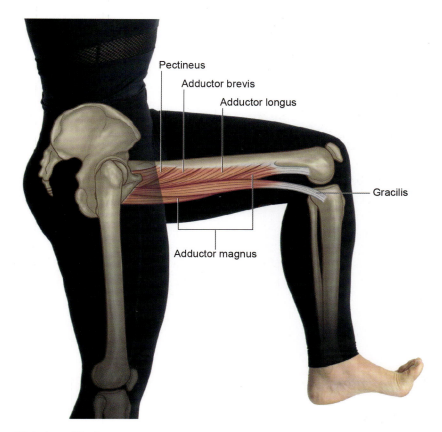

Figure 19.1. Inner Hip Compartment.

The Inner Compartment

We most commonly refer to this as the inner thigh. This includes the adductor muscles (fig. 7.8) which work to move the leg across the midline of the body.

The Outer Compartment

This group includes all the muscles that cross the hip joint from behind and/or the side (lateral). These muscles extend, abduct, internally rotate, and externally rotate the thigh. See the hip extensor muscles (fig. 7.6), abductors (fig. 7.9), medial rotators (fig. 7.11), and lateral rotators (fig. 7.10).

PART THREE | THE POSTURES

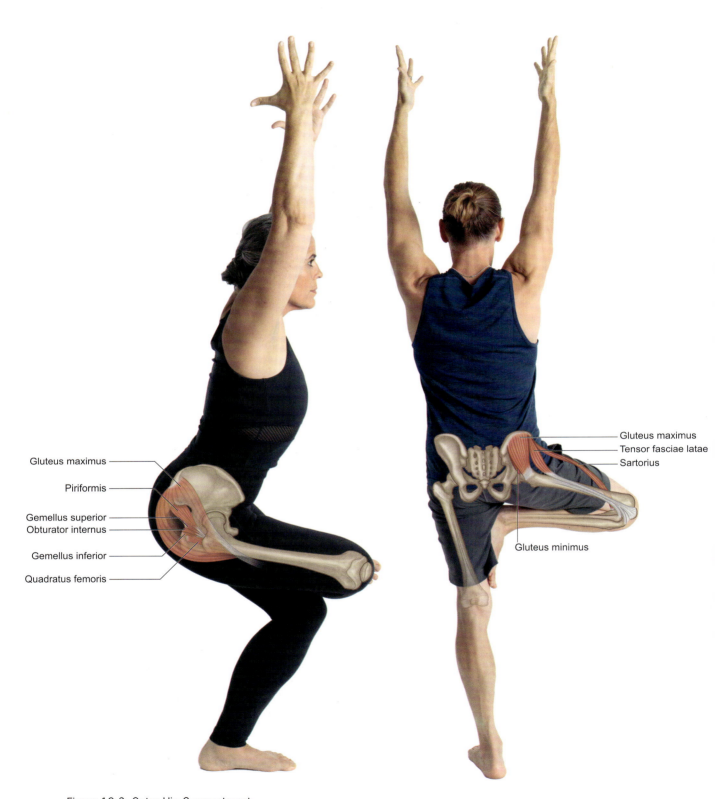

Figure 19.2. Outer Hip Compartment.

HIP OPENERS | CHAPTER 19

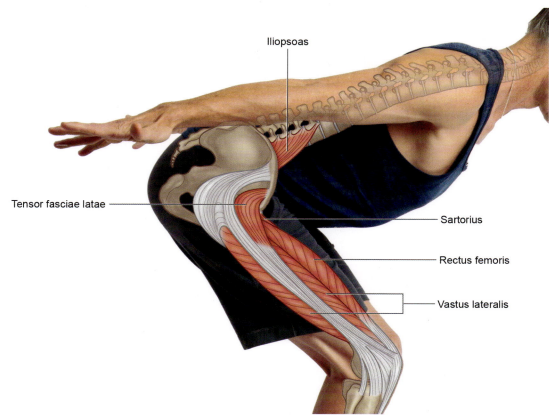

Figure 19.3. Front Hip Compartment.

The Front Compartment

This muscle group flexes the thigh toward the front hip or the front hip toward the thigh. It includes the muscles we refer to as hip flexors (fig. 7.5).

Varying the Pose

Because these muscles and tendons cross the hip joint, one end attaches to the leg, and one end attaches to the pelvis. The location, amount, and intensity of stretch will depend on the relationship between the pelvis and the leg(s). How we shift the pelvis in relation to the legs or vice versa is going to change where the stretch is predominantly happening. For example, taking the thighs closer or farther apart in Full Pigeon (fig. 19.8) will change the location and quality of the stretch within the Outer Compartment. Aim to maintain balance by continuously varying your approach. Instead of finding your "right" alignment and repeating it over and over, change it up daily, perhaps by varying the angle of the pelvis or the legs. "Correct" posture alignment is a broad spectrum. I will give you pose variations incorporating this idea. Keep in mind that experiences will be unique from mat to mat with students' varying anatomical structures.

PART THREE | THE POSTURES

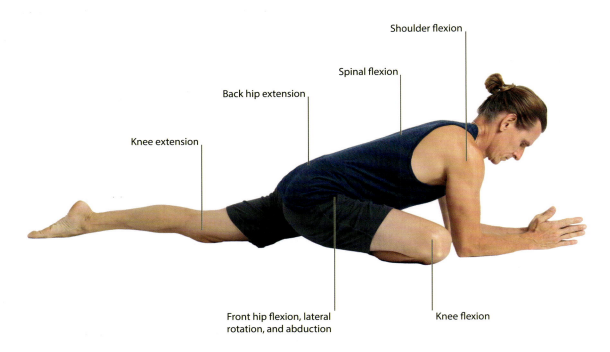

Figure 19.4. The anatomical actions of Half Pigeon.

Half Pigeon

Half Pigeon
Sleeping Pigeon
Eka Pada Rajakapotasana variation

Half Pigeon falls mainly in the **Outer Compartment** category, but it can facilitate **Front Compartment** opening as well when the torso is upright.

Start on your hands and knees. Slide your right knee toward your right hand, and slide your right foot out from beneath your body. Extend your left leg straight back behind you, keeping your back knee facing down if possible. Untuck your back toes, allowing the top of your foot to touch the floor. Stay upright with your hands pressing into the floor. Engage both of your legs while lifting up through your chest. Aim to keep your hips square, lifting up and away to access a front-hip stretch on the left side. Stay here a few breaths. As you walk your hands forward and lower your torso down, you are moving away from left front-hip stretch and into outer-hip stretch on the right side. Lower to your elbows. Allow the weight of your legs and hips to be held by the floor.

HIP OPENERS | CHAPTER 19

Half Pigeon. What am I feeling?

HOW DO I GET THERE?	WHAT IS STRENGTHENING?	WHERE COULD I NOTICE TIGHTNESS?	IS COMPRESSION POSSIBLE?
Front-leg hip flexion	Passive	**Front-leg hip extensors, fig. 7.6**	✓ Fig. 7.4
Front-leg hip lateral rotation	Passive	**Front-leg hip medial rotators, fig. 7.11**	✓ Fig. 7.10
Front-leg hip abduction	Passive	Front-leg hip adductors, fig. 7.8	
Front-leg knee flexion	Passive	Knee extensors, fig. 8.2	
Back-leg knee extension	Passive	Back-leg knee flexors, fig. 8.3	
Back-leg hip extension	Passive	**Back-leg hip flexors, fig. 7.5** When torso is upright	
Spinal flexion	Passive	**Spinal extensors, fig. 5.3**	
Shoulder flexion	Passive	Shoulder extensors, fig. 6.5	

My discoveries:

I have highlighted the most common tendencies I see in my students. It is possible to feel strengthening or to notice tightness in any of the muscle groups listed within their respective columns.

311

PART THREE | THE POSTURES

Special Considerations

Because of the deep hip flexion combined with lateral rotation, it is important to be aware of any sensation deep within the hip joint. Be cautious with any pinchy, catchy, or compressive sensations; back out for relief if they are present. *Review information on impingement (p. 66).*

If you have a compressive sensation in your front hip or an excessive, localized, strong stretching sensation in the outer hip, it's best to do this pose propped on your elbows as described above, rather than completely releasing down and forward with your chest and arms. Remember, a little stretch goes a long way.

Align this pose so that you have no pain at your knees, feet, or ankles. If you have back kneecap pain, tuck your back toes under to relieve pressure, or place padding under your knee.

Modifications

Stay more upright with extended arms and claw fingertips to the floor, or put blocks under your forearms if you have front hip-crease compression or knee pressure, or if you need to lessen the degree of stretch.

If you can't find comfort in the pose, try doing it seated upright or reclined.

Teachers commonly offer a variation of placing a block under the hip if it is off the ground. This may or may not be helpful to you. Sometimes, this can completely take away any stretch. Other times, it offers just enough support for a practitioner to be able to relax in the pose.

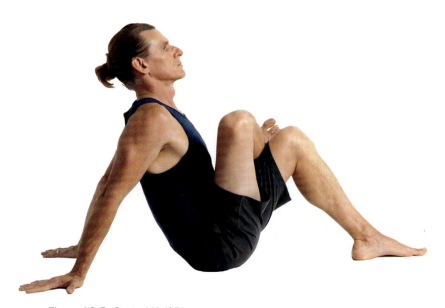

Figure 19.5. Seated Half Pigeon.

Variations

Add a back-leg bind for a quadricep stretch.

Exploration/Possible Cues

Try changing the relationship between your pelvis and front leg. Angle your torso in different directions. Angle your front leg in different directions. Feel the location of the stretch shift.

Try flexing and then pointing your front foot. Feel this shift in stretch sensation.

Stay up high, tuck your back toes under, and shift your hips toward square. Now untuck your toes, and release your weight into the floor.

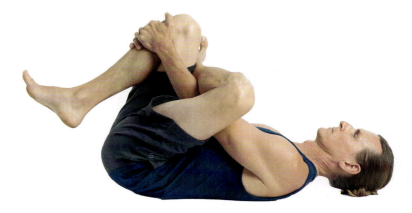

Figure 19.6. Reclined Half Pigeon.

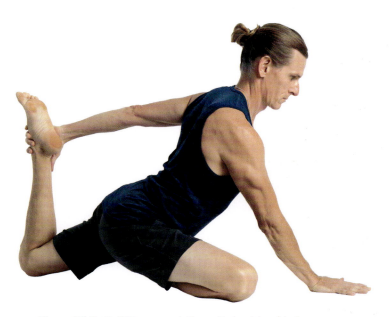

Figure 19.7. Half Pigeon variation with back-leg bind.

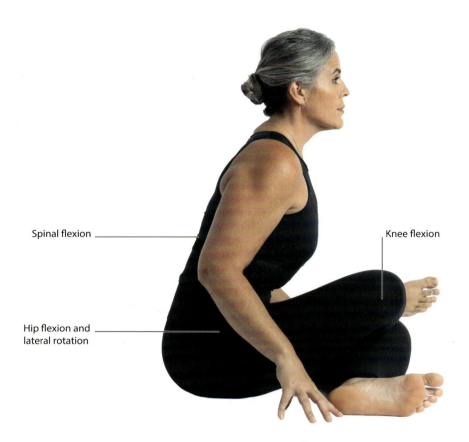

Figure 19.8. The anatomical actions of Full Pigeon.

Full Pigeon

Full Pigeon
Double Pigeon
Fire Log
Box Pose
Agnistambhasana

Full Pigeon is the pose that comes to mind most quickly when the phrase "hip opening" is mentioned. It offers **Outer Compartment** opening.

Begin seated. Bend both legs, stacking your right leg on top of your left. Looking down at your thigh bones, move them *toward* parallel. If you can comfortably place your top ankle on your bottom knee, do so. This will leave your foot barely hanging off the edge of your knee. Placing your hands on the floor for support, lift your seat off the ground and slightly back to unanchor your sitting bones. Sit nice and tall, and then slowly hinge forward as needed for comfortable stretch. As you hinge forward, maintain a tall spine. The stretch will land predominantly in your top-leg outer hip.

HIP OPENERS | CHAPTER 19

Full Pigeon. What am I feeling?

HOW DO I GET THERE?	WHAT IS STRENGTHENING?	WHERE COULD I NOTICE TIGHTNESS?	IS COMPRESSION POSSIBLE?
Hip flexion	Passive	Hip extensors, fig. 7.6	✓ Fig. 7.4
Hip lateral rotation	Passive	Hip medial rotators, fig. 7.11	✓ Fig. 7.10
Knee flexion	Passive	Knee extensors, fig. 8.2	
Axial extension or spinal flexion See Special Considerations below.	Axial extensors, fig. 5.10	Entire trunk	
Spinal flexion	Passive	Spinal extensors, fig. 5.3	

My discoveries:

Special Considerations

Knee, hip, or spine injury can limit this pose.

Instructors often emphasize maintaining axial extension in forward-folding postures. This is not necessarily right or wrong. With the spine in axial extension, these postures will be felt predominantly in the lower body, in the hips for Full Pigeon. *Axial extension will also keep the spinal discs in a neutral position rather than in the forward-flexion shape with discs pushing back toward the spinal cord.*

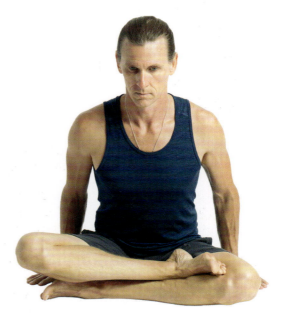

Figure 19.9. Full Pigeon modification with knees wider.

PART THREE | THE POSTURES

Consequently, axial extension is an important safeguard for anyone with disc injury (p. 32).

If we allow for some forward rounding in the spine with this sort of posture, it can give a nice posterior stretch, much like in Child's pose. *As long as you have no spinal disc issues, a bit of forward flexion is fine.* Just know that with spinal flexion, part of the range of motion is gathered from the spine, moving some of the sensation away from the lower body.

If you are teaching, you should always understand the why behind what you are asking your students to do or not to do.

Modifications

If you have skeletal compression with hip flexion in Full Pigeon, as always, the solution is playing with the angles of how the joints articulate. Play with taking the knees wider until the pressure lessens in the front hip crease so you can access a posterior hip stretch.

Placing the top foot on the floor or on a block can help relieve either hip compression or excessive tightness in your hips.

If none of these modifications work, simply do Half Pigeon (fig. 19.4) or Half Pigeon variation (fig. 19.5) instead.

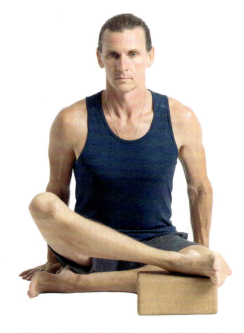

Figure 19.10. Full Pigeon modification with top foot on block.

Variations

Cow Face is a variation of Full Pigeon pose in which the legs are adducted, creating an added stretch for the hip abductors.

Full Pigeon setup is the perfect place to add a spinal twist.

Full Pigeon anchors the bottom leg well for a lateral side-body stretch or twist.

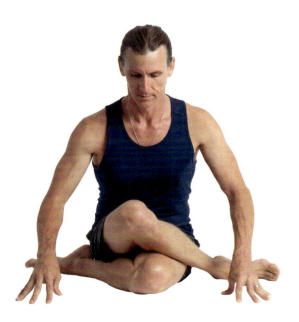

Figure 19.11. Cow Face pose.

HIP OPENERS | CHAPTER 19

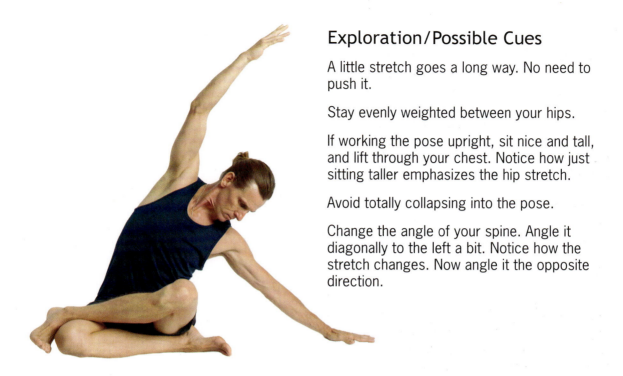

Exploration/Possible Cues

A little stretch goes a long way. No need to push it.

Stay evenly weighted between your hips.

If working the pose upright, sit nice and tall, and lift through your chest. Notice how just sitting taller emphasizes the hip stretch.

Avoid totally collapsing into the pose.

Change the angle of your spine. Angle it diagonally to the left a bit. Notice how the stretch changes. Now angle it the opposite direction.

Figure 19.12. Full Pigeon with lateral side stretch.

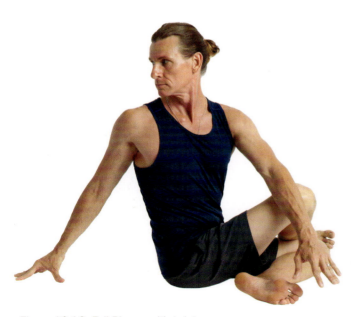

Figure 19.13. Full Pigeon with twist.

PART THREE | THE POSTURES

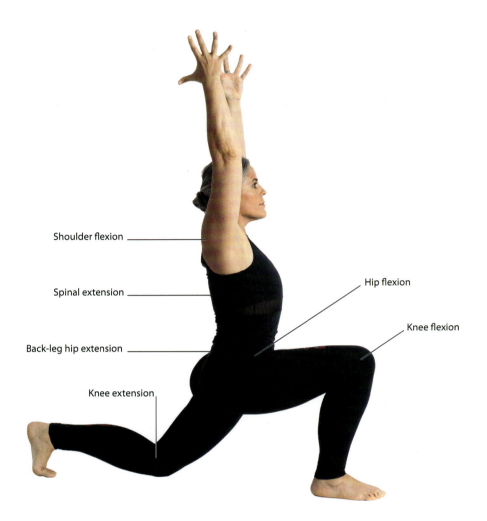

Figure 19.14. The anatomical actions of Low Lunge.

Low Lunge

Low Lunge
Upright Low Lunge
Anjaneyasana
Dragon

Low Lunge counters the biomechanics of sitting, targeting the **Front Compartment** of the hip.

Begin in Downward-Facing Dog. Step your right foot to your right hand, and lower your back knee to the ground. Leave the top of your back foot flat on the floor, or tuck your toes if needed for comfort or balance. Keep your front knee near stacked over your front heel; you may need to wiggle your front foot forward to achieve this. Lift your arms straight up into the air while drawing your sacrum toward the ground and lifting your front hip pointers upward toward your chest.

HIP OPENERS | CHAPTER 19

Low Lunge. What am I feeling?

HOW DO I GET THERE?	WHAT IS STRENGTHENING?	WHERE COULD I NOTICE TIGHTNESS?	IS COMPRESSION POSSIBLE?
Spinal extension *Minimal*	Spinal extensors, fig. 5.3	Spinal flexors, fig. 5.5	
Front-leg hip flexion	**Hip extensors, fig. 7.6** Front-leg hip extensors work eccentrically and/or isometrically to oppose gravity.		
Front-leg knee flexion	**Knee extensors, fig. 8.2** Even though the knee is bent, the extensors work eccentrically and/or isometrically to oppose gravity.		
Back-leg hip extension	**Back-leg hip extensors, fig. 7.6**	**Back-leg hip flexors, fig. 7.5**	
Back-leg knee extension	Back-leg knee extensors, fig. 8.2	Back-leg knee flexors, fig. 8.3	
Shoulder flexion	**Shoulder flexors, fig. 6.4**	Shoulder extensors, fig. 6.5	✓ Fig. 6.3

My discoveries:

Special Considerations

If you have knee tenderness that causes discomfort, place padding under your back knee, and/or tuck your back toes to help relieve any pressure.

Sometimes this pose is practiced by allowing the front knee to go forward toward the front toes. In this alignment, a lot of lumbar extension (backward bend) tends to happen. As more range of motion is gathered from the spine, stretch/sensation is taken away from the hip flexor. This is neither right nor wrong. Just be aware that this variation does not typically target the hip flexor stretch in the same way. The two different alignments simply offer unique experiences.

Hip flexor (Front Compartment) stretch depends on the relationship between the pelvis and the legs. In a Low Lunge variation where the hands or forearms are on the floor, the pelvis is tilted toward the leg; therefore, hip flexor stretch is diminished. Opening the angle between the pelvis and the hip (lifting the torso upright) is required to stretch the hip flexors.

Modifications

Place your hands in Prayer.

Variations

Try varying arm positions or binds.

Depending on your unique body composition, taking your hands or arms to the floor may shift the pose away from being primarily a Front Compartment opener, turning it into a combination of Front and Inner Compartment stretch.

When the front foot is rolled onto its outer edge, the posture may bring additional Outer Compartment opening.

Exploration/Possible Cues

Play with tilting your pelvis differently to feel the shift in sensation. Can you feel how an anterior tilt (fig. 14.6) brings you more into backward bend while a posterior tilt (fig. 14.5) lands more in hip flexor stretch?

Draw your belly in and up as you reach.

Breathe into the whole front side of your body.

HIP OPENERS | CHAPTER 19

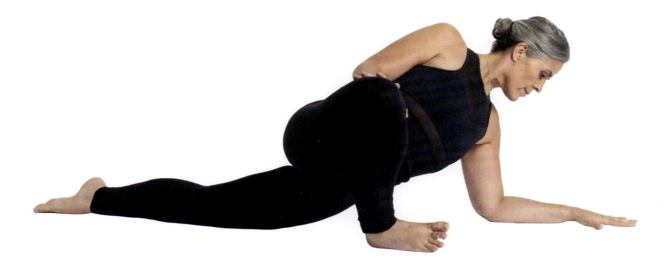

Figure 19.15. Low Lunge variation hands/elbows on floor.

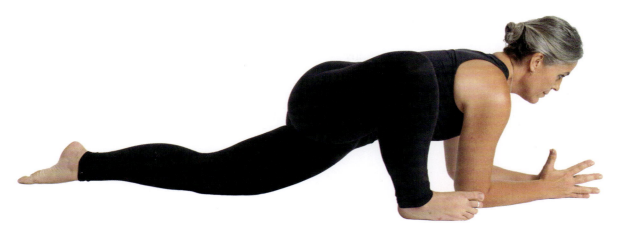

Figure 19.16. Low Lunge variation foot rolled to outer edge.

PART THREE | THE POSTURES

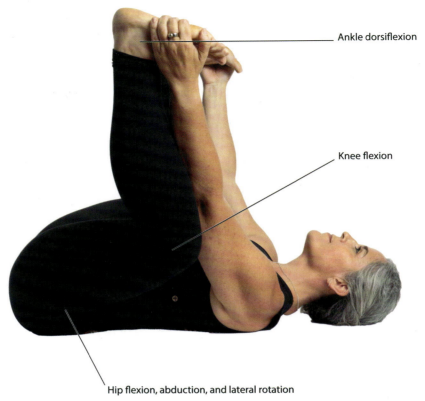

Figure 19.17. The anatomical actions of Happy Baby.

Happy Baby

Happy Baby
Dead Bug
Ananda Balasana

Happy Baby pose reminds us of the freedom and flexibility we had as little children. It is an **Inner Compartment** hip opener. This pose also helps bring an overall awareness of the femoroacetabular hip joint (fig. 7.1).

Start on your back. Hold on to the outer edges of both feet, keeping your feet directly over your knees. Bring your knees toward the floor beside your body with the soles of your feet facing the ceiling. Gently draw your knees down. Lengthen your sacrum away from your shoulders to add an easy back stretch.

Special Considerations

You must access the full range of flexion in your hip joints for poses like Crow and Running Man, and also for transitioning into inversions such as Headstand and Handstand. If you are having difficulty finding your way into any of these postures, spend some time daily with Happy Baby.

HIP OPENERS | CHAPTER 19

Happy Baby. What am I feeling?

HOW DO I GET THERE?	WHAT IS STRENGTHENING?	WHERE COULD I NOTICE TIGHTNESS?	IS COMPRESSION POSSIBLE?
Hip flexion	Passive	Hip extensors, fig. 7.6	✓ Fig. 7.4
Hip abduction	Passive	**Hip adductors, fig. 7.8**	✓ Fig. 7.7
Hip lateral rotation	Passive	Hip medial rotators, fig. 7.11	✓ Fig. 7.10
Knee flexion	Passive	Knee extensors, fig. 8.2	
Ankle dorsiflexion	Ankle dorsiflexors, fig. 9.3	Ankle plantar flexors, fig. 9.4	

My discoveries:

Modifications

Place a strap around the soles of your feet if they are difficult to reach.

Variations

Take one leg and then the other out straight for a stretch variation.

Exploration/Possible Cues

Play with a mini pelvis tilt as in Cat/Cow; notice the shift in sensation.

Rock the pose gently from side to side.

PART THREE | THE POSTURES

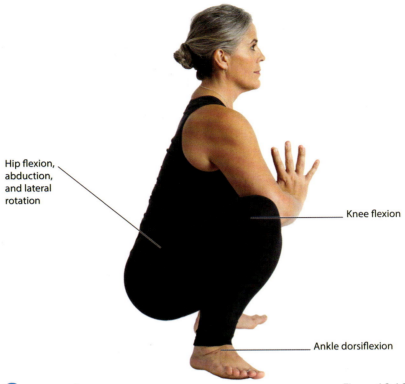

Figure 19.18. The anatomical actions of Yogi Squat.

Yogi Squat

Yogi Squat
Malasana
Garland Pose

Yogi Squat is a good reminder of the importance of maintaining mobility in our lower-body joints. Being able to fully use our ankles, knees, and hips will help us remain active and playful for the long haul. This is mainly an **Inner Compartment** hip opener.

Begin standing with your feet a little wider than hip-width distance apart. Externally rotate your hips by turning your toes slightly outward. Lower your hips toward the floor. Readjust your feet as needed for comfort and support. Place your hands in Prayer position, and use your elbows to gently brace your inner knees. Stay lifted through your chest and crown. Remain here for several breaths, and sense your lower-body mobility.

Special Considerations

Hip, knee, or ankle injury will limit this pose.

Those with uniquely shaped hips and ankles may find this pose challenging. If you are unable to lower enough to find comfort in this pose, you are likely meeting compression in the hip and/or ankle.

If you can't "sit" all the way into Yogi Squat, your knee extensors will be working fiercely to oppose gravity.

HIP OPENERS | CHAPTER 19

Yogi Squat. What am I feeling?

HOW DO I GET THERE?	WHAT IS STRENGTHENING?	WHERE COULD I NOTICE TIGHTNESS?	IS COMPRESSION POSSIBLE?
Hip flexion	Passive	Hip extensors, fig. 7.6	✓ Fig. 7.4
Hip abduction	Passive	**Hip adductors, fig. 7.8**	✓ Fig. 7.7
Hip lateral rotation	Passive	Hip medial rotators, fig. 7.11	✓ Fig. 7.10
Knee flexion	Passive	Knee extensors, fig. 8.2	
Ankle dorsiflexion	Passive	Ankle plantar flexors, fig. 9.4	✓ Fig. 9.2

My discoveries:

Modifications

If ankle compression is an issue for you, simply allow your heels to lift.

Lifting your hips higher can also minimize ankle flexion.

Sitting on one or two blocks can lift your hips just enough for any needed support.

Keep in mind that as your hips lift higher, flexion in the hips, knees, and ankles is lessened.

Variations

Move your spine as in Cat/Cow to shift the overall sensation.

Try varying your arm positions to change and shift where the predominant sensation lands.

Exploration/Possible Cues

This pose truly helps you feel your lower-body range of motion. Go into it slowly, and feel from within. Can you feel what is stopping you when you can't go farther? Can you get a good sense of your joints moving from within?

Maintain Mountain alignment in your torso.

As you press your hands together, lift your chest higher.

Snug your shoulder blades slightly back and down.

PART THREE | THE POSTURES

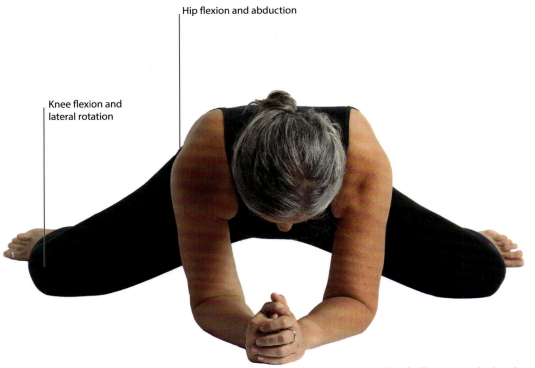

Figure 19.19. The anatomical actions of Frog.

Frog

Frog
Mandukasana

Frog is an **Inner Compartment** hip opener that you either love or hate. If you are in the latter category, it could simply mean you haven't found the right variation for your body. Yoga poses should offer a sensory experience, but they should not be painful.

Begin in Tabletop position (fig. 13.5). Slide your knees wide apart until you land in a gentle inner-thigh stretch. Send each shin out to form a near-90-degree angle with your thighs. Turn your toes out laterally. Prop your elbows under your shoulders, and relax your head and neck. Lengthen your sacrum away from your crown, bringing space into the lumbar spine; *this is a posterior tilt of the pelvis.*

Special Considerations

Knee tenderness can make this pose uncomfortable. Placing padding under your knees can help.

Some attempting this pose may experience pinching or pressure on the posterior hip socket where the femur meets the acetabulum (fig. 7.7). This usually results in not feeling any inner-thigh stretch at all because the practitioner is getting caught in compression. The solution here is to play with the angles. See Modifications below.

HIP OPENERS | CHAPTER 19

Frog. What am I feeling?

HOW DO I GET THERE?	WHAT IS STRENGTHENING?	WHERE COULD I NOTICE TIGHTNESS?	IS COMPRESSION POSSIBLE?
Hip flexion	Passive	Hip extensors, fig. 7.6	✓ Fig. 7.4
Hip abduction	Passive	**Hip adductors, fig. 7.8**	✓ Fig. 7.7
Knee flexion	Passive	Knee extensors, fig. 8.2	
Knee lateral rotation	Passive	**Knee medial rotators, fig. 8.4**	

My discoveries:

If relaxing completely into this pose is too intense, activating the hip adductors as if drawing the knees together will provide lift and support.

Modifications

Change the angles of the pose by moving your hips farther back toward your feet. Also try shifting the direction of your feet, and/or draw your feet closer together. Experiment until the compression sensation in the back of your hips diminishes and/or you feel an inner stretch.

If none of this works, try Happy Baby pose instead (fig. 19.17).

Variations

Place a block under your chest.

Place a bolster under your chest.

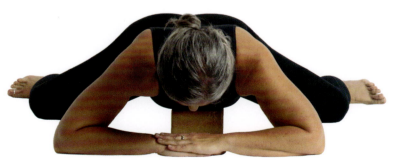

Figure 19.20. Frog Variation with block.

Exploration/Possible Cues

This pose can bring up a lot of sensation. Notice where you are feeling it most. Send some breath there. Learn to distinguish between when to stay and when to shift. This is a perfect pose to practice increasing your time between stimulus and response. Being mindfully aware of when to stay and when to move gives us access to this skill within all of our life actions.

PART THREE | **THE POSTURES**

Chapter 20
Arm Balances and Inversions

An Approach to Arm Balances and Inversions

Everywhere you look on social media, you can find photos of flawless yoga bodies in awe-inspiring arm balances or inversions. Some might argue that these pictures have led to confusion about what yoga truly is, defining it as a practice whose goal is aesthetic perfection and beauty rather than awareness. Others would say that these pictures inspire and encourage, and that just like any other postures, practicing these poses also provides the opportunity to cultivate mindful awareness. In an embodied approach to yoga, it depends on the practitioner's intention and the viewer's perspective.

I happen to enjoy some of these poses, and they have been pivotal in my personal growth and in my cultivation of awareness. However, you never have to do any of these postures to practice *advanced* yoga. Advancing your practice arises from an inner experience only known by you, the practitioner; it cannot be judged by the appearance of a pose. The postures are simply vehicles for the practice of yoga.

Practicing these postures requires exploring new relationships with your body and space. Increased **interoception** and **proprioception** are vital. Once you begin to practice and learn more than one of these poses, you will see that they all share the following important elements.

Body Physics

When attempting to balance your body weight on your hands, you are dealing with the physics of matter, gravity, and motion. To lift your weight successfully off the ground, something must counterbalance it in the other direction. Furthermore, the overall physics and experience of the pose are significantly influenced by body proportions, such as

ARM BALANCES AND INVERSIONS | CHAPTER 20

having longer legs and a shorter torso, or vice versa. Learning how to navigate your own center of gravity and how to make minor shifts of weight distribution, as well as how to activate particular actions/forces, will be very useful. So, going into your practice with an awareness of physics is often beneficial.

Patience with Neuroplasticity

The main reason these poses can be challenging is simply that you've never done them before. Your brain doesn't contain the neural wiring to achieve these shapes in your body. This is why many of the yogis you see easily mastering inversions have a history of gymnastics or tumbling. They already have some previously established neural wiring that makes these poses much easier for them.

I recently led a workshop called, "Forty Days to Handstand in the Middle of the Room." We had close to fifty people sign up. The first thing I asked the group was, "How many of you did gymnastics when you were young?" None of them raised their hands. Yogi gymnasts didn't attend the workshop; they already know how to do Handstand.

The good news is that our brains are neuroplastic. In other words, you can learn new things and grow new neural pathways. It just takes a lot of patience. It is worthwhile when approaching these poses to understand that it is not only a physical rewiring, but also a mental rewiring. Again, be patient. When you are practicing a certain skill, if you repetitively keep doing it "wrong," stop, pause, and change what you are doing. That way, you aren't wiring in the wrong information over and over again.

Sthira Sukham Asanam

Sthira sukham asanam is a phrase taken from the *Yoga Sutras of Patanjali*, an ancient text of yoga teachings. *Sthira* means steadiness, and *sukham* means ease. An **asana** is a posture. This idea is that yoga posture should be a blend of steadiness and ease. While obviously important for all postures, it is vital to mention this here since these postures typically test one's strength and overall balance. The *effort* aspect of these poses is commonly overdone, diminishing the body's innate capacity to balance and align. Simply keep this in mind when practicing. Approach your pose with the intention of finding your perfect balance of strength and ease.

PART THREE | THE POSTURES

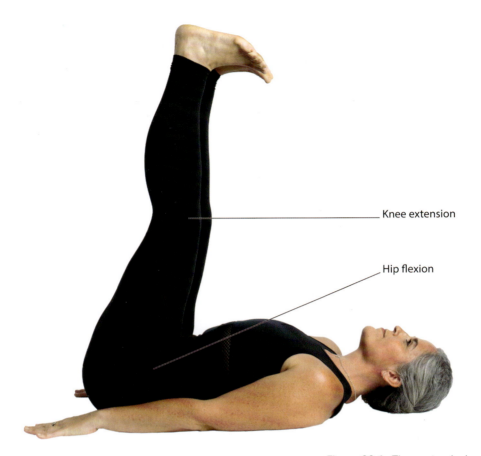

Figure 20.1. The anatomical actions of Waterfall.

Waterfall

Waterfall
Legs-Up-the-Wall Pose
Viparita Karani

Waterfall is the perfect option for a restorative inversion.

Lie down on your back, and lift your legs straight up with the soles of your feet facing the ceiling. Allow a soft bend to remain in your knees. Only activate enough to hold the pose. Your arms can rest in any comfortable position. Relax and breathe deeply.

Special Considerations

Since the torso rests on the floor in Waterfall, it is less of an inversion than the other poses in this group. Consequently, it may be more suitable for those who can't do full inversions for medical reasons.

ARM BALANCES AND INVERSIONS | CHAPTER 20

Waterfall. What am I feeling?

HOW DO I GET THERE?	WHAT IS STRENGTHENING?	WHERE COULD I NOTICE TIGHTNESS?	IS COMPRESSION POSSIBLE?
Hip flexion	Hip flexors, fig. 7.5	Hip extensors, fig. 7.6	
Knee flexion	Knee extensors, fig. 8.2	Knee flexors, fig. 8.3	

My discoveries:

Modifications

Rest your raised legs on a wall to make the pose even more restorative.

Holding the ends of a strap, loop it around the soles of your feet to minimize the effort required by your legs.

Variations

Place a block underneath your hips for a small shift in perspective and an added low back stretch. Be sure to place the block under the hip bones and not under the lumbar spine. Using the block lengthwise, left to right, is typically best for full support of the pelvis.

Exploration/Possible Cues

Enjoy the sensation of your feet being up in the air.

Your legs have been holding you all day; now let them rest.

Breathe deeply while you give your body a much-needed break.

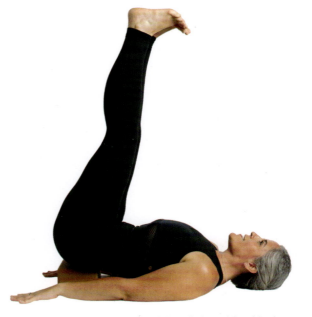

Figure 20.2. Waterfall variation with a block.

PART THREE | THE POSTURES

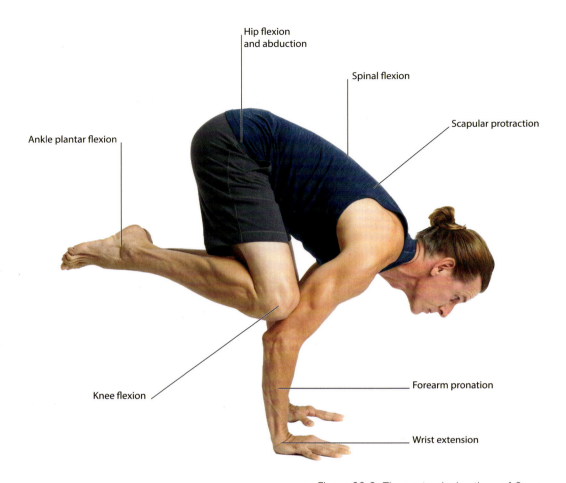

Figure 20.3. The anatomical actions of Crow.

Crow

Crow
Bakasana

For most practitioners, Crow is typically the first experience of balancing body weight on the hands. It cultivates a sense of playfulness, strength, and balance.

Begin in Rag Doll (fig. 17.3). Move your feet back just enough so that you can place your hands flat on the floor a little wider than shoulder width. Activate your hands, and press evenly through all ten fingertips. Snug your knees into your arms while keeping your hips high in the air. Depending on your body proportions, your knees will connect to the backs or sides of your upper arms; get them as close to your armpits as possible. Wiggle your feet together, connecting the inner rims from big toes to heels. Reach your chest slightly forward while engaging your abdominals as if rounding into Cat pose (fig. 13.6). Squeeze your feet together while activating in and up. Lift your feet off the ground, and balance your body weight evenly in your hands. Land your gaze six to twelve inches in front of you on the floor, and breathe.

ARM BALANCES AND INVERSIONS | CHAPTER 20

Crow. What am I feeling?

HOW DO I GET THERE?	WHAT IS STRENGTHENING?	WHERE COULD I NOTICE TIGHTNESS?	IS COMPRESSION POSSIBLE?
Spinal flexion	Spinal flexors, fig. 5.5	Spinal extensors, fig. 5.3	
Knee flexion	Knee flexors, fig. 8.3	Knee extensors, fig. 8.2	
Hip flexion	Hip flexors, fig. 7.5	Hip extensors, fig. 7.6	✓ Fig. 7.4
Hip abduction	Hip adductors, fig. 7.8 *Although legs are often placed in abduction, adduction is necessary to lift in and up, opposing gravity.*		
Scapular protraction	Protractors of the scapulae, p. 54	Retractors of the scapulae, p. 54	
Wrist extension	Wrist extensors, fig. 11.2	Wrist flexors, fig. 11.3	✓ Fig. 11.1
Forearm pronation	Forearm pronators, fig. 10.5	Forearm supinators, fig. 10.4	
Ankle plantar flexion	Ankle plantar flexors, fig. 9.4	Ankle dorsiflexors, fig. 9.3	

My discoveries:

Special Considerations

If you have wrist injury or weakness, weight bearing in your hands will probably be problematic.

Be careful not to take your wrist joints too far into extension, especially while bearing weight, since this may strain them (fig. 13.23).

If you need relief, change the angle of your wrists with padding to minimize extension. You can do this for any pose that requires weight bearing in the hands.

Modifications

Beginners can build strength and confidence by lifting one foot.

Try placing a block underneath your feet to make it easier to get your knees higher on your arms.

Variations

One-legged Crow is a fun variation to add to a sturdy Crow foundation.

Place a block between your feet to change the physics of the pose and to emphasize feet and core activation.

Exploration/Possible Cues

Reach your chest forward, as if you had a flashlight on it shining onto the floor in front of you.

Push the floor away while rounding your spine toward the ceiling.

Spread the spaces between your toes, and fire up your feet.

As you squeeze the inner rims of your feet together, let that activate your core.

Don't take yourself too seriously. It's only yoga.

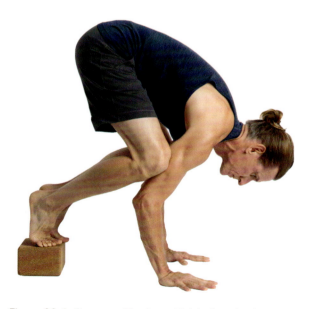

Figure 20.4. Crow modification with block under feet.

ARM BALANCES AND INVERSIONS | CHAPTER 20

Imperfection is not our personal problem—it is a natural part of existing.
—Tara Brach

PART THREE | THE POSTURES

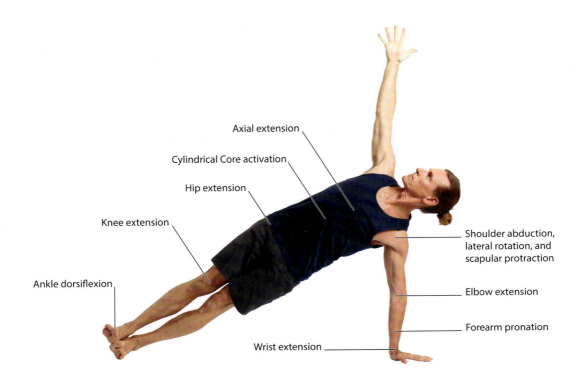

Figure 20.5. The anatomical actions of Side Plank.

Side Plank

Side Plank
Vasisthasana

Some might think of Side Plank as an upper-body strengthener, but actually it is a full-body strengthener when approached properly.

Begin in Plank (fig. 13.18). Maintain Plank pose activation through your legs and Cylindrical Core. Position your feet together so that your ankles are touching. Leave your left hand where it is on the floor. Slide your left shoulder blade strongly toward your left hand (protraction) for joint stability. While reaching your right hand up and out of your shoulder, spin onto the outer edge of your left foot, stacking your right foot on top of it. With the inner rims of your feet together, keep your feet very active as if standing on the ground. Do not disengage your legs or core. Maintain Mountain alignment through your body as you actively reach your right hand up toward the ceiling. Gaze toward or beyond your lifted hand.

ARM BALANCES AND INVERSIONS | CHAPTER 20

Side Plank. What am I feeling?

HOW DO I GET THERE?	WHAT IS STRENGTHENING?	WHERE COULD I NOTICE TIGHTNESS?	IS COMPRESSION POSSIBLE?
Cylindrical Core activation	Cylindrical Core, fig. 13.17		
Axial extension	Axial extensors, fig. 5.10	Entire trunk	
Shoulder abduction	Shoulder abductors, fig. 6.7	Shoulder adductors, p.45	
Shoulder lateral rotation	Shoulder lateral rotators, fig. 6.14	Shoulder medial rotators, fig. 6.11	
Scapular protraction *Bottom arm*	Protractors of the scapulae, p. 54	Retractors of the scapulae, p. 54	
Hip extension	Hip extensors, fig. 7.6 Even though hips are in neutral, hip extensors work isometrically to hold body in space.	Hip flexors, fig. 7.5	
Knee extension	Knee extensors, fig. 8.2	Knee flexors, fig. 8.3	
Bottom-arm wrist extension	Wrist extensors, fig. 11.2	Wrist flexors, fig. 11.3	✓ Fig. 11.1
Elbow extension	Elbow extensors, fig. 10.2	Elbow flexors, fig. 10.3	
Forearm pronation *Bottom arm*	Forearm pronators, fig. 10.5	Forearm supinators, fig. 10.4	
Ankle dorsiflexion	Ankle dorsiflexors, fig. 9.3	Ankle plantar flexors, fig. 9.4	

My discoveries:

Special Considerations

Shoulder, wrist, or back injury can limit this pose.

It is always important to pay close attention to the weight-bearing joints in any pose. Aim to stay active in the rest of your body, as needed, to minimize weight collapse into the load-bearing joint. In Side Plank, weight is on the bottom shoulder and wrist. All alignment points should support keeping these joints healthy. This pose is often taught with a vertical stack of the arm; in other words, the wrist is directly under the shoulder. This can be effective for some, as long as the rest of the body stays active to minimize the weight dropping into the shoulder and wrist. Another approach to Side Plank is to slightly angle the bottom arm by sliding the hand a few inches forward of the shoulder. When combined with a sense of pushing the ground away while "hollowing out" the armpits, this activates the muscles that hug the scapula into the thorax, providing a sense of strong support and lift.

If you have wrist injury, one of the most troublesome positions is wrist extension with weight bearing. Make sure your wrist is never hyperextended in any pose in which the hands are bearing weight. You may need to avoid this pose altogether, or place your elbow and forearm on the floor to take the weight completely out of your wrist and hand.

Modifications

Place your bottom knee on the ground for more stability or while building strength. Your bottom foot can act as a kickstand behind the body for even more support. Or line up your bottom foot under the top leg for a balance challenge.

Staggering your feet instead of stacking them will distribute your weight differently, making the pose slightly easier.

Variations

Many playful variations of this pose involve changing the top leg.

You can grab the top knee or foot for a challenge.

Try Dancer with the top leg for a strength and balance challenge.

ARM BALANCES AND INVERSIONS | CHAPTER 20

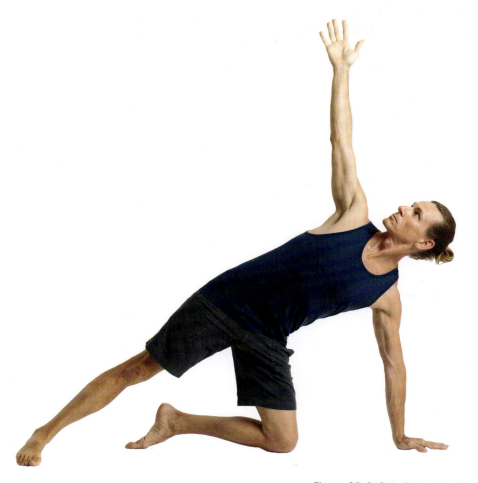

Figure 20.6. Side Plank modification.

Exploration/Possible Cues

Shine bright in all directions.

Push the floor away to activate your entire body.

Try stacking your hand directly under your bottom shoulder, and then try angling your bottom arm. Which option feels sturdier?

Keep your legs strong and active.

Brighten up the soles of your feet by reaching through them.

If you are building strength toward the full pose, try it for a bit, and then lower your bottom knee as soon as you feel instability.

PART THREE | THE POSTURES

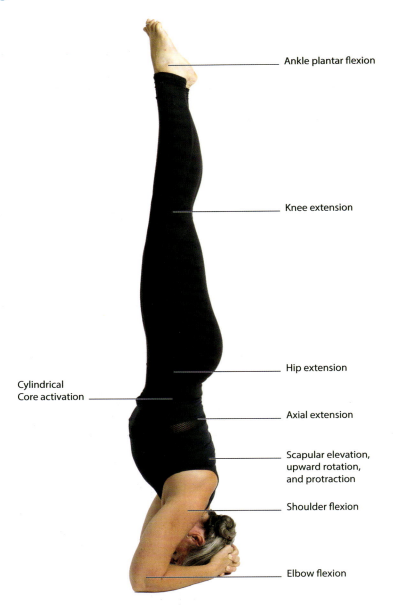

Figure 20.7. The anatomical actions of Headstand.

Headstand

Headstand
Classical Headstand
Sirsasana
Salamba Sirsasana
King of Asanas

Headstand can be empowering and refreshing both physically and mentally. It offers overall strengthening and heightened awareness of body integration. *Even though it is called Headstand, you are not balancing your weight on your head.* You must remember this to keep your cervical spine safe.

Begin standing in Mountain. Establish the sensory experience of standing tall with a **neutral** spine. Notice what a neutral neck (cervical spine) feels like. Feel how your head is positioned to maintain a neutral neck (fig. 20.8). This is how you will want to be in Headstand.

ARM BALANCES AND INVERSIONS | CHAPTER 20

Headstand. What am I feeling?

HOW DO I GET THERE?	WHAT IS STRENGTHENING?	WHERE COULD I NOTICE TIGHTNESS?	IS COMPRESSION POSSIBLE?
Cylindrical Core activation	**Cylindrical Core, fig. 13.17**		
Shoulder flexion	**Shoulder flexors, fig. 6.4**	**Shoulder extensors, fig. 6.5**	✓ Fig. 6.3
Scapular elevation and upward rotation *Natural position with arm placement*	Elevators and upward rotators of the scapulae, p. 54	Depressors and downward rotators of the scapulae, p. 54	
Scapular protraction *This action presses elbows into the floor.*	**Protractors of the scapulae, p. 54**	Retractors of the scapulae, p. 54	
Hip flexion *In the setup*	Hip flexors, fig. 7.5	**Hip extensors, fig. 7.6** *In the setup*	✓ Fig. 7.4
Hip extension	**Hip extensors, fig. 7.6** Even though legs are in neutral, hip extensors work isometrically to hold body in space.	**Hip flexors, fig. 7.5**	
Hip adduction *To hold legs together*	**Hip adductors, fig. 7.8**	Hip abductors, fig. 7.9	
Knee extension	**Knee extensors, fig. 8.2**	**Knee flexors, fig. 8.3** *In the setup*	
Elbow flexion	Elbow extensors, fig. 10.2 *Elbow extensors work eccentrically and/or isometrically.*		
Ankle plantar flexion or dorsiflexion	Ankle plantar flexors, fig. 9.4 Ankle dorsiflexors, fig. 9.3	Ankle dorsiflexors, fig. 9.3 Ankle plantar flexors, fig. 9.4	

My discoveries:

PART THREE | THE POSTURES

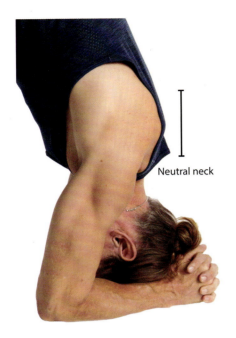

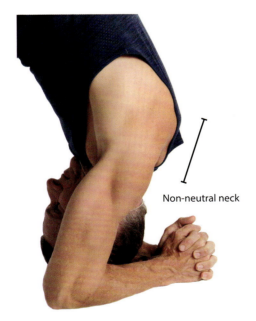

Figure 20.8. Neutral neck vs. non-neutral neck setup.

Come to Tabletop. Lower your elbows to the floor near shoulder-width distance apart. Clasp your hands together, and tuck your bottom pinky under so that your hands meet the floor evenly. Hold your hands as if you have a lemon between them (fig. 20.9). Place the top of your head on the floor so that your neck is in a neutral position. Your hands can touch your head, but avoid pressing into the back of your head as this can lead to collapse and weight bearing in the neck. Strongly press your elbows into the floor, staying very light on your head. Tuck your toes under, and lift your lower body as in Downward-Facing Dog. Stay very active in your upper body while you tippy-toe your feet closer toward your arms. Aim to get your hips over your shoulders. Take one leg straight up into the air, and draw the other bent leg into your chest. Spread the spaces between your toes, and stay actively engaged in your legs. Once steady, draw both legs straight up and together. Remain light in your head while actively pushing your elbows down and reaching up through your toes toward the ceiling. To come down, stay actively engaged, and lower one leg at a time. You will need to shift your hips slightly forward to counterbalance the weight of your legs lowering.

Special Considerations

This posture should be avoided if you have any neck injury or weakness.

Inversions should be avoided if you have glaucoma. Going upside down increases intraocular pressure which is hazardous with this condition.[43]

This pose has a bad reputation in some yoga circles, with good reason. If done improperly, it can put the neck at risk. The cervical spine is the most mobile and fragile part of the spine. If Headstand is not approached with neck safety as the number-one priority, it shouldn't be attempted at all.

Avoid the temptation to throw (kick) yourself up with momentum at a wall because this almost always leads to collapse and weight bearing in the neck. Learn to use your strength to lift up while remaining very light on your head. This is the perfect

ARM BALANCES AND INVERSIONS | CHAPTER 20

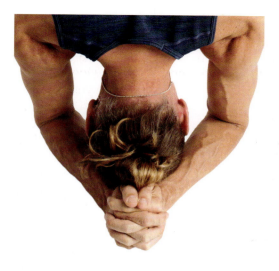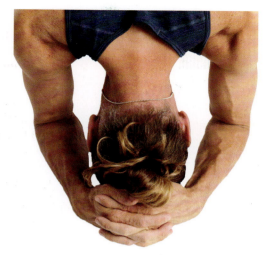

Figure 20.9. Close-up comparison of hand position options for Headstand.

opportunity to practice a heightened awareness of your body.

In my many years of guiding students, I find that there are two different approaches to getting into Headstand. Depending on your unique body dynamics, one or the other will be more natural for you. One way is as described above, lifting one leg up first. This entry requires enough flexibility to lift your leg. The other approach is what I call Bunny Lift. The initial setup is the same, but you take a controlled, micro bunny hop, lifting both knees up together.

Although it is rare, I have had a few students with body proportions that prevent safe headstands. Their humeri (upper-arm bones) are not long enough, so the tops of their heads touch first, keeping their forearm base from reaching the floor to support them in the pose. Consequently, they cannot do the pose without compressing their cervical spines. If you do Headstand arm setup while standing in Mountain, you can see where your elbows will land relative to the top of your head. For these students, their elbows were lower than the tops of their heads. Read more on body proportions in chapter 12, "Navigating the Posture."

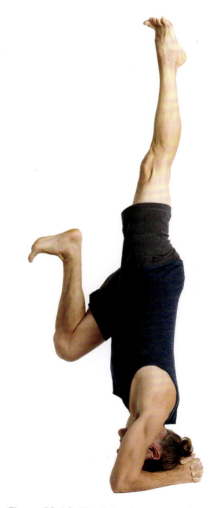

Figure 20.10. Headstand setup one knee in.

PART THREE | THE POSTURES

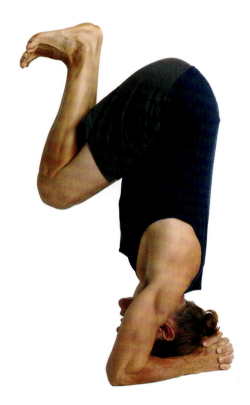

Figure 20.11. Headstand setup with two knees in.

The action of scapular protraction (fig. 6.17) typically causes a slight doming of the upper back. This action shifts in postures like Headstand and Forearm Stand. Instead of the upper back doming, the muscular action of scapular protraction sends force down through the elbows for a stronger press and a sturdier center of gravity.

Modifications

Do the beginning stages without lifting off.

Try using a wall either with your back facing it, or with your feet pressing into it for L-Stand. When doing the pose with your back to the wall, don't throw your body up. Don't lean on the wall. Use it for mental support, or have just one heel touching it.

Dolphin pose helps build strength for Headstand. It is a mixture of Headstand setup and Downward-Facing Dog.

ARM BALANCES AND INVERSIONS | CHAPTER 20

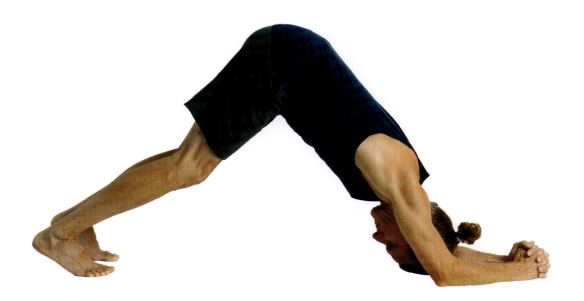

Figure 20.12. Dolphin pose.

Variations

Try varying leg positions once you establish a very stable foundation. Continue to prioritize neck safety. Always remain neutral in your neck and spine.

Exploration/Possible Cues

Activate a line of energy from your forearms to your toes.

Get lighter and lighter on your head.

Increase the space between your shoulders and ears.

Stay lifted out of your shoulder joints.

Spread your toes, and reach up as if you were going to grab something above you.

PART THREE | THE POSTURES

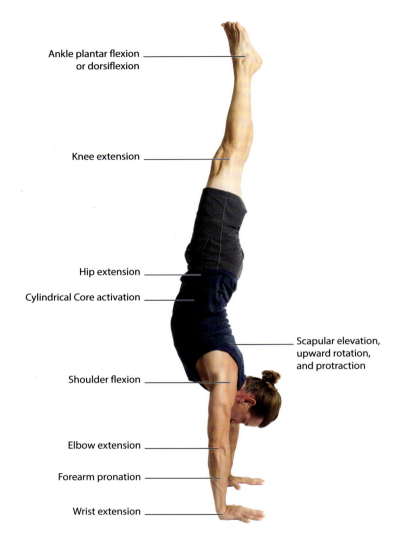

Figure 20.13. The anatomical actions of Handstand.

Handstand

Handstand
Adho Mukha Vrksasana

I've noticed that merely mentioning anything connected to Handstand creates a tightening response in my classes. Breath stops short, and I can literally hear the wheels turning. If this pose invokes fear for you, you are not alone. The fear of falling is a valid concern when practicing Handstand. I'd like to say that I can offer you a few simple steps to master the pose with ease, but the truth is for most people it takes time to develop. Here we will look at doing the pose using the wall for support.

ARM BALANCES AND INVERSIONS | CHAPTER 20

Handstand. What am I feeling?

HOW DO I GET THERE?	WHAT IS STRENGTHENING?	WHERE COULD I NOTICE TIGHTNESS?	IS COMPRESSION POSSIBLE?
Cylindrical Core activation	**Cylindrical Core, fig. 13.17**		
Shoulder flexion	**Shoulder flexors, fig. 6.4**	**Shoulder extensors, fig. 6.5**	✓ Fig. 6.3
Scapular elevation and upward rotation	**Elevators and upward rotators of the scapulae, p. 54**	Depressors and downward rotators of the scapulae, p. 54	
Scapular protraction	**Protractors of the scapulae, p. 54**	Retractors of the scapulae, p. 54	
Hip flexion *In the setup*	Hip flexors, fig. 7.5	**Hip extensors, fig. 7.6** *In the setup*	✓ Fig. 7.4
Hip extension	**Hip extensors, fig. 7.6** Even though legs are in neutral, hip extensors work isometrically to hold body in space.	**Hip flexors, fig. 7.5**	
Knee extension	**Knee extensors, fig. 8.2**	**Knee flexors, fig. 8.3** *In the setup*	
Wrist extension	**Wrist extensors, fig. 11.2**	**Wrist flexors, fig. 11.3**	✓ Fig. 11.1
Elbow extension	**Elbow extensors, fig. 10.2**	Elbow flexors, fig. 10.3	
Forearm pronation	Forearm pronators, fig. 10.5	Forearm supinators, fig. 10.4	
Ankle plantar flexion or dorsiflexion	Ankle plantar flexors, fig. 9.4 Ankle dorsiflexors, fig. 9.3	Ankle dorsiflexors, fig. 9.3 Ankle plantar flexors, fig. 9.4	

My discoveries:

I have highlighted the most common tendencies I see in my students. It is possible to feel strengthening or to notice tightness in any of the muscle groups listed within their respective columns.

PART THREE | THE POSTURES

Find a clear wall space. Before setting up, remember the alignment for Handstand is the same as Mountain. We are just turning it upside down. Come into Downward-Facing Dog with your fingertips about five inches away from the wall. Activate your hands, and press evenly through all ten fingers. Firmly activate your arms as if pressing the floor away from you. Gaze at the floor between your hands. Begin tippy-toeing your feet toward your hands to walk your hips above your shoulders. Take one leg up, and maintain a squared hip position. Remain very active in both legs all the way through your toes. Now begin taking little hops up. Think of lifting from your hips rather than simply kicking your legs. Once you are able, take both legs up with your heels touching the wall. Activate Mountain alignment. Elongate your armpits bringing your biceps toward your ears. Draw your tailbone toward your heels, and snug your front lower ribs into your belly. Activate your Cylindrical Core. With this activation, aim to come down slowly and lightly, one foot at a time.

Special Considerations

Inversions should be avoided if you have glaucoma. Going upside down increases intraocular pressure which is hazardous with this condition.[43]

If you are a Handstand beginner, first practice using the wall, eventually progressing to the middle of the room. Practicing at the wall will help build strength and wire in the neural circuitry required to hold your weight in your hands, wrists, and shoulders. Once proficient at getting up at the wall, you can practice taking one foot, then two, away from the wall. When you are ready to move to the middle of the room, you will want to employ all the foundational pieces described above. You will also need to learn how to balance your weight in your hands to keep from falling out. Pressing into your fingertips is the braking action to keep you from going over forward; pressing into the base of your hands can keep you from landing back on your feet.

The other key is feeling confident about your exit strategy. You will never "let" your body go all the way up into stacked balance if you are fearful about what is going to happen once you are there. The most effective exit strategy is to cartwheel or round-off when you are losing your balance going forward. This requires learning to take a hand step forward while your hips rotate and your feet land. If you did cartwheels or round-offs when you were younger, this will come quite easily. If you have no experience with this, be patient while your brain and body learn the new action.

Head positioning is variable. As a beginner, it is easier to pick a gaze point between your hands. As you gain confidence and proficiency, you can practice dropping your head more and more until you have a neutral neck. This will allow you to maintain axial extension and a "hollow" belly.

Modifications

Walking your feet up a wall while your hands are on the floor can be a great way to experience the initial sensation of bearing weight in your hands. Begin in Downward Dog with your heels near the wall. Walk your hands in closer to your feet, and then press one foot, then the other, into the wall. Eventually work toward holding your hips directly above your shoulders with legs parallel to the ground and feet on the wall. You will find this requires just as much or more strength as holding the pose in the middle of the room.

ARM BALANCES AND INVERSIONS | CHAPTER 20

Variations

Try varying leg positions once you are stable. You may find that shifting the physics of the pose a bit helps you balance more easily.

Exploration/Possible Cues

Five Tips:

    1. Elbows: Keep them straight and strong.

    2. Hands: Spread your hands actively, and grip the ground. Use your fingers! They are your brakes to keep you from going over.

    3. Torso and core: get to know the relationship between your ribs and hips; feel how they move together, how they move separately, and how to integrate them with core.

    4. Shoulders: Stand on your feet, and take your arms up into the air like you are doing Handstand upside down. You will need the mobility to take your arms straight up in line with your body to access this pose. If you don't have this, work on more openness in the shoulder fronts and chest with any poses that extend the shoulders or stretch and release the front of the body. Remember, the natural position of your scapulae with your arms overhead is upward rotation and elevation. While in Handstand, actively lift your shoulders toward your ears. Try to make your armpits longer and deeper as you go up; this will protract your scapulae, activating your serrati muscles, and providing stability at your shoulders.

    5. Legs and toes: Squeeze your quadriceps strongly, and spread your toes as if you are trying to grab something on the ceiling.

Visualize yourself in the pose before going up.

Use your breath to calm your mind.

Create a strong line of energy from your hands to your feet.

Play with how you are holding your head. Because it is quite heavy, it will affect the overall physics of the pose. Pick a spot between your hands to look at rather than lifting your head to gaze forward on the floor. Soften the back of your neck.

Squeeze your legs like crazy. Firm legs are much easier to balance than soft legs.

Hold your arms like strong, tall pillars; don't soften or collapse.

Try ease. Sometimes less is more.

PART THREE | THE POSTURES

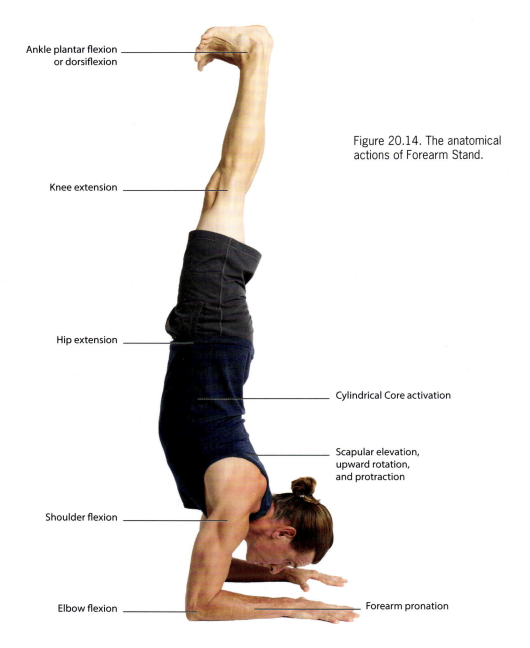

Figure 20.14. The anatomical actions of Forearm Stand.

Forearm Stand

Forearm Stand
Pincha Mayurasana

This empowering inversion can be a good option for those needing to avoid Headstand. The physics of this pose is quite different from Handstand because the fulcrum point of the hips is much closer to the floor. You will find that you need less momentum to get up because of this. As in the other inversions, aim for Mountain alignment and Cylindrical Core activation.

ARM BALANCES AND INVERSIONS | **CHAPTER 20**

Forearm Stand. What am I feeling?

HOW DO I GET THERE?	WHAT IS STRENGTHENING?	WHERE COULD I NOTICE TIGHTNESS?	IS COMPRESSION POSSIBLE?
Cylindrical Core activation	Cylindrical Core, fig. 13.17	Entire trunk	
Shoulder flexion	Shoulder flexors, fig. 6.4	Shoulder extensors, fig. 6.5	✓ Fig. 6.3
Scapular elevation and upward rotation *Natural position with arm placement*	Elevators and upward rotators of the scapulae, p. 54	Depressors and downward rotators of the scapulae, p. 54	
Scapular protraction *This action presses elbows into the floor.*	Protractors of the scapulae, p. 54	Retractors of the scapulae, p. 54	
Hip flexion *In the setup*	Hip flexors, fig. 7.5	Hip extensors, fig. 7.6 *In the setup*	✓ Fig. 7.4
Hip extension	Hip extensors, fig. 7.6 *Even though legs are in neutral, hip extensors work isometrically to hold body in space.*	Hip flexors, fig. 7.5	
Knee extension	Knee extensors, fig. 8.2	Knee flexors, fig. 8.3 *In the setup*	
Forearm pronation	Forearm pronators, fig. 10.5	Forearm supinators, fig. 10.4	✓ Fig. 10.5
Elbow flexion	Elbow extensors, fig. 10.2 *Elbows are bent, but the extensors work to oppose collapse with gravity.*		
Ankle plantar flexion or dorsiflexion	Ankle plantar flexors, fig. 9.4 Ankle dorsiflexors, fig. 9.3	Ankle dorsiflexors, fig. 9.3 Ankle plantar flexors, fig. 9.4	

My discoveries:

PART THREE | THE POSTURES

Begin in Tabletop (fig. 13.5). Place your forearms on the floor with elbows about shoulder-width distance apart and palms facing down. Look between your hands while tippy-toeing your feet forward to move your hips over your shoulders. Take one leg up, and maintain a squared hip position. Remain very active in both legs all the way through your toes. Now begin little hops up. Think of lifting from your hips rather than simply kicking your legs. Once you are able, take both legs up and together. Activate Mountain alignment. Elongate your armpits to avoid collapsing. Draw your tailbone toward your heels, and snug your front lower ribs into your belly. Come down slow and controlled, one leg at a time.

Special Considerations

Your body proportions will greatly influence how easily you can do this pose. This is true for many poses, especially arm balances and inversions.

Because the hands and elbows are anchored to the floor in this pose, skeletal shoulder flexion and skeletal forearm pronation can be challenging for certain body structures. If it seems like your bones "just don't go that way," try taking your elbows slightly farther apart, and position your hands differently. This is an example of where you can navigate around skeletal compression by playing with the angles.

If upper-body range of motion is an issue, you might have more success with "Headless Headstand" pose. It has the same setup and positioning as Headstand (fig. 20.7), but the head is off the floor. This hand positioning bypasses the forearm pronation and encourages external rotation of the upper-arm bones at the shoulder joint. This can increase mobility if you have compression with shoulder flexion (fig. 6.3).

Just like in Handstand, head positioning is variable. As a beginner, it is easier to pick a gaze point between your hands. As you gain confidence and proficiency, you can practice dropping your head more and more until you have a neutral neck. This will allow you to maintain axial extension and a "hollow" belly.

Inversions should be avoided if you have glaucoma. Going upside down increases intraocular pressure which is hazardous with this condition.[43]

Modifications

Practice the pose at a wall, touching your feet to the wall, then slowly finding the stability to take them away.

Dolphin pose (fig. 13.10) helps build strength for Forearm Stand. It is a mixture of Headstand setup and Downward-Facing Dog.

Use a block or two for stabilization.

For some people, holding one block lengthwise between the hands places the elbows too close together on the floor to accommodate the shoulders. If this is the case, then blocks may not be a good guide for you.

ARM BALANCES AND INVERSIONS | CHAPTER 20

Variations

Try varying leg positions once you establish a stable foundation.

Exploration/Possible Cues

Play with all the different ways of setting up your hands/arms until you find the one that works for your body.

Press the floor away while reaching up with your toes.

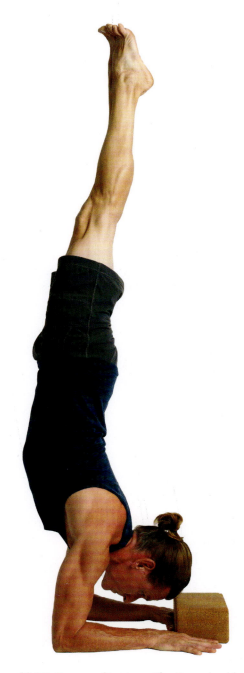

Figure 20.15. Forearm Stand modification using block.

PART THREE | THE POSTURES

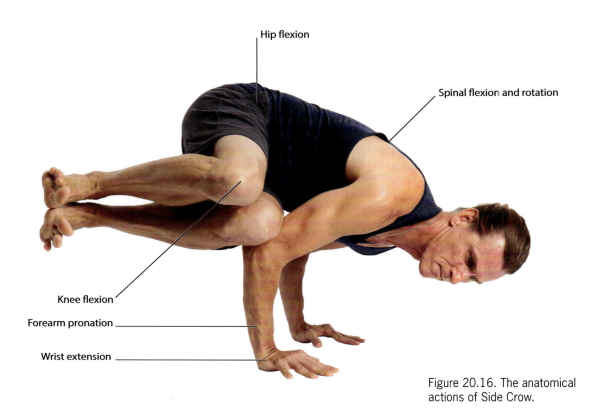

Figure 20.16. The anatomical actions of Side Crow.

Side Crow

Side Crow
Parsva Bakasana

Side Crow is yet another way to take flight and experience balancing your body weight on your hands. It requires varying degrees of core strength, depending on your body physics. Interestingly, your body's unique proportional structure and ranges of motion will determine your ease or challenge in accessing certain poses, including Side Crow. Consequently, some practitioners say this pose requires much less strength than regular Crow, but some argue quite the opposite.

Begin in Chair Twist to the left (fig. 15.3). Bend your knees until you are in a full squat with the twist. Place your hands on the floor outside your left thigh. Your hands and arms will be similar to Low Plank (fig. 13.21). Lean your body into your arms, using the backs of your upper arms as a tabletop support. Reach forward through your chest, and lift your legs off the floor. Actively reach your toes away as you balance evenly between both hands.

ARM BALANCES AND INVERSIONS | CHAPTER 20

Side Crow. What am I feeling?

HOW DO I GET THERE?	WHAT IS STRENGTHENING?	WHERE COULD I NOTICE TIGHTNESS?	IS COMPRESSION POSSIBLE?
Spinal flexion	Spinal flexors, fig. 5.5	Spinal extensors, fig. 5.3	
Spinal rotation	Spinal rotators, fig. 5.9	Opposing spinal rotators, fig. 5.9	✓ Fig. 5.7 ✓ Fig. 5.8
Knee flexion	Knee flexors, fig. 8.3	Knee extensors, fig. 8.2	
Hip flexion	Hip flexors, fig. 7.5	Hip extensors, fig. 7.6 On side twisting toward	✓ Fig. 7.4
Wrist extension	Wrist extensors, fig. 11.2	Wrist flexors, fig. 11.3	✓ Fig. 11.1
Forearm pronation	Forearm pronators, fig. 10.5	Forearm supinators, fig. 10.4	

My discoveries:

Special Considerations

As with many yoga poses, the ease with which you can access Side Crow depends on your body structure. I've seen brand-new students easily drop into it while long-time practitioners can have difficulty. Body proportions, range of motion with spine rotation, and leg size all influence this. Using blocks in various ways, as described in Modifications, sometimes helps with body-structure barriers.

As in any other twist, once the spinal-rotation range of motion is maxed out, the knees/hips will become uneven if rotation is pushed further.

PART THREE | THE POSTURES

Modifications

Stay in the pose setup, keeping your toes on the floor.

Put a block under your feet for more lift and accessibility.

Place blocks under your hands to change the physics for lifting off.

Variations

Twisted Scissor variation is another example of playing with the physics of the pose. Extending your legs out will shift the overall feel, balance, and playfulness.

Exploration/Possible Cues

Reach through your chest, and oppose this with active toes.

Engage your core to lift up and away from the ground.

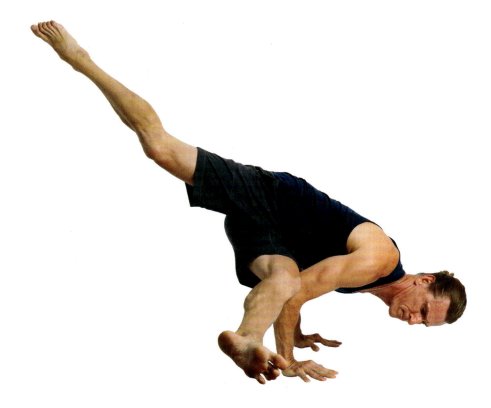

Figure 20.17. Side Crow with Scissor legs.

ARM BALANCES AND INVERSIONS | CHAPTER 20

Not until we are lost do we begin to understand ourselves.
—Henry David Thoreau

PART THREE | THE POSTURES

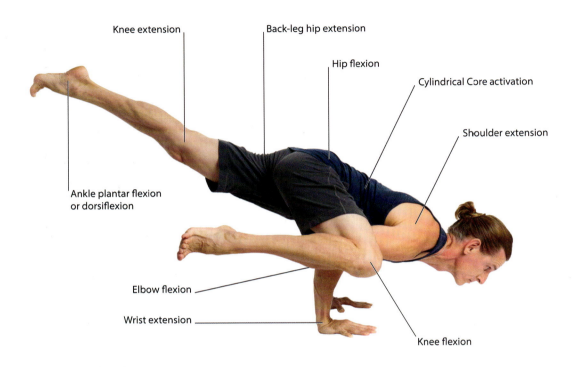

Figure 20.18. The anatomical actions of Running Man.

Running Man

Running Man
Eka Pada Koundinyasana II
Mountain Climber Variation

This fun pose almost always elicits giggles and conversation when I teach it in class, probably because finding it for the first time is such a new experience. Running Man offers overall body strengthening and heightened awareness of body weight balancing.

Begin in Downward-Facing Dog. Take a shortened stance so that your feet are slightly closer to your hands than usual. Lift your right leg up into the air. With active energy, draw your right knee to the back or side of your right arm. Lean into Chaturanga arms (fig. 13.21) while reaching your chest forward. Your left elbow can support the left side of your body somewhere between your ribs and hip. You might find that angling your left hand out to the left slightly helps. Keep a dynamic squeeze between your right knee and arm, activate your core, and lift your left leg up into the air behind you. Keep a fiery reach through all ten toes.

ARM BALANCES AND INVERSIONS | CHAPTER 20

Running Man. What am I feeling?

HOW DO I GET THERE?	WHAT IS STRENGTHENING?	WHERE COULD I NOTICE TIGHTNESS?	IS COMPRESSION POSSIBLE?
Cylindrical Core activation	**Cylindrical Core, fig. 13.17**		
Shoulder extension	**Shoulder flexors, fig. 6.4** *Although the shoulders are extended, the flexors work eccentrically and/or isometrically to oppose gravity and hold the body in space.*		
Wrist extension	**Wrist extensors, fig. 11.2**	**Wrist flexors, fig. 11.3**	✓ Fig. 11.1
Front-leg hip flexion	Hip flexors, fig. 7.5	**Front-leg hip extensors, fig. 7.6**	✓ Fig. 7.4
Front-leg knee flexion	**Knee flexors, fig. 8.3**	Knee extensors, fig. 8.2	
Back-leg hip extension	**Hip extensors, fig. 7.6**	**Hip flexors, fig. 7.5**	
Back-leg knee extension	**Knee extensors, fig. 8.2**	Knee flexors, fig. 8.3	
Elbow flexion	**Elbow extensors, fig. 10.2** *Although the elbows are bent, the extensors work eccentrically and/or isometrically to hold the body in space.*		
Ankle plantar flexion or dorsiflexion	Ankle plantar flexors, fig. 9.4 Ankle dorsiflexors, fig. 9.3	Ankle dorsiflexors, fig. 9.3 Ankle plantar flexors, fig. 9.4	

My discoveries:

Special Considerations

In a typical flow class, I see this pose quickly thrown into a sequence that consists of moving repetitively through some upper-body strength moves. This can be fine, but if you are new to the pose, you might have more success if you do it as a stand-alone pose. Instead of entering straight from Downward Dog, step your right foot forward into a Low Lunge, and begin from there. This can be a much more accessible entry for many people.

Modifications

Have an assistant/teacher/friend press into your back foot to help you achieve liftoff. Press your foot strongly into their hand while reaching forward with your chest.

Place blocks under your hands to change the physics of the pose.

Place your ear on the floor for support and easier liftoff.

Variations

Bending your back leg will change the physics of the pose, making it easier to lift as well as adding a bit more playfulness.

Exploration/Possible Cues

Create an active line of energy from your chest to your reaching toes.

Play with your body weight. Allow your head or ear to get a little lower to the floor to provide the forward counterweight for lifting your leg.

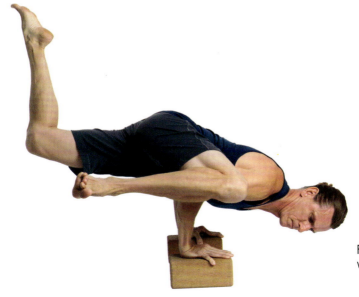

Figure 20.19. Running Man variation with back leg bent.

ARM BALANCES AND INVERSIONS | CHAPTER 20

Do the best you can until you know better. Then when you know better, do better.
—Maya Angelou

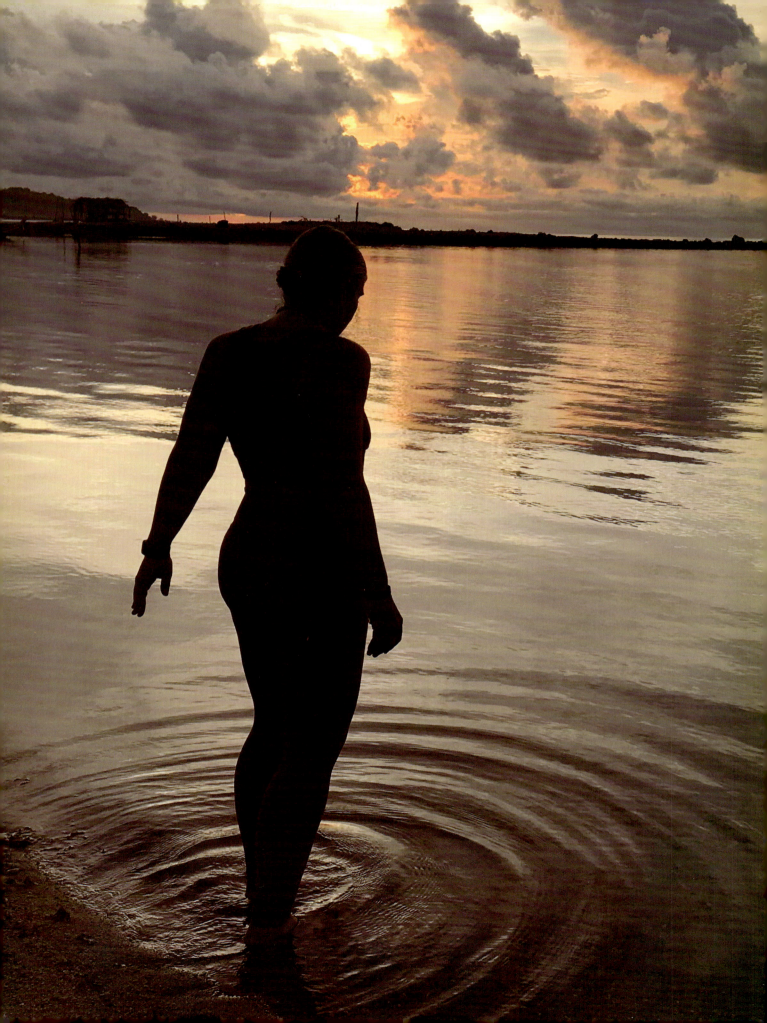

PART FOUR
The Gifts

PART FOUR | THE GIFTS

Chapter 21

Teaching Embodiment and Portable Gifts

Thoughts on Teaching Embodiment

Yoga postures give us the opportunity to stay and feel. Put very simply, yoga teaches us to pay attention, and paying attention to what we are feeling within our own bodies is a doorway back into a true sense of self. This has been a tremendous gift in my own life. Sharing this with others is my greatest aim in teaching the practice of embodiment through yoga.

If you want to teach anything, first aim to keep it alive within yourself. Cultivate your own increased interoception, the awareness of what's happening on the inside. Feel your yoga poses from within while you are on the mat. Then practice feeling the parade of sensations that ebb and flow within your body throughout your day. Feel what arises when you have moments of fear, anger, sadness, and joy. Practice staying still with what is. Gain an intimate understanding of how your own mind and body respond to your life circumstances. Aim to increase self-understanding and compassion. The more familiar you become with yourself, the better you can understand others. The more you can access love and compassion for yourself, the more you can find love and compassion for others. *Your personal journey with embodiment will be your primary instruction for teaching it.*

TEACHING EMBODIMENT AND PORTABLE GIFTS | CHAPTER 21

As you step into your classes, make connectivity your priority. Mutual respect, clear communication, and trust naturally arise through connectivity,

Never stop learning. Since you are asking your students to do things with their bodies, learn as much as possible about the body. Use this book to go beyond the typical bullet-point list of posture alignment cues and to deepen your understanding of the body in posture. Know the *hows* and *whys* behind your instruction. Understand that bodies are variable, breath is variable, individual experiences are unique, and poses will look and feel different from mat to mat. Learn to think critically about the body and biomechanics. Expand your ability as a helpful resource for your students. Remember, you don't have to know everything; it's OK to say, "I'm not sure." But intentionally expand your knowledge of the body and the physical discipline you are teaching. As your competency begins to grow in one or two areas, general concepts will more easily reveal themselves, and your knowledge and confidence will increase exponentially.

Stick with common language that is relatable to everyone. *When you use anatomical terms, teach your students what they mean.*

Keep your teaching simple and straightforward. If you choose to use anatomy to teach body awareness, use one concept per class rather than overcrowding your class with excessive information. Be patient with yourself and with your teaching. Leave space around your instruction so that your students have time to be curious and feel.

As you begin to think critically about yoga alignment, teach your students to do the same. Empower them to find their own way. Instill a sense of agency.

Teach your students about mindful awareness. Let them know that when they are paying attention to what they are feeling in the moment, without judgement, they are mindfully aware and present. Assure them that the part of them that notices and feels the breath is the same part that notices thought. Noticing thought is acute awareness. It is not failure, as many believe it to be. De-mystify the practices of awareness and presence for your students, so they can trust that they can do this. Remind them that if they have breath, they are fully capable of practicing mindful awareness. This is not a practice reserved for certain types or groups of people. It is for everyone.

View the classroom as a place to collaborate. Teach by sharing what you understand. Then be open to learning something new from your students. They are your greatest teachers.

Lastly, and most of all, enjoy this incredible opportunity you have been given to share the life-transforming practice of yoga.

PART FOUR | THE GIFTS

Ideas for Teaching Embodiment/Embodied Posture Teaching Themes

I don't believe that themes are always needed for a yoga class to be effective, but if you are looking for ways to be more intentional about teaching body awareness, themes are incredibly helpful. Personally, I enjoy sharing new and intriguing information for my students to explore on their mats, providing an easily accessible doorway into the experience of presence.

This book is a valuable resource for class theme ideas. These are just a few of the ideas within the pages of *Embodied Posture*:

I. The Spine

    A. Primary and secondary curves

    B. Spinal extension

    C. Spinal flexion

    D. Spinal rotation

    E. Axial extension

    F. Lateral flexion

    G. Intervertebral discs and their response to movement

    H. Reciprocal inhibition

    I. The agonist-antagonist relationship

II. The Shoulder

    A. Getting to know your skeletal structure/Finding your natural ranges of motion

    B. Shoulder flexion

    C. Shoulder extension

    D. Shoulder abduction

    E. Shoulder adduction

    F. Scapular protraction and retraction

    G. Scapular elevation and depression

    H. Scapular upward and downward rotation

III. The Hip

    A. Hip flexion

    B. Hip extension

    C. Hip medial rotation

    D. Hip lateral rotation

    E. Hip abduction

TEACHING EMBODIMENT AND PORTABLE GIFTS | CHAPTER 21

    F. Hip adduction

    G. Comparing passive anatomical actions and active anatomical actions

IV. The Knee

    A. Knee flexion

    B. Knee extension

    C. Knee medial rotation

    D. Knee lateral rotation

    E. Balancing the flexors and extensors for knee stability

V. The Ankle

    A. Dorsiflexion

    B. Plantar flexion

    C. Weight-bearing vs. non-weight-bearing ankle anatomical actions (foot on the floor vs. foot in the air)

    D. Dorsiflexion range of motion in lunge poses

VI. The Elbow

    A. Elbow extension

    B. Elbow flexion

    C. Forearm supination

    D. Forearm pronation

    E. Distinguishing between actions at the shoulder, elbow, or forearm

    F. Avoiding hyperextension of the elbows in hand weight-bearing postures

VII. The Wrist

    A. Wrist extension

    B. Wrist flexion

    C. Redistributing center of gravity to minimize weight bearing in hands

VIII. Navigating the Posture

    A. Deciphering between tension and compression

    B. Navigating tension

    C. Navigating compression

    D. Awakening to how body proportions affect posture

    E. Playing your edge with strength

PART FOUR | THE GIFTS

    F. The biomechanics of breath

    G. The ebb and flow of victorious breath

    H. Victorious breath as a tool for strength and stamina

    I. Longer, slower, deeper breaths to invoke parasympathetic response

    J. The steady power of drishti

IX. Foundation Postures

    A. The sensory experience of balanced, symmetrical poses

    B. Finding Mountain alignment in all postures

    C. Approaching posture with curiosity

    D. Neuroplasticity in posture

    E. Awakening to moments of autopilot

    F. Cylindrical Core—when is it most relevant?

    G. Finding fluidity and softness in strong postures

X. Standing Postures

    A. Closed-hip postures

    B. Open-hip postures

    C. Hip abduction with open-hip postures

    D. Getting to know your natural hip range of motion

    E. Pelvic tilt vs. torso tilt

    F. Anterior pelvic tilt

    G. Posterior pelvic tilt

XI. Twists

    A. The anatomy of the spine and twists (lumbar vs. thoracic)

    B. Using the exhalation to find the rotation

    C. Softness with twist

    D. Unanchored vs. anchored pelvis

    E. Considering the questions, "How is this serving me?" or "What is my aim?" in your approach to posture

XII. Standing Balance

    A. Open-hip balance postures

    B. Closed-hip balance postures

    C. Using gaze as an anchor for mind and body

XIII. Forward Folds
   A. Where am I accessing range of motion for the fold?
   B. Hip flexion in folding
   C. Spinal flexion in folding
   D. Engaging the front body to release the back body
   E. Releasing back-body tightness with knee bend

XIV. Backward Bends
   A. Hip extension in backbends
   B. Spinal extension in backbends
   C. Finding mobility in the entire spine
   D. Limiting lumbar spinal extension
   E. Increasing thoracic mobility
   F. Finding just the right foot placement
   G. Longer, not higher, backbends
   H. Shoulder mobility in backbending
   I. Using breath to stretch from the inside out
   J. Countering the biomechanics of sitting and "tech-ing"
   K. Using extensor muscles to backbend

XV. Hip Openers
   A. The 360° of the hip joint
   B. Front compartment
   C. Inner compartment
   D. Outer compartment
   E. Variability with hip opening
   F. A little stretch goes a long way.

XVI. Arm Balances and Inversions
   A. If it's not working, change something.
   B. Take the time to wire in the foundations.
   C. Patience with neuroplasticity
   D. Sthira Sukham Asanam

PART FOUR | THE GIFTS

Gifts

My Saturday morning class is the one class I have been teaching consecutively since our studios opened in 2005. The studio is always filled with chattiness, laughter, and connectivity. I'm sure many of you can relate. I wake up every Saturday morning excited to get there and teach. During a recent, hectic pre-class check-in, I overheard one of my long-time students say something that stopped me in my tracks. A woman who was there for her first time appeared hesitant and nervous as she set her mat up among all the other chatty practitioners. This long-time student walked right up to her and said, "Showing up today will be the best thing you have ever done for yourself and for your life." With a huge smile, she excitedly replied, "Really?" Her entire body softened, and she immediately seemed more at ease from his kind gesture. It wasn't only what he said but how he said it that was so impactful. He had such conviction and enthusiasm that there was no way she couldn't believe him. Yoga had supported him on a 75-pound weight-loss journey, increasing his cardiovascular health after a heart attack. His practice has indeed transformed his life. He was speaking from his personal truth. In these moments, I have no doubts about this practice.

Yoga is not a panacea, and it is certainly not a perfect practice. Yet, I have witnessed its positive effects in many lives, and I have experienced its gifts on a deep personal level. In closing, I share with you a few of the portable gifts that I have received while on my mat. I hope that you also have a life-long practice of receiving and giving these beautiful gifts.

The Ability to Feel

I spent many years of my life not feeling, or worse, thinking I was wrong for what I felt. Strong feelings were a trigger to lash out, go numb, run away, find distraction, or place blame. Embodiment of posture has created a safe space for me to get reacquainted with what I am feeling on the inside. As I wire my mind to feel how my bones and muscles are taking shape within a posture, I wire my mind to awaken to the sensory experiences of being alive. I am learning to stay with the uncomfortable feelings of anxiousness, sadness, fear, and shame as they arrive. As I acknowledge, allow, stay with, and investigate what is present in my body and mind, my feelings simply become information along my path toward living a wholehearted life.

Increased Space Between Stimulus and Response

Holding a long Warrior II brings up feelings in my body and mind. As soon as I cross over into expansion and growth, sensation kicks into high gear. Instead of immediately dropping out of the pose, I can use my breath to anchor into the moment for just a little bit longer. In the clear space of breath, the urgency of the moment dissipates. Then before I know it, it's time for the next pose. Holding a yoga pose increases my ability to pause and get grounded. It increases the space between stimulus and response, the only place I can find access to clear choice.

TEACHING EMBODIMENT AND PORTABLE GIFTS | CHAPTER 21

Self-Compassion and Kindness

Being with myself in a yoga pose is being in a vulnerable place. It's just me, my body, and my breath. With steady practice, I am learning that the only effective way to be in a pose is to simply meet myself where I am. I've discovered that seeing myself with love, forgiveness, and acceptance is much more energizing and life giving than meeting myself with dissatisfaction and self-blame. Observing myself with this awareness helps me see things I didn't see before. This clarity shows me that many of my thoughts and beliefs about myself are simply non-truths I am carrying from past experiences. Only when I see these things clearly can I begin to let them go with compassion. The kindness and self-compassion I am learning on my mat not only affect the way I treat myself, but they shift my ability to truly see those around me.

Balance

As I set the intention to do my postures with a blend of strength and ease, I observe myself more closely. I notice places in my body that are overworking along with places that are sleepy. Noticing this is usually all it takes to rebalance my physical energy and efforts. This practice on the mat is giving me the gift of realizing where I am overdoing or overextending myself in the moments of my life. I am awakening to areas of my life that have lost vitality and spark, and little by little, I am learning to say no to the things that deplete me. As on my mat, the first and most important step toward balance is always self-observation.

Anchoring in the Now

For years, I read books, listened to podcasts and even took courses on the topic of being present. Even though I *sort* of "got it," I never *really* "got it"—until yoga. For me, the physicality was the easiest doorway. In yoga posture, I aim to focus on concrete sensations within my body, breath, and surroundings. These concrete sensations are always happening in the now, and they are right there for me at any point in time. I am literally rewiring my brain to be in the present moment. Like exercising any muscle in my body, my ability to be present—anchoring into the now as it is happening in this moment—grows stronger as I practice it. This gift of presence affords me the beautiful reality of fully living my life as it is happening now. What an amazing gift to receive. I am incredibly grateful.

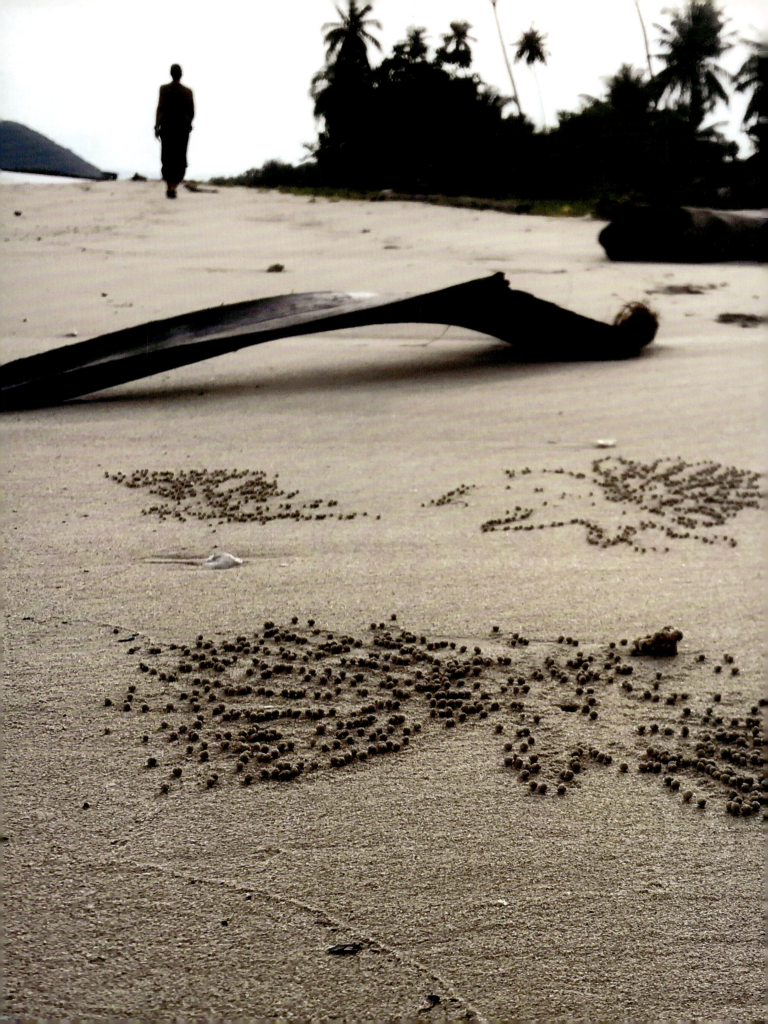

The best and most beautiful things in the world cannot be seen or even touched—they must be felt with the heart.

—Helen Keller

Glossary

abduction: Moving a limb away from the centerline of the body.

acetabulum: The socket of the hip ball-and-socket joint.

adduction: Moving a limb toward the centerline of the body.

agonist: The prime mover muscles of any joint action.

anatomical position: The upright, standing position of the human body with face forward and palms forward, used for describing the relationship between parts of the body.

annulus fibrosus: The tough, outer portion of an intervertebral disc.

antagonist: The opposing muscles of the agonists; also the muscles being stretched in any joint action.

anterior: In anatomy, referring to the front of the body.

asana: Sanskrit word for physical yoga posture.

autonomic balance: Balanced tone of the sympathetic nervous system and the parasympathetic nervous system.

autonomic nervous system (ANS): The part of the nervous system responsible for bodily functions that are happening automatically or autonomically.

bursitis: Inflammation of small, fluid-filled sacs near a joint.

compression: When two objects meet; skeletal compression: when two bones meet.

concentric: When a muscle shortens while working.

Cylindrical Core: The muscular core as a cylindrical container that has a front, sides, and back, including rectus abdominis, external and internal obliques, transverse abdominis, quadratus lumborum, erector spinae, and Iliopsoas muscles.

deep: In anatomy, toward the center of the body, below the surface.

depression: As in scapular depression, lowering the scapula downward, away from the ears.

diaphragm: One of the main muscles of ventilation, an umbrella-shaped muscle that separates the thoracic and abdominal cavities.

distal: In anatomy, referring to a muscle, bone, or limb, that part farthest away from the attachment.

drishti: Sanskrit word for gaze point.

eccentric: When a muscle lengthens while working.

elevation: As in scapular elevation, lifting the scapula upward toward the ears.

Embodied Posture Methodology (EPM): Yoga alignment methodology which encourages aligning your postures from within. It is a practice of combining awareness, information, and exploration.

embodiment: Being in the felt sense of the body, as in "feeling from my heart, my skin, my muscles, and my bones."

extension: Increasing the angle between two corresponding bones in a joint. This can be thought of as opening the joint.

exteroceptive awareness: Noticing our surroundings.

fascia: A thin sheet of connective tissue surrounding muscles and internal organs.

flexion: Decreasing the angle between two corresponding bones in a joint. This can be thought of as closing the joint.

front hip compartment: The group of muscles on the front of the hip, including the hip flexors.

impingement: When soft tissues get caught between two or more articulating bones at a joint.

inferior: In anatomy, toward the feet, or relationally below.

inner hip compartment: The group of muscles on the inner thigh, including the hip adductors.

insertion: The tendinous attachment farther away from the midline of the body.

interoceptive awareness: Noticing physical sensations within the body.

intervertebral disc: A shock-absorbing cartilage structure that separates the vertebral bodies of the spine.

isometric: When a muscle does not shorten or lengthen while working; it remains static.

kyphosis: A chronically rounded, flexed spine.

kyphotic: Primary curvature of the spine; the curves that round away from the center of the body.

labrum: Cartilage lining of the hip socket or the acetabulum.

lateral: In anatomy, the side of the body.

lordotic: Secondary curvature of the spine; the curves that round toward the center of the body.

medial: In anatomy, toward the middle of the body.

midline: An invisible line down the middle of the body.

Glossary (continued)

mindfulness: "Awareness that arises through paying attention, on purpose, in the present moment, non-judgmentally," as defined by Jon Kabat-Zinn.[1]

myofascial connectivity: The continuous connection between fascia and muscle.

neuropathy: Traveling nerve sensation.

neutral: A neutral joint is one that is not in flexion, extension, abduction, adduction, medial rotation, lateral rotation, etc.

nucleus pulposus: The softer, inner material of an intervertebral disc.

origin: The tendinous attachment of a muscle closer to the midline of the body.

outer hip compartment: This group includes all the muscles that cross the hip joint from behind and/or the side (lateral). These muscles extend, abduct, internally rotate, and externally rotate the thigh.

parasympathetic nervous system (PNS): A branch of the autonomic nervous system (ANS) responsible for slowing the effects of the stress response or sympathetic branch, also referred to as the rest-and-digest branch of the autonomic system.

piriformis syndrome: An injury in which the piriformis muscle puts pressure on the sciatic nerve resulting in sciatica.

posterior: In anatomy, the backside of the body.

pranayama: Breath control exercises.

pronation: In reference to the hand, turning the palm backward from anatomical position or palm down.

proprioceptive awareness: Noticing the position of the body in space.

protraction: As in scapular protraction, sliding the scapula laterally on the thorax.

proximal: In anatomy, when referring to a muscle, bone, or limb, that part closest to the attachment.

reciprocal inhibition: The theory that muscles work in pairs, and when we activate muscles on one side of a joint, those on the opposite side release.

retraction: Drawing the scapula medially on the thorax, or drawing the scapulae toward each other.

soft tissue: Tissues that surround and support the bones and vital organs, including muscles, tendons, ligaments, fascia, fat, nerves, membranes, and blood vessels.

sprain: Torn or overstretched ligament.

superficial: In anatomy, toward the skin or relationally less deep.

superior: In anatomy, toward the head or relationally above.

supination: In reference to the hand, turning the palm forward as in anatomical position or palm up.

sympathetic nervous system (SNS): A branch of the autonomic nervous system (ANS) responsible for activating the fight-or-flight stress response.

tendinopathy: Disease of a tendon.

thoracolumbar junction: Where the thoracic spine merges with the lumbar spine.

tibiotalar joint: The primary joint of the ankle.

ujjayi breath: Slightly audible breath used in yoga, done by restricting air at the glottis—much like whispering.

victorious breath: Another name for ujjayi breath.

vinyasa: A style of yoga that emphasizes synchronizing breath with movement.

Endnotes

1. Kabat-Zinn, Jon. *Wherever You Go, There You Are: Mindfulness Meditation in Everyday Life.* 1st ed. New York: Hyperion, 1994.

2. Anatomy for Yoga DVD by Paul Grilley. 1st ed. Pranamaya.

3. Fisher, James P., Colin N. Young, and Paul J. Fadel. "Central Sympathetic Overactivity: Maladies and Mechanisms." *Autonomic Neuroscience: Basic & Clinical* 148, no. 1–2 (June 15, 2009): 5–15. https://doi.org/10.1016/j.autneu.2009.02.003.

4. Komori, Teruhisa. "The Relaxation Effect of Prolonged Expiratory Breathing." *Mental Illness* 10, no. 1 (May 16, 2018). https://doi.org/10.4081/mi.2018.7669.

5. Fisher, James P., Colin N. Young, and Paul J. Fadel. "Central Sympathetic Overactivity: Maladies and Mechanisms." *Autonomic Neuroscience: Basic & Clinical* 148, no. 1–2 (June 15, 2009): 5–15. https://doi.org/10.1016/j.autneu.2009.02.003.

6. Serpa, J. Greg, Stephanie L. Taylor, and Kirsten Tillisch. "Mindfulness-Based Stress Reduction (MBSR) Reduces Anxiety, Depression, and Suicidal Ideation in Veterans." *Medical Care* 52, no. 12 Suppl 5 (December 2014): S19-24. https://doi.org/10.1097/MLR.0000000000000202.

7. Myers, Thomas W. *Anatomy Trains: Myofascial Meridians for Manual and Movement Therapists.* 3rd ed. Edinburgh: Elsevier, 2014.

8. Martini, Frederic, Judi Lindsley Nath, and Edwin F. Bartholomew. *Fundamentals of Anatomy & Physiology.* Tenth edition. Boston: Pearson, 2015.

9. Myers, Thomas W. *Anatomy Trains: Myofascial Meridians for Manual and Movement Therapists.* p. 45.

10. Schoenfeld, Andrew J, and Bradley K Weiner. "Treatment of Lumbar Disc Herniation: Evidence-Based Practice." *International Journal of General Medicine* 3 (July 21, 2010): 209–14.

11. Billy, Gregory G., Susan K. Lemieux, and Mosuk X. Chow. "Lumbar Disc Changes Associated with Prolonged Sitting." *PM & R: The Journal of Injury, Function, and Rehabilitation* 6, no. 9 (September 2014): 790–95. https://doi.org/10.1016/j.pmrj.2014.02.014.

12. Han, Suk Ku, Yong Sik Kim, Tae Hyeon Kim, and Soo Hwan Kang. "Surgical Treatment of Piriformis Syndrome." *Clinics in Orthopedic Surgery* 9, no. 2 (June 2017): 136–44. https://doi.org/10.4055/cios.2017.9.2.136.

13. Fredericson, M., S. U. Lee, J. Welsh, K. Butts, A. Norbash, and E. J. Carragee. "Changes in Posterior Disc Bulging and Intervertebral Foraminal Size Associated with Flexion-Extension Movement: A Comparison between L4-5 and L5-S1 Levels in Normal Subjects." *The Spine Journal: Official Journal of the North American Spine Society* 1, no. 1 (February 2001): 10–17.

14. Raj, Marc A., and Scott C. Dulebohn. "Pain, Sacroiliac Joint." In *StatPearls*. Treasure Island (FL): StatPearls Publishing, 2018. http://www.ncbi.nlm.nih.gov/books/NBK470299/.

15. Aragão, José Aderval, Leonardo Passos Silva, Francisco Prado Reis, and Camilla Sá dos Santos Menezes. "Analysis on the Acromial Curvature and Its Relationships with the Subacromial Space and Types of Acromion." *Revista Brasileira de Ortopedia* 49, no. 6 (October 31, 2014): 636–41. https://doi.org/10.1016/j.rboe.2013.10.005.

16. "Rotator Cuff Tears - OrthoInfo - AAOS." Accessed September 6, 2018. https://www.orthoinfo.org/en/diseases–conditions/rotator-cuff-tears/.

17. Zeng, Yiming, You Wang, Zhenan Zhu, Tingting Tang, Kerong Dai, and Shijing Qiu. "Differences in Acetabular Morphology Related to Side and Sex in a Chinese Population." *Journal of Anatomy* 220, no. 3 (March 2012): 256–62. https://doi.org/10.1111/j.1469-7580.2011.01471.x.

18. Bogusiewicz, Michał, Katarzyna Rosinska-Bogusiewicz, Andrzej Drop, and Tomasz Rechberger. "Anatomical

Variation of Bony Pelvis from the Viewpoint of Transobturator Sling Placement for Stress Urinary Incontinence." *International Urogynecology Journal* 22, no. 8 (August 2011): 1005–9. https://doi.org/10.1007/s00192-011-1421-4.

19. Martin, Charys M, James G Turgeon, Aashish Goela, Charles L Rice, and Timothy D Wilson. "A Three-Dimensional Measurement Approach for the Morphology of the Femoral Head." *Journal of Anatomy* 225, no. 3 (September 2014): 358–66. https://doi.org/10.1111/joa.12207.

20. Beck, M., M. Kalhor, M. Leunig, and R. Ganz. "Hip Morphology Influences the Pattern of Damage to the Acetabular Cartilage: Femoroacetabular Impingement as a Cause of Early Osteoarthritis of the Hip." *The Journal of Bone and Joint Surgery. British Volume* 87, no. 7 (July 2005): 1012–18. https://doi.org/10.1302/0301-620X.87B7.15203.

21. Lempainen, Lasse, Kristian Johansson, Ingo J. Banke, Juha Ranne, Keijo Mäkelä, Janne Sarimo, Pekka Niemi, and Sakari Orava. "Expert Opinion: Diagnosis and Treatment of Proximal Hamstring Tendinopathy." *Muscles, Ligaments and Tendons Journal* 5, no. 1 (March 27, 2015): 23–28.

22. Kiapour, A. M., and M. M. Murray. "Basic Science of Anterior Cruciate Ligament Injury and Repair." *Bone & Joint Research* 3, no. 2 (February 1, 2014): 20–31. https://doi.org/10.1302/2046-3758.32.2000241.

23. Lee, Beom Koo, and Shin Woo Nam. "Rupture of Posterior Cruciate Ligament: Diagnosis and Treatment Principles." *Knee Surgery & Related Research* 23, no. 3 (September 2011): 135–41. https://doi.org/10.5792/ksrr.2011.23.3.135.

24. Haddad, M. Alex, Justin M. Budich, and Brian J. Eckenrode. "Conservative Management of an Isolated Grade III Lateral Collateral Ligament Injury in an Adolescent Multi-sport Athlete: A Case Report." *International Journal of Sports Physical Therapy* 11, no. 4 (August 2016): 596–606.

25. Chen, Lan, Paul D. Kim, Christopher S. Ahmad, and William N. Levine. "Medial Collateral Ligament Injuries of the Knee: Current Treatment Concepts." *Current Reviews in Musculoskeletal Medicine* 1, no. 2 (December 7, 2007): 108–13. https://doi.org/10.1007/s12178-007-9016-x.

26. DeClaire, Jeffrey H., Tatjana T. Savich, B. S. Adrienne LeGasse Montgomery, and Olayinka K. Warritay. "Significant Weight Loss May Delay or Eliminate the Need for Total Knee Replacement." *International Journal of Preventive Medicine* 5, no. 5 (May 2014): 648–52.

27. Hubbard, Tricia J, and Erik A Wikstrom. "Ankle Sprain: Pathophysiology, Predisposing Factors, and Management Strategies." *Open Access Journal of Sports Medicine* 1 (July 16, 2010): 115–22.

28. Lavery, Kyle P., Kevin J. McHale, William H. Rossy, and George Theodore. "Ankle Impingement." *Journal of Orthopaedic Surgery and Research* 11, no. 1 (September 9, 2016). https://doi.org/10.1186/s13018-016-0430-x.

29. Kaux, J. F., F. Delvaux, B. Forthomme, F. D. Marguerite, D. François, J. M. Crielaard, and J. L. Croisier. "Eccentric Training for Elbow Hypermobility." *Br J Sports Med* 48, no. 7 (April 1, 2014): 617–617. https://doi.org/10.1136/bjsports-2014-093494.154.

30. pmhdev. "Carpal Tunnel Syndrome - National Library of Medicine." PubMed Health. Accessed September 6, 2018. https://www.ncbi.nlm.nih.gov/pubmedhealth/PMHT0023117/.

31. Fufa, Duretti T., and Charles A. Goldfarb. "Sports Injuries of the Wrist." *Current Reviews in Musculoskeletal Medicine* 6, no. 1 (December 12, 2012): 35–40. https://doi.org/10.1007/s12178-012-9145-8.

32. Jerath, Ravinder, John W. Edry, Vernon A. Barnes, and Vandna Jerath. "Physiology of Long Pranayamic Breathing: Neural Respiratory Elements May Provide a Mechanism That Explains How Slow Deep Breathing Shifts the Autonomic Nervous System." *Medical Hypotheses* 67, no. 3 (2006): 566–71. https://doi.org/10.1016/j.mehy.2006.02.042.

Endnotes (*continued*)

33. *Breathing: The Master Key to Self Healing: The Benefits of Breathwork.* Boulder, CO: Sounds True, 1999.

34. "Biomechanics of Respiration." Accessed September 6, 2018. https://ouhsc.edu/bserdac/dthompso/web/namics/respire.htm.

35. "The Vital Capacity of The Lungs—Its Significance In Disease." *Journal of the American Medical Association* LXIX, no. 18 (November 3, 1917): 1528–1528. https://doi.org/10.1001/jama.1917.02590450048019.

36. Kim, Eun-Kyung. "The Effect of Gluteus Medius Strengthening on the Knee Joint Function score and Pain in Meniscal Surgery Patients." *Journal of Physical Therapy Science* 28, no. 10 (October 2016): 2751–53. https://doi.org/10.1589/jpts.28.2751.

37. Sinclair, Marybetts. "The Use of Abdominal Massage to Treat Chronic Constipation." *Journal of Bodywork and Movement Therapies* 15, no. 4 (October 2011): 436–45. https://doi.org/10.1016/j.jbmt.2010.07.007.

38. Sung, Youn-Bum, Jung-Ho Lee, and Young-Han Park. "Effects of Thoracic Mobilization and Manipulation on Function and Mental in Chronic Lower Back Pain." *Journal of Physical Therapy Science* 26, no. 11 (November 2014): 1711–14. https://doi.org/10.1589/jpts.26.1711.

39. Lee, Joon-Hee. "Effects of Forward Head Posture on Static and Dynamic Balance." *Journal of Physical Therapy Science* 28, no. 1 (January 2016): 274–77. https://doi.org/10.1589/jpts.28.274.

40. Billy, Gregory G., Susan K. Lemieux, and Mosuk X. Chow. "Lumbar Disc Changes Associated with Prolonged Sitting." *PM & R: The Journal of Injury, Function, and Rehabilitation* 6, no. 9 (September 2014): 790–95. https://doi.org/10.1016/j.pmrj.2014.02.014.

41. Cho, Juchul, Eunsang Lee, and Seungwon Lee. "Upper Thoracic Spine Mobilization and Mobility Exercise versus Upper Cervical Spine Mobilization and Stabilization Exercise in Individuals with Forward Head Posture: A Randomized Clinical Trial." *BMC Musculoskeletal Disorders* 18 (December 12, 2017). https://doi.org/10.1186/s12891-017-1889-2.

42. Nadler, S. F., G. A. Malanga, J. H. Feinberg, M. Prybicien, T. P. Stitik, and M. DePrince. "Relationship between Hip Muscle Imbalance and Occurrence of Low Back Pain in Collegiate Athletes: A Prospective Study." *American Journal of Physical Medicine & Rehabilitation* 80, no. 8 (August 2001): 572–77.

43. Weinreb, R. N., J. Cook, and T. R. Friberg. "Effect of Inverted Body Position on Intraocular Pressure." *American Journal of Ophthalmology* 98, no. 6 (December 15, 1984): 784–87.

Additional Sources

Adams, M. A., S. May, B. J. Freeman, H. P. Morrison, and P. Dolan. "Effects of Backward Bending on Lumbar Intervertebral Discs. Relevance to Physical Therapy Treatments for Low Back Pain." *Spine* 25, no. 4 (February 15, 2000): 431–437; discussion 438.

"Bone Photos – Yin Yoga Teacher Training." Accessed September 12, 2018. http://paulgrilley.com/bone-photos/.

Brach, Tara. *Radical Acceptance: Embracing Your Life with the Heart of a Buddha*, 2004.

Brown, C. Brené. *The Gifts of Imperfection: Let Go of Who You Think You're Supposed to Be and Embrace Who You Are*. Center City, Minn: Hazelden, 2010.

Desikachar, T. K. V. *The Heart of Yoga: Developing a Personal Practice*. Rev. ed. Rochester, Vt: Inner Traditions International, 1999.

Faulds, Danna. *Go in and in: Poems from the Heart of Yoga*. Greenville, Va.: Peaceable Kingdom Books, 2002.

Jalal al-Din Rumi, and Coleman Barks. *The Essential Rumi*. San Francisco, CA: Harper, 1995.

Koopman, Frieda A, Susanne P Stoof, Rainer H Straub, Marjolein A van Maanen, Margriet J Vervoordeldonk, and Paul P Tak. "Restoring the Balance of the Autonomic Nervous System as an Innovative Approach to the Treatment of Rheumatoid Arthritis." *Molecular Medicine* 17, no. 9–10 (2011): 937–48. https://doi.org/10.2119/molmed.2011.00065.

Mannor, Dana A., and Thomas N. Lindenfeld. "Spinal Process Apophysitis Mimics Spondylolysis: Case Reports." *The American Journal of Sports Medicine* 28, no. 2 (March 1, 2000): 257–60. https://doi.org/10.1177/03635465000280022001.

Quinlan, Erin, Tari Reinke, and William C. Bogar. "Spinous Process Apophysitis: A Cause of Low Back Pain Following Repetitive Hyperextension in an Adolescent Female Dancer." *Journal of Dance Medicine & Science: Official Publication of the International Association for Dance Medicine & Science* 17, no. 4 (December 2013): 170–74.

Siegel, Daniel J. *Mind: A Journey to the Heart of Being Human*. First edition. New York: W.W. Norton & Company, 2017.

Siegel, D. J. (2010). *Mindsight: The new science of personal transformation*. New York, NY: Bantam.

Weinreb, R. N., J. Cook, and T. R. Friberg. "Effect of Inverted Body Position on Intraocular Pressure." *American Journal of Ophthalmology* 98, no. 6 (December 15, 1984): 784–87.

Index of Postures

A

Airplane, 133, 134, 166, 167, 263, 274, 302-304

B

Boat, 240, 250-252

Bridge, 60, 261, 282-285, 297

C

Camel, 261, 286-289

Chair, 50, 146-149, 189-193, 218, 354

Chair Twist, 189-193, 354

Child's, 37, 79, 111, 114-117, 125, 316

Cobra, 270-272, 280

Crescent Twist, 28, 30, 194-197, 208

Crow, 96, 106, 322, 332-334, 354-356

D

Dancer, 42, 48, 50, 292, 298-301, 338

Downward-Facing Dog, 9, 96, 105, 117, 122-127, 318, 342, 344, 348, 352, 358

E

Eagle, 46-47, 61-62, 174-175, 217-221

Easy Pose, 150-152, 212

F

Final Rest, 154-155

Floor Bow, 290-293

Forearm Stand, 344, 350-353

Frog, 326-327

Full Pigeon, 37, 48, 104, 309, 314-317

H

Half Moon, 5, 81, 82, 198, 199, 200, 217, 236-239

Half Pigeon, 79, 310-313, 316

Halfway Lift, 58, 59, 96, 132-134, 169, 240, 263

Handstand, 5, 96, 322, 329, 346-352

Happy Baby, 322-323, 327

Headstand, 73, 75, 83, 84, 106, 322, 340-345, 350, 352

High Lunge, 10, 12, 135, 157, 158, 161, 167, 194, 222, 263

L

Locust, 8, 263, 274-277, 302

Low Lunge, 81, 318-321, 360

Low Push-Up, 8, 53, 54, 89, 95, 102, 103, 140-144, 354

M

Mountain, 31, 43, 50, 88, 90, 113, 127-130, 132, 136, 146, 154, 163, 168, 176, 178, 186, 202, 205, 218, 20, 226, 227, 230, 232, 240, 242, 250, 252, 298, 302, 325, 336, 340, 343, 348, 350, 352, 358, 368

P

Plank, 8, 53-55, 86, 89, 92, 95-97, 103, 136-144, 163, 280, 336-339, 354

Pyramid, 157, 168-171, 208

R

Reverse Warrior, 157, 180-183

Revolved Half Moon, 198-201

Revolved Supported Leg Raise, 202-205

Revolved Triangle, 206-209

Running Man, 322, 358-360

S

Seated Forward Fold, 27, 240, 254-257

Seated Twist, 210-212

Side Angle, 48, 157, 163, 176-179

Side Crow, 354-356

Side Plank, 55, 92, 96, 336-339

Sphinx, 35, 266-269, 272, 280

Standing Forward Fold, 102, 240, 242-245, 248

Standing Wide-Leg Forward Fold, 240, 246-249

Supine Twist, 214-216

Supported Front Leg Raise, 217, 226-228

Supported Side Leg Raise, 202, 217, 228-230

T

Tabletop, 117-122, 125, 134, 136, 326, 342, 352

Tree, 61, 63, 217, 232-234

Triangle, 73, 74, 84, 184-187, 206-209

U

Upward-Facing Dog, 22, 23, 270, 278-281

W

Warrior I, 39, 41, 55, 155, 157, 160, 164-168, 206

Warrior II, 5, 44, 45, 47, 50, 53, 55, 91, 92, 96, 136, 157, 172-176, 178, 180, 182, 184, 370, 236, 370

Warrior III, 134, 217, 222-225, 263, 302

Waterfall, 9, 330-331

Wheel, 260, 261, 294-297

Y

Yogi Squat, 81, 324-325

Index of Anatomical Actions

A

anterior tilt of the pelvis, 69, 152, 160-163, 241, 260, 263, 320

B

backward bending, 22, 30, 35, 160, 167, 185, 187, 259, 260, 268, 284, 298. See also spinal extension

D

dorsiflexion, 80-84,
    in posture, 119, 123, 137, 141, 147, 159, 165, 169, 191, 195, 199, 203, 207, 227, 228, 237, 238, 255, 287, 323, 325, 337, 341, 347, 351, 359, 367

E

elbow extension, 88-89,
    in posture, 119, 123, 127, 129, 135, 137, 147, 159, 165, 173, 185, 191, 195, 199, 203, 207, 223, 237, 251, 367, 279, 283, 287, 291, 295, 299, 303, 337, 347, 367

elbow flexion, 88, 89,
    in posture, 141, 219, 247, 267, 341, 351, 359, 367

F

forward rounding, 22, 24, 30, 35, 163, 187, 192, 229, 251, 316. See also spinal flexion

H

hip abduction, 61, 63,
    in posture, 151, 173, 175, 177, 181, 185, 217, 229, 233, 237, 245, 288, 323, 325, 327, 333, 366, 368

hip adduction, 61, 62,
    in posture, 147, 193, 211, 219, 288, 341, 367

hip extension, 12, 22, 60, 105,
    in posture, 159, 165, 195, 199, 237, 259, 261, 267, 270, 271, 275, 279, 283, 287, 291, 295, 301, 337, 341, 347, 351, 366, 369

hip flexion, 12, 58-60, 67, 69,
    in posture, 102, 115, 117, 123, 133, 147, 151, 159, 163, 165, 169, 173, 177, 178, 181, 185, 186, 191, 195, 199, 203, 207, 208, 211, 215, 219, 227, 229, 233, 240, 241, 243, 247, 251, 255, 257, 264, 311, 312, 315, 316, 319, 323, 325, 327, 331, 333, 341, 347, 351, 355, 359, 366, 369

hip lateral rotation, 65,
    in posture, 237, 315, 323, 325, 366

hip medial rotation, 64,
    in posture, 366

K

knee extension, 12, 22, 73-74,
    in posture, 123, 129, 133, 135, 137, 139, 141, 159, 165, 169, 173, 177, 181, 185, 195, 199, 203, 207, 223, 227, 229, 233, 237, 243, 247, 251, 255, 261, 267, 271, 275, 279, 283, 287, 291, 295, 299, 303, 337, 341, 347, 351, 365, 367

knee flexion, 12, 73, 75, 79,
    in posture, 115, 117, 119, 147, 151, 159, 165, 173, 177, 181, 191, 195, 211, 215, 219, 233, 241, 315, 323, 325, 327, 331, 333, 355, 367

knee lateral rotation, 77

knee medial rotation, 76

L

lateral spinal flexion, 25, 26,
    in posture, 181, 186

P

plantar flexion, 22, 80, 81, 83, 84,
    in posture, 117, 119, 169, 185, 186, 207, 219, 238, 267, 271, 275, 279, 287, 333, 341, 347, 351, 359, 367

posterior tilt of the pelvis, 119, 160, 161, 163, 260, 263, 286, 297, 300, 320, 326

pronation (forearm), 18, 22, 80, 86, 90, 91,
    in posture, 123, 137, 173, 267, 271, 279, 295, 333, 336, 347, 351, 352, 355, 367, 376

S

scapular depression, 18, 55,
    in posture, 142, 266, 267, 270, 271, 274, 275, 278, 279, 286, 287, 302, 303, 374

scapular downward rotation, 18, 55

scapular elevation, 12, 18,
    in posture, 115, 123, 147, 159, 223, 341, 347, 351, 366

scapular protraction, 18, 53, 54,
    in posture, 136, 341, 347, 351, 366

scapular retraction, 18, 54,
    in posture, 142, 266, 267, 270, 271, 274, 275, 278, 279, 286, 287, 302, 303

scapular upward rotation, 18,
    in posture, 114, 115, 122, 123, 147, 158, 159, 222, 223, 341, 347, 351, 366

shoulder extension, 22, 41, 43,
    in posture, 264, 271, 275, 279, 283, 287, 291, 292, 303, 359, 366

shoulder flexion, 41, 42, 43, 55,
    in posture, 105, 115, 117, 119, 123, 137, 145, 147, 157, 159, 165, 219, 223, 227, 229, 233,

Index of Anatomical Actions (*continued*)

247, 251, 295, 299, 311, 319, 341, 347, 351, 352, 366

shoulder horizontal abduction, 44, 45

shoulder horizontal adduction, 46, 47, 219

shoulder lateral adduction, 44, 45

shoulder lateral abduction, 44, 45,
   in posture, 180, 181, 190, 191, 236, 237, 336, 337

shoulder lateral rotation, 50,
   in posture, 129, 173, 177, 185, 275, 299, 303, 337

shoulder medial rotation, 48, 49

spinal extension, 22, 22, 35,
   in posture, 163, 239, 259, 260, 267, 268, 271, 272, 275, 279, 280, 283, 284, 287, 288, 291, 295, 298, 299, 301, 302, 303, 319, 366, 369. *See also* backward bending.

spinal flexion, 22, 24, 25, 26,
   in posture, 115, 161, 163, 169, 186, 188, 189, 240, 241, 243, 247, 255, 263, 311, 315, 316, 333, 355, 366, 369. *See also* forward rounding

spinal rotation, 27, 29,
   in posture, 188, 189, 191, 195, 199, 201, 203, 207, 208, 211, 215, 355, 366. *See also* twisting

supination (forearm), 80, 86, 90, 91,
   in posture, 129, 177, 181, 275, 303, 367, 377

T

torso tilt, 163, 177, 185, 240, 241, 254, 368

twisting, 7, 27, 28, 188, 189, 193, 196, 197, 198, 208, 244, 355. *See also* spinal rotation

W

wrist extension, 22, 95, 96,
   in posture, 119, 123, 135, 137, 139, 141, 143, 279, 295, 333, 338, 347, 355, 359, 367

wrist flexion, 95, 96,
   in posture, 367

Index of The Body

A

acetabulum, 56-66, 326, 374, 375

acromion, 40, 41, 42, 43-45, 51

adductor brevis, 62-63

adductor longus, 62-63

adductor magnus, 59-63

anconeus, 88-89

ankle, 10, 12, 22, 80-85, 96,
    dorsiflexors of, 82
    injuries of, 84-85
    plantar flexors of, 83
    skeletal diagrams, 80, 81

B

biceps brachii, 42-43, 88-91, 264

brachialis, 88-89

brachioradialis, 88-89

C

cervical spine, 20, 33, 106, 287, 340, 342-343

clavicle, 40, 41, 42, 44

coccyx, 20, 163, 251

coracobrachialis, 42, 43, 45, 46

Cylindrical Core, 7, 96, 133, 134, 135, 136, 137, 139, 140, 141, 160, 163, 167, 187, 199, 222, 223, 224, 236, 237, 238, 250, 251, 368, 304, 305, 336, 337, 341, 347, 348, 350, 351, 359, 370, 374

D

deltoid, 42, 43, 44, 45, 46, 49, 50

diaphragm, 107, 108, 109, 135, 374

E

elbow, 10, 124, 86-89
    extensors of, 88
    flexors, 89
    injuries of, 92
    pronators, 91
    skeletal diagram, 87
    supinators, 90

erector spinae, 23, 24, 26, 31, 203, 227, 229, 374

extensor carpi radialis brevis, 95, 96

extensor carpi radialis longus, 95

extensor carpi ulnaris, 95, 96

extensor digitorum longus, 82, 83

extensor hallucis longus, 82, 83

F

femoroacetabular joint, 56, 157,
    impingement in, 66, 379

femur, 56, 57, 58, 59, 60, 62, 63, 64, 65, 66, 72, 73, 76, 77, 104, 157, 178, 186, 217, 230, 238, 240, 248, 326

flexor carpi radialis, 95, 96

flexor carpi ulnaris, 95, 96

flexor digitorum longus, 82, 83

flexor digitorum superficialis, 82, 83

flexor hallucis longus, 82, 83

G

gastrocnemius, 73, 82, 83

glenoid fossa, 40, 41, 44, 51, 52, 53

gluteus maximus, 59, 60, 64, 65

gluteus medius, 62, 63, 64, 65, 217

gluteus minimus, 62, 63, 64, 65, 217

gracilis, 62, 63, 73, 76, 77

H

hamstrings, 16, 17, 27, 59, 60, 69, 274

hip, 58-69, 76, 79, 80, 96
    abductors of, 63
    adductors of, 62
    extensors of, 60
    flexors of, 59
    injuries of, 66-70
    lateral rotators of, 65
    medial rotators of, 64
    skeletal diagrams, 56, 57, 58

humerus, 6, 40, 41, 42, 43, 44, 45, 46, 48, 49, 50, 51, 52, 53, 86, 88, 89, 124, 161

I

iliopsoas, 23, 24, 59, 60, 135, 264, 265

iliotibial band, 194, 206, 209, 210, 217

inferior gemellus, 64

intervertebral disc, 32, 35, 37, 169, 241, 256, 374, 375, 376
    herniation of, 32, 33

K

knee, 10, 12, 22, 27, 69, 72-80,
    extensors of, 73, 74
    flexors of, 73, 75
    injuries of, 78, 79,
    lateral rotators of, 77
    medial rotators of, 76
    overview diagram, 72

L

labrum of the hip, 52, 66, 375

latissimus dorsi, 42, 43, 45, 49, 50, 54, 264

lumbar spine, 20, 22, 24, 28, 29, 33, 35, 133, 135, 146, 160, 163, 166, 172, 174, 188, 189, 204, 208, 210, 239, 241, 256, 259, 260, 261, 268, 272, 280, 284, 288, 298, 300, 320, 326, 369, 373, 377
    facet joint of, 28, 29, 188

Index of The Body (*continued*)

M

meniscus, 78, 79

multifidus, 29

O

obliques, 23, 24, 26, 29, 374

obturator externus, 64, 65

obturator internus, 64, 65

olecranon process, 88

P

palmaris longus, 95, 96

pectineus, 62, 63

pectoralis major, 42, 43, 45, 46, 49, 50, 54, 264, 276

pelvis, 38, 39, 56, 58, 69, 104, 113, 162, 163

piriformis, 33, 64, 65, 376

plantaris, 82, 83

popliteus, 73, 76, 77

pronator quadratus, 90, 91

pronator teres, 90, 91

psoas, 26

Q

quadratus femoris, 64, 65

quadratus lumborum, 26, 37, 374

quadriceps, 27, 73, 144, 168, 184, 247, 261, 282, 284, 289, 290, 294, 297, 349

R

radius, 86, 89, 90, 91, 94, 95, 96

rectus abdominis, 23, 24, 31, 135, 374

rectus femoris, 59, 60, 73

rotator cuff, 51, 52, 53, 160

rotatores brevis, 29

S

sacroiliac joint, 38, 216

sacrum, 20, 38, 128, 136, 146, 160, 163, 166, 168, 172, 189, 190, 194, 196, 208, 260, 274, 282, 284, 290, 294, 300, 318, 322, 326

sartorius, 59, 60, 62, 63, 64, 65, 73, 76, 77

scapula, 18, 40, 41, 42, 44, 53, 55, 138, 338, 374, 376

serratus, 42, 43, 54, 55

shoulder, 10, 22, 41-55
    extensors, 43
    flexors, 42
    horizontal abductors, 46, 47
    horizontal adductors, 46, 47
    injuries of, 51-53
    lateral abductors of, 45
    lateral adductors of, 45
    lateral rotators of, 50
    medial rotators of, 48
    skeletal diagrams, 40, 41

soleus, 82, 83

spine, 7, 10, 11, 20-39
    axial extensors of, 31
    extensors of, 23
    flexors of, 25
    injuries of, 32-39
    lateral flexors of, 26
    rotators of, 30
    skeletal diagrams, 21, 22, 24, 28, 29

spinous processes, 22, 23, 24, 160, 259, 260, 296

subscapularis, 49, 50, 51

superior gemellus, 64, 65

supinator, 10, 91

supraspinatus, 44, 45, 51, 52

T

talus, 80, 81, 82, 83, 84

tensor fasciae latae, 59, 60, 62, 63, 64, 65

teres major, 42, 43, 45, 49, 50

teres minor, 49, 50, 51

thoracic, 20, 27, 28, 29, 37, 108, 109, 188, 189, 212, 215, 259, 260, 261, 287, 296, 368, 369, 374, 377, 380,
    facet joint of, 27, 28, 29, 189

thoracolumbar junction, 259, 377

tibia, 69, 72, 73, 76, 77, 80, 81, 82, 83, 84

tibialis anterior, 82, 83

tibialis posterior, 82, 83

tibiotalar joint, 80, 84, 377

transverse abdominis, 135, 374

triceps brachii, 42, 43, 87, 89

U

ulna, 86-96

W

wrist, 10, 22, 94, 95, 96, 97,
    extensors of, 95, 96
    flexors of, 95, 96
    injuries of, 97
    skeletal diagram, 94

Index of Other Content

A

agonist, 13, 19, 27, 366, 374

ankle impingement, 84, 379

antagonist, 13, 24, 27-28, 112

autonomic balance, 8, 108, 374

autonomic nervous system (ANS), 5, 8, 108, 154, 374, 376-377

C

carpal tunnel syndrome, 97, 379

closed-hip, 157, 158, 167, 168, 217, 218, 222, 226, 238

E

Embodied Posture, 2, 3, 4, 10, 124, 366, 110, 366, 364, 375

Embodied Posture Methodology, 10, 20, 112, 375

Embodiment, 2, 3, 364, 366, 370

EPM, 10, 11, 102, 375

exteroception (exteroceptive awareness), 5, 375

F

functional strength, 6, 7, 8, 69, 274

H

hyperextension, 365, 367

hypermobility, 92, 375, 379

I

impingement, 52, 84, 312, 375, 379

interoception, 5, 6, 124, 328, 364

interoceptive awareness, 5, 102, 261, 375

K

kyphosis, 240, 375

kyphotic, 20, 375

L

lordotic, 20, 375

M

mindful awareness, 4, 5, 6, 9, 106, 127, 328, 364

musculoskeletal wellness, 5, 8, 9, 20, 67, 105

myofascial connectivity, 13, 17, 23, 24, 376

O

open-hip, 157, 164, 172, 176, 180, 184, 217, 228, 232, 236, 238, 368

P

parasympathetic, 8, 9, 108, 368, 374, 376

proprioception, 5, 328

proximal biceps tendinopathy, 52

R

range of motion, 6, 8, 11, 48, 58, 69, 76, 79, 84, 85, 103, 104, 112, 117, 127, 148, 170, 172, 174, 178, 186, 188, 196, 197, 201, 204, 211, 214, 215, 226, 234, 238, 240, 243, 259, 260, 280, 296, 301, 316, 320, 325, 352, 355, 367, 368, 369

reciprocal inhibition, 27, 105, 376

S

skeletal compression, 6, 13, 103, 105, 112, 179, 240, 248, 257, 271, 275, 296, 316, 352, 374

soleus, 82, 83

sprain, 376, 78, 84, 92, 97, 372

sympathetic, 7, 9, 374, 376, 377

U

ujjayi breath, 111

V

victorious breath, 11, 110, 111, 368, 377

To be yourself in a world that is constantly trying to make you something else is the greatest accomplishment.

—Ralph Waldo Emerson